The International Politics of Ebola

The outbreak of Ebola virus disease that gripped Liberia, Guinea and Sierra Leone through much of 2014 and 2015 was undoubtedly a health emergency, yet it was also a global political event. This book examines the international politics of the Ebola outbreak in all of its dimensions, critically assessing the global response, examining what the outbreak can tell us about contemporary global health governance and examining the inequalities and injustices that were laid bare. In doing so, the book shows how some of the concepts, debates and findings from the growing field of global health research in International Relations can help both in furthering understanding of the Ebola crisis and also in improving policy responses to future infectious disease outbreaks. This book was originally published as a special issue of *Third World Quarterly*.

Anne Roemer-Mahler is a Lecturer in International Relations and a Fellow at the Centre for Global Health Policy at the University of Sussex, UK. Her research focuses on the role of pharmaceutical companies in global governance and the pharmaceuticalisation of global health.

Simon Rushton is a Lecturer in the Department of Politics at the University of Sheffield, UK. He has written widely on international responses to HIV/AIDS and other diseases; the links between health and security; the changing nature of global health governance; and issues surrounding health, conflict and post-conflict reconstruction.

T0174754

ThirdWorlds

Edited by
Shahid Qadir, *University of London, UK*

ThirdWorlds will focus on the political economy, development and cultures of those parts of the world that have experienced the most political, social, and economic upheaval, and which have faced the greatest challenges of the postcolonial world under globalisation: poverty, displacement and diaspora, environmental degradation, human and civil rights abuses, war, hunger, and disease.

 ThirdWorlds serves as a signifier of oppositional emerging economies and cultures ranging from Africa, Asia, Latin America, Middle East, and even those 'Souths' within a larger perceived North, such as the U.S. South and Mediterranean Europe. The study of these otherwise disparate and discontinuous areas, known collectively as the Global South, demonstrates that as globalisation pervades the planet, the south, as a synonym for subalterity, also transcends geographical and ideological frontier.

For a complete list of titles in this series, please visit https://www.routledge.com/series/TWQ

Recent titles in the series include:

Negotiating Well-being in Central Asia
Edited by David W. Montgomery

New Actors and Alliances in Development
Edited by Lisa Ann Richey and Stefano Ponte

Emerging Powers and the UN
What Kind of Development Partnership?
Edited by Thomas G. Weiss and Adriana Erthal Abdenur

Corruption in the Aftermath of War
Edited by Jonas Lindberg and Camilla Orjuela

Everyday Energy Politics in Central Asia and the Caucasus
Citizens' Needs, Entitlements and Struggles for Access
Edited by David Gullette and Jeanne Féaux de la Croix

The International Politics of Ebola

Edited by
Anne Roemer-Mahler and Simon Rushton

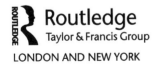
Routledge
Taylor & Francis Group

LONDON AND NEW YORK

First published 2017 by Routledge

2 Park Square, Milton Park, Abingdon, Oxfordshire OX14 4RN
52 Vanderbilt Avenue, New York, NY 10017

Routledge is an imprint of the Taylor & Francis Group, an informa business

First issued in paperback 2018

British Library Cataloguing in Publication Data
A catalogue record for this book is available from the British Library

ISBN 13: 978-1-138-29358-8 (hbk)
ISBN 13: 978-0-367-13907-0 (pbk)

Typeset in MyriadPro
by diacriTech, Chennai

Publisher's Note
The publisher accepts responsibility for any inconsistencies that may have
arisen during the conversion of this book from journal articles to book chapters,
namely the possible inclusion of journal terminology.

Disclaimer
Every effort has been made to contact copyright holders for their permission to
reprint material in this book. The publishers would be grateful to hear from any
copyright holder who is not here acknowledged and will undertake to rectify
any errors or omissions in future editions of this book.

Contents

CONTENTS

Citation Information

The chapters in this book were originally published in *Third World Quarterly*, volume 37, issue 3 (March 2016). When citing this material, please use the original page numbering for each article, as follows:

Chapter 1
Introduction: Ebola and International Relations
Anne Roemer-Mahler and Simon Rushton
Third World Quarterly, volume 37, issue 3 (March 2016) pp. 373–379

Chapter 2
Crisis! What crisis? Global health and the 2014–15 West African Ebola outbreak
Colin McInnes
Third World Quarterly, volume 37, issue 3 (March 2016) pp. 380–400

Chapter 3
WHO's to blame? The World Health Organization and the 2014 Ebola outbreak in West Africa
Adam Kamradt-Scott
Third World Quarterly, volume 37, issue 3 (March 2016) pp. 401–418

Chapter 4
Public health emergencies: a new peacekeeping mission? Insights from UNMIL's role in the Liberia Ebola outbreak
Sara E. Davies and Simon Rushton
Third World Quarterly, volume 37, issue 3 (March 2016) pp. 419–435

Chapter 5
Ebola respons-ibility: moving from shared to multiple responsibilities
Clare Wenham
Third World Quarterly, volume 37, issue 3 (March 2016) pp. 436–451

Chapter 6

Ebola at the borders: newspaper representations and the politics of border control
Sudeepa Abeysinghe
Third World Quarterly, volume 37, issue 3 (March 2016) pp. 452–467

Chapter 7

Infectious injustice: the political foundations of the Ebola crisis in Sierra Leone
Emma-Louise Anderson and Alexander Beresford
Third World Quarterly, volume 37, issue 3 (March 2016) pp. 468–486

Chapter 8

The race for Ebola drugs: pharmaceuticals, security and global health governance
Anne Roemer-Mahler and Stefan Elbe
Third World Quarterly, volume 37, issue 3 (March 2016) pp. 487–506

Chapter 9

Personal Protective Equipment in the humanitarian governance of Ebola: between individual patient care and global biosecurity
Polly Pallister-Wilkins
Third World Quarterly, volume 37, issue 3 (March 2016) pp. 507–523

Chapter 10

Ebola, gender and conspicuously invisible women in global health governance
Sophie Harman
Third World Quarterly, volume 37, issue 3 (March 2016) pp. 524–541

Chapter 11

Ebola and the production of neglect in global health
João Nunes
Third World Quarterly, volume 37, issue 3 (March 2016) pp. 542–556

For any permission-related enquiries please visit:
http://www.tandfonline.com/page/help/permissions

Notes on Contributors

Sudeepa Abeysinghe is a Lecturer in Global Health Policy in the School of Social and Political Science, University of Edinburgh, Scotland, UK.

Emma-Louise Anderson is a Lecturer in International Development at the University of Leeds, UK. Her research focuses on the structural determinants of health in Africa.

Alexander Beresford is a Lecturer in the Politics of African Development at the University of Leeds, UK, and a Senior Research Associate in the Centre for Social Change at the University of Johannesburg, South Africa.

Sara E. Davies is an Associate Professor in the Centre for Governance and Public Policy, Griffith University, Queensland, Australia. She is also an Adjunct Associate Professor at the School of Social Sciences, Monash University, Victoria, Australia.

Stefan Elbe is the Director of the interdisciplinary Centre for Global Health Policy and Professor of International Relations at the University of Sussex, UK.

Sophie Harman is a Reader in the School of Politics and International Relations at Queen Mary University of London, UK, where she teaches and conducts research into global health politics, global governance, and Africa and international relations.

Adam Kamradt-Scott is based at the Centre for International Security Studies, Department of Government and International Relations, University of Sydney, Australia. His research and teaching explores how governments and multilateral organisations respond to adverse health events.

Colin McInnes holds the UNESCO chair in HIV/AIDS Education and Health Security in Africa and is the Director of the Centre for Health and International Relations at Aberystwyth University, Wales, UK.

João Nunes is a Lecturer in International Relations at the University of York, UK. His research interests include global health, international security, food politics and Brazilian health and foreign policies.

Polly Pallister-Wilkins is based at the Department of Politics, University of Amsterdam, The Netherlands. She specialises in the intersection of humanitarian intervention and border control.

NOTES ON CONTRIBUTORS

Anne Roemer-Mahler is a Lecturer in International Relations and a Fellow at the Centre for Global Health Policy at the University of Sussex, UK. Her research focuses on the role of pharmaceutical companies in global governance and the pharmaceuticalisation of global health.

Simon Rushton is a Lecturer in the Department of Politics at the University of Sheffield, UK. He has written widely on international responses to HIV/AIDS and other diseases; the links between health and security; the changing nature of global health governance; and issues surrounding health, conflict and post-conflict reconstruction.

Clare Wenham is a Research Fellow in the department of Infectious Disease Epidemiology at the London School of Hygiene and Tropical Medicine, UK

Introduction: Ebola and International Relations

Anne Roemer-Mahler[a] and Simon Rushton[b]

[a]Centre for Global Health Policy, University of Sussex, Brighton, UK; [b]Department of Politics, University of Sheffield, UK

ABSTRACT
The outbreak of Ebola Virus Disease (EVD) that gripped Liberia, Guinea and Sierra Leone through much of 2014 and 2015 was an enormous and in many ways unprecedented health emergency. Yet the outbreak was not only a global health event – it was also a global political event. In this introduction to the special issue we discuss the contribution that International Relations scholarship can make to analysing and understanding the Ebola outbreak and the global response to it. We group our comments around four key themes: (1) allocating responsibility in a diffuse global health governance system; (2) the causes and effects of Ebola being perceived as a global crisis; (3) the downsides of a security-driven approach to global health emergencies; and (4) issues of inequality both between and within countries, including those around gender, resources and power.

The outbreak of Ebola Virus Disease (EVD) that gripped Liberia, Guinea and Sierra Leone through much of 2014 and 2015 was an enormous and in many ways unprecedented health emergency. At the time of writing (early November 2015) Liberia and Sierra Leone have been officially declared by the World Health Organization (WHO) to be Ebola free, although a small number of cases continue to be diagnosed in Guinea. Although the emergency appears to be passing, no-one is yet declaring with any confidence that the outbreak is over. In all over 11,000 people have died, making this the most deadly Ebola outbreak in history. Indeed, it surpasses the combined total of deaths caused by all of the previous Ebola outbreaks since the discovery of the virus in 1976. The West African outbreak of 2014–15 was the first to occur in the region, and the first to take hold in densely populated urban areas. It also received a level of global public and media attention far beyond that of most global health crises.

Harrowing stories and images from the region were beamed around the world, but despite the efforts of Médecins sans Frontières (MSF) and others working in the region to raise the alarm, concerted international efforts to provide assistance were slow to materialise. As late as September 2014 (almost six months into the outbreak), Joanne Liu, International President of MSF, was still condemning the global response as 'lethally inadequate'. The proof of that statement was clear for all to see in the regular updates of new cases and deaths.

This was an outbreak that was out of control, with huge consequences for individuals and communities in the region.

As examined in several of the papers in this issue, however, it was when consequences began to be felt outside the region that the international response began to take on a new urgency. The repatriation of infected health workers to the USA, the UK and Spain raised fears of the disease spreading beyond West Africa. The discovery of cases in Nigeria, Mali and the USA demonstrated the ease with which the virus could cross state boundaries. In response, neighbouring countries in the region attempted to close their borders – an action condemned by the WHO, the UN Security Council and others. By September 2014 it was becoming increasingly apparent that the ongoing outbreak was not only a global health problem but also a global political problem.

Understanding Ebola: what can International Relations offer?

In November 2014 a group of scholars working on various aspects of the global politics of health gathered for a one-day workshop at the University of Sussex, hosted by the Centre for Global Health Policy as part of an ESRC-sponsored seminar series on Global Health Security. The aim of the workshop was to allow researchers from International Relations (IR) and cognate disciplines to share their thoughts and reflections on the responses to the Ebola outbreak. Some of the discussion papers presented at the workshop were then developed into the articles gathered together in this special issue of *Third World Quarterly*.

As these articles show, the engagement of IR with the Ebola outbreak – and indeed with global health politics more generally – is both broad and varied, crossing sub-disciplinary boundaries and encompassing a wide range of theoretical, conceptual and methodological approaches. Some of the papers in this issue explicitly tackle policy questions, some pursue a more conceptual and theoretical approach. Indeed, this special issue is deliberately eclectic, illustrating the different dimensions of an 'International Relations response' to the outbreak, while showcasing the richness and diversity of what IR research has to offer to our understanding of global health politics.

IR has had a long engagement with charting the emergence of a new global health governance architecture over the past two decades, and in critically examining the political and economic interests and motivations that have underpinned that process.[1] Driven by the idea that tackling disease is important not only for people's well-being but also for economic development and security reasons, global political attention and financial resources for health both increased rapidly after 1990. Development assistance for health has more than quadrupled in that time;[2] a host of new organisations – public, private and hybrid – were created *de novo* to perform key roles in global health governance,[3] alongside such bodies as the WHO, which had been the lead international health agency in the post-Second World War global institutional architecture. In addition, bodies such as the UN Security Council and the G8, which had not previously seen health issues as being part of their mandate, began to pay attention to the impact that disease could have on their 'core business'.

Yet, despite two decades of political attention and significant investment in global health, the international response to the outbreak of Ebola in West Africa was slow and uncoordinated; neither a vaccine nor a cure were available despite years of research. The Ebola crisis, therefore, could be seen as having revealed the limits or, as some have argued, the outright failure of global health governance. Several articles in this issue explore the question of what light the Ebola crisis can shed on our understanding of contemporary global health governance. Kamradt-Scott examines the roles played by the WHO – a body that came in for significant criticism over its handling of the outbreak. Setting the WHO's performance in the broader context of recent reform pressures and other constraints on the organisation, Kamradt-Scott examines the politically sensitive issue of the WHO's role in ensuring global health security, and its responsibility for the underwhelming early response to the outbreak. Davies and Rushton, meanwhile, examine another body which some have argued should have done more: the UN's peacekeeping mission in Liberia (UNMIL). The UNMIL mission, which was beginning a process of 'drawdown' at the time Ebola struck, was a well-established presence in Liberia and had an extensive track record in delivering healthcare services to parts of the Liberian population. When the outbreak began, however, the mission largely withdrew to its barracks – in large part because of the fear of Troop Contributing Countries that their personnel would become infected. Davies and Rushton use this example as a way into examining the question of the appropriate role of peacekeeping forces in cases of health emergency. What can they practically contribute, what roles are appropriate for them to play, and how much responsibility should they have for assisting host governments in addressing such crises?

Clare Wenham also picks up on the notion of responsibility in global health governance from a more theoretical vantage point, exploring the norm of 'shared responsibility' for combating infectious disease threats championed by a growing number of global health practitioners and organisations. She argues that, while attractive in theory, this notion of shared responsibility makes it difficult in practice to hold international actors accountable for their actions (or inaction). Wenham argues that 'shared responsibility' should be reframed as 'multiple responsibilities' for individual actors, with a far clearer division of labour between the different governance actors involved in responding to such events.

Language, and the way that global health issues are 'framed', has been another focus of scholars examining the global politics of health.[4] This is reflected in a second theme touched upon by several articles in this issue: the causes and consequences of portraying the Ebola outbreak as a 'crisis' and/or as a threat to international security. McInnes contributes to the rich literature on agenda setting in global health.[5] He does so by grappling with the question of why some issues (including, eventually, Ebola) receive global political attention while others do not. Taking a constructivist theoretical angle, he highlights the fact that the global attention to the outbreak was not a 'natural' response to an objective crisis event but was based on the *perception* of a crisis – a perception rooted in a process of social construction. Such an understanding of Ebola as a crisis became possible, McInnes argues, not merely because of the material facts of a fast spreading (but regional) epidemic (although that was an important condition), but because it resonated with a broader and well-established narrative of 'global health'.

A key element of this narrative is the interpretation of diseases (especially rapidly spreading infectious diseases) as potential threats to national and international security. Drawing on 'securitisation theory',[6] IR scholarship has devoted considerable attention to exploring the implications of this 'health security' agenda.[7] Among other things, this literature has shown how viewing health as a security threat has helped mobilise political attention and resources – a phenomenon also observed in the Ebola outbreak. Yet some have raised concerns about the possible downsides of addressing health in security terms.[8] One concern is that global health issues only become a priority when the West feels threatened. In examining the portrayal of Ebola in the print media in Australia, the UK and the USA Abeysinghe shows how the Ebola epidemic was transformed from a problem of West Africa to a problem of the West. The context of West Africa and affected populations was largely hidden to the extent that 'Ebola cease[d] being an issue of global health'. Rather, it became a prism through which domestic party politics in Australia, the UK and the USA were played out. To a great extent, therefore, the Ebola outbreak as read through Western newspaper coverage became a story about the West and the West's security – a reading that may have increased the pressure on Western political leaders to act, but which portrayed the outbreak in a way that was fundamentally detached from the ongoing human catastrophe in West Africa.

Though approaching the subject from a very different angle, Anderson and Beresford's article also speaks to the relationship between West Africa and the wider world. In doing so, it addresses an area that is comparatively under-developed in IR: the relationship between domestic politics (especially within developing countries) and international-level responses to health crises. Through this, Anderson and Beresford highlight another of the downsides of seeing health as a security threat: a tendency for security-driven responses to be reactive in nature, with too little attention being paid to the underlying structural causes of insecurity. As Anderson and Beresford show, aid intended to help strengthen the post-conflict health system in Sierra Leone did little to tackle the political causes of that country's chronically weak health system, which include acute external dependency, patron–client politics, endemic corruption and weak state capacity. Their conclusions draw our attention to the concern that the security-driven emergency modality of the international Ebola response, focused as it was on rapidly putting in place treatment facilities and searching for a pharmaceutical solution, overlooked important socioeconomic and political underpinnings of the 'crisis'.

This technical, quick-fix approach of the international Ebola response is also interrogated in the articles by Roemer-Mahler and Elbe, and by Pallister-Wilkins. Roemer-Mahler and Elbe explore why the international Ebola response focused so much energy and resources on the attempt to develop drugs and vaccines, even though they would most probably not become available in time to contain the outbreak. The authors argue that in this respect the international Ebola response followed a common pattern seen in the responses to other 'health security threats'. This 'pharmaceuticalisation' of global health policy, they show, is linked to the 'securitisation' of health.[9] First, securitisation encourages technological policy responses; second, it creates an exceptional political space in which pharmaceutical development can be freed from constraints; and third, the securitisation of health has created an institutional architecture that facilitates further pharmaceutical policy responses.

Pallister-Wilkins' article looks into a different 'technical fix', that of Personal Protective Equipment (PPE) – the 'space suits' that quickly became emblematic of the Ebola outbreak and were used to illustrate almost every media story from the region. Pallister-Wilkins' preoccupation is with the relationship between the individual medical treatment of Ebola patients and the wider system of global health security, in which PPE became an important mediator, with 'its wearers both *at* risk of catching the virus and simultaneously *a* risk as a possible transmission vector'. At the same time, she argues, PPE became a symbol of the hierarchical relationship between the technically capable West and the most affected countries, which lacked even the most basic resources necessary for fighting the epidemic.

This brings us to our fourth theme – that of inequality, and what the Ebola outbreak revealed about inequalities both within and between countries. Many of the articles in this issue tackle the subject of inequalities between countries in one form or another. Harman focuses instead on the issue of gender inequality, highlighting the 'conspicuous invisibility' of women not only in the dominant narratives on Ebola and the international response but also in global health governance more widely. Harman argues that, despite the fact that healthcare around the world rests to a significant extent on the 'free' labour of women, women frequently become invisible in policy discussions. Examining this in the Ebola case, the article demonstrates how the discussions over both the emergency response to Ebola and longer-term efforts to strengthen health systems paid little regard to gender or women – a fact that will, Harman argues, be to the detriment of women's health and well-being.

Again drawing attention to the politics of inequality, Nunes' article in many ways links all the four themes discussed here together. He argues that, notwithstanding the attention it received throughout 2014, Ebola should be seen as a 'neglected' issue in global health. Addressing issues of responsibility, Western interests, security concerns and global inequalities, Nunes argues that, despite the media spectacle that Ebola became, its framing as an 'African problem' (a framing which brought with it a good deal of colonial and racist baggage) served to re-inscribe neglect, and reinforce the 'preference for short-term, crisis-management responses that detracted from long-term structural solutions'.

While IR therefore has much to contribute to discussion of the Ebola outbreak, it certainly does not have all the answers, nor all the necessary conceptual and methodological tools at its disposal. Global Health is, and must be, a fundamentally interdisciplinary field, bringing together scholars from International Relations, Anthropology, Sociology, Public Health, Medicine, and many other disciplines besides. Our collective purpose in this issue is to show how some of the concepts, debates and findings from the growing field of global health research in IR can help both in furthering understanding of the Ebola crisis and also in improving policy responses to future infectious disease outbreaks.

Disclosure statement

No potential conflict of interest was reported by the authors.

Funding

We are grateful to the Economic & Social Research Council for sponsoring the seminar which led to this special issue [Grant reference ES/L000326/1].

Acknowledgements

We are grateful to Professor Stefan Elbe and the Centre for Global Health Policy at the University of Sussex for hosting the workshop that led to this special issue, and to Shahid Qadir and Sean Rothman of *Third World Quarterly* for their help and support throughout the process of putting this Special Issue together.

Notes

1. Youde, *Global Health Governance*; Kay and Williams, *Global Health Governance*; Harman, *Global Health Governance*; and Cooper et al., *Governing Global Health*.
2. Ravishankar et al., "Financing of Global Health."
3. Rushton and Williams, *Partnerships and Foundations in Global Health Governance*; Buse and Harmer, "Power to the Partners?"; Buse and Walt, "Global Public–Private Partnerships: Part I"; and Buse and Walt, "Global Public–Private Partnerships: Part II."
4. McInnes and Roemer-Mahler, "Competition and Cooperation in Global Health Governance"; McInnes and Lee, "Framing Global Health Governance"; and Rushton and Williams, "Frames, Paradigms and Power."
5. Hafner and Shiffman, "The Emergence of Global Attention"; Shiffman and Smith, "Generation of Political Priority"; and Shiffman, "A Social Explanation."
6. Buzan et al., *Security*.
7. Aldis, "Health Security"; Elbe, *Security and Global Health*; Enemark, "Is Pandemic Flu a Security Threat?"; Enemark, *Disease and Security*; McInnes, "HIV/AIDS and Security" ; McInnes and Rushton, "HIV/AIDS and Securitization Theory"; McInnes and Lee, "Health, Security and Foreign Policy"; and Rushton and Youde, *Routledge Handbook of Global Health Security*.
8. Elbe, "Should HIV/AIDS be Securitized?"; and Rushton, "Global Health Security."
9. Elbe et al., "Medical Countermeasures"; Elbe et al., "Securing Circulation"; and Roemer-Mahler, "The Rise of Companies from Emerging Markets."

Bibliography

Aldis, William L. "Health Security as a Public Health Concept: A Critical Analysis." *Health Policy and Planning* 23, no. 6 (2008): 369–375.
Buse, Kent, and Andrew Harmer. "Power to the Partners? The Politics of Public-Private Health Partnerships." *Development* 47, no. 2 (2004): 49–56.
Buse, Kent, and Gill Walt. "Global Public-Private Partnerships: Part I – A New Development in Health?" *Bulletin of the World Health Organization* 78, no. 4 (2000): 549–561.
Buse, Kent, and Gill Walt. "Global Public-Private Partnerships: Part II – What are the Health Issues for Global Governance?" *Bulletin of the World Health Organization* 78, no. 5 (2000): 699–709.
Buzan, Barry, Ole Wæver, and Jaap de Wilde. *Security: A New Framework for Analysis*. Boulder, CO: Lynne Rienner, 1998.
Cooper, Andrew, John Kirton, and Ted Schrecker (eds.). *Governing Global Health: Challenge, Response. Innovation*. Aldershot: Ashgate, 2007.
Elbe, Stefan. *Security and Global Health*. Cambridge: Polity, 2010.
Elbe, Stefan. "Should HIV/AIDS be Securitized? The Ethical Dilemmas of linking HIV/AIDS and Security." *International Studies Quarterly* 50, no. 1 (2006): 119–144.

Elbe, Stefan, Anne Roemer-Mahler, and Christopher Long. "Medical Countermeasures for National Security: A New Government Role in the Pharmaceuticalization of Society." *Social Science & Medicine* 131 (2014): 263–271.

Elbe, Stefan, Anne Roemer-Mahler, and Christopher Long. "Securing Circulation Pharmaceutically: Antiviral Stockpiling and Pandemic Preparedness in the European Union." *Security Dialogue* 45, no. 5 (2014): 440–457.

Enemark, Christian. *Disease and Security*. Abingdon: Routledge, 2007.

Enemark, Christian. "Is Pandemic Flu a Security Threat?" *Survival* 51, no. 1 (2009): 191e–214.

Hafner, Tamara, and Jeremy Shiffman. "The Emergence of Global Attention to Health Systems Strengthening." *Health Policy and Planning* 28 (2013): 41–50.

Harman, Sophie. *Global Health Governance*. London: Routledge, 2012.

Kay, Adrian, and Owain Williams (eds.). *Global Health Governance: Crisis*. Institutions and Political Economy. London: Palgrave Macmillan, 2009.

McInnes, Colin. "AIDS and Security." *International Affairs* 82, no. 2 (2006): 315–326.

McInnes, Colin, and Kelley Lee, eds. "Framing Global Health Governance." *Global Public Health* (special supplement) 7 (2012).

McInnes, Colin, and Kelley Lee. "Health, Security and Foreign Policy." *Review of International Studies* 32, no. 1 (2006): 5e–23.

McInnes, Colin, and Anne Roemer-Mahler, "Competition and Co-operation in Global Health Governance: The Impact of Multiple Framing." In *Law and Global Health*, edited by Michael Freeman, Sarah Hawkes and Belinda Bennett, 513–531. Current Legal Issues 16. Oxford: Oxford University Press, 2013.

McInnes, Colin, and Simon Rushton. "HIV/AIDS and Securitization Theory." *European Journal of International Relations* 19, no. 1 (2011): 115–138.

Ravishankar, Nirmala, Paul Gubbins, Rebecca J. Cooley, Katherine Leach-Kemon, Catherine M. Michaud, Dean T. Jamison, and Christopher J. L. Murray. "Financing of Global Health: Tracking Development Assistance for Health fromto 2007." *Lancet* 373 2009: 2113–2124.

Roemer-Mahler, Anne. "The Rise of Companies from Emerging Markets in Global Health Governance: Opportunities and Challenges." *Review of International Studies* 40, no. 5 (2014): 897–918.

Rushton, Simon. "Global Health Security: Security for Whom? Security from What?" *Political Studies* 59, no. 4 (2011): 779–796.

Rushton, Simon, and Owain Williams. "Frames, Paradigms and Power: Global Health Policy-making under Neoliberalism." *Global Society* 26, no. 2 (2012): 147–167.

Rushton, Simon, and Owain Williams. *Partnerships and Foundations in Global Health Governance*. Basingstoke: Palgrave Macmillan, 2011.

Rushton, Simon, and Jeremy Youde (eds.). *Routledge Handbook of Global Health Security*. Abingdon: Routledge, 2014.

Shiffman, Jeremy. "A Social Explanation for the Rise and Fall of Global Health Issues." *Bulletin of the World Health Organization* 87 (2009): 608–613.

Shiffman, Jeremy, and Stephanie Smith. "Generation of Political Priority for Global Health Initiatives: A Framework and Case Study of Maternal Mortality." *Lancet* 370 (2007): 1370–1379.

Youde, Jeremy. *Global Health Governance*. Cambridge: Polity Press, 2012.

Crisis! What crisis? Global health and the 2014–15 West African Ebola outbreak

Colin McInnes

Department of International Politics, Aberystwyth University, UK

ABSTRACT
This article examines why the 2014–15 outbreak of Ebola in West Africa, which subsequently spread more widely, was understood as a crisis. It begins from the basis that there was nothing 'natural' about it being considered a crisis; rather it was socially constructed as such. Specifically it suggests that the outbreak could be understood as a crisis because of the way in which it resonated with the global health narrative. The article examines how the elements which constitute this narrative – the effects of globalisation, the emergence of new risks and the requirement for new political responses – are fundamental to how Ebola was understood as a crisis.

In West Africa, what began as a health crisis quickly escalated into a humanitarian, social, economic, and security crisis. (WHO Director-General Margaret Chan, 25 January 2015)[1]

In March 2014 the World Health Organization (WHO) alerted the world to an outbreak of Ebola in West Africa, at that time confined to Guinea but soon spreading to the neighbouring states of Liberia and Sierra Leone. As the outbreak developed over the course of the year it was increasingly framed in terms of a crisis. Some of the more extreme estimates suggested that cases might exceed a million; fears were expressed over wider social consequences (including state failure) in the region; and concerns emerged over its possible spread to Europe and North America. This article, however, suggests that the framing of the outbreak as a crisis had less to do with these rationalist concerns, which dominated explanations both at the time and subsequently; rather such framing was because of the manner in which this resonated with a narrative on global health that had been developing, especially since the millennium. The significance of this is that it suggests attention and action on global health issues are determined less by levels of mortality and morbidity – although material factors such as these are not discounted – but by the success with which a disease or condition can be constructed as a global health threat by resonating with this narrative.

The Ebola crisis

The 2014–15 outbreak of Ebola in West Africa was the most severe on record.[2] By the beginning of June 2015 the WHO estimated that there had been 27,181 cases and 11,162 deaths from Ebola, almost all in West Africa.[3] This was more than in all of the previous outbreaks of the disease combined.[4] The WHO had announced an Ebola outbreak in Guinea on 23 March 2014 through its Africa Regional Office. The next month, at a press conference in Geneva, it described the outbreak as 'one of the most challenging…that we have ever faced', and in June declared it a level 3 emergency, the highest level possible.[5] With the disease having also spread to Liberia and Sierra Leone (and later to Nigeria), Médecins Sans Frontières (MSF), which was by then heavily engaged in treating cases of the disease in West Africa, warned that the outbreak was out of control.[6] MSF was subsequently widely praised for its efforts, in stark contrast to the WHO, whose response was described as 'anemic'.[7] Over the summer a range of social distancing measures were introduced in the three most affected West African states, including school closures, curfews and limits on border crossings. In late July and early August, two US aid workers – Kent Brantly and Nancy Writebol – became infected with Ebola and were airlifted to the USA, beginning a small but steady flow of medical evacuations for infected health workers back to the USA or Europe. On 8 August, for only the third time in its history, the WHO declared the outbreak a Public Health Emergency of International Concern (PHEIC) under the 2005 revisions to the International Health Regulations. On 14 August it announced that field reports may have underestimated the severity of the outbreak and on 28 August released its 'roadmap' to coordinate the response.[8] In September 2014 WHO Director-General Margaret Chan described the outbreak as 'the largest, most complex and most severe we've ever seen'.[9] With numbers of deaths still rising, the UN Security Council passed Resolution 2177, declaring the outbreak a threat to international peace and security,[10] and the General Assembly authorised the Secretary General's request for the establishment of the UN Mission for Emergency Ebola Relief (UNMEER).[11] Fears that the disease was 'raging out of control' in West Africa were supported by a US Centers for Disease Control and Prevention (CDC) estimate at the end of September that the number of cases in Liberia and Sierra Leone might, by the end of January 2015, exceed 1.4 million.[12] On 30 September CDC announced that Thomas Edward Duncan had become the first case of Ebola identified within the USA, quickly followed by two further cases involving medical workers treating Duncan.[13] This led to concerns over the ability of the USA to contain the disease, concerns echoed in Europe when a nursing assistant, Maria Teresa Romero Ramos, was also diagnosed as having caught the disease while working at a hospital in Spain. World leaders queued up to express their concern, offer aid and in a limited number of cases, to dispatch troops to assist in the aid effort.[14] The BBC reported that by mid-October 2014, when the first cases had appeared in Europe and North America, fear of the virus was spreading 'faster than the virus itself' through the use of social media.[15]

What is striking is the manner in which the outbreak of Ebola in West Africa was described and understood as a crisis – sometimes literally, on other occasions in terms evoking crisis such as 'emergency', 'catastrophe' or 'disaster'.[16] Although some organisations had criteria for such judgments (including the WHO in declaring a PHEIC), for many these terms appeared to be less a rigorous application of previously identified criteria than an indication of substantial concern.[17] Various arguments were used to justify this description, some envisaging potential state collapse, others an uncontrolled spread of the disease, with its unusually high levels of both morbidity and mortality and lack of proven vaccine, beyond West Africa. Neither of these arguments had much foundation, either in retrospect or at the time: state failure through a disease outbreak is extremely unlikely, even for weak states,[18] while previous outbreaks of Ebola had demonstrated that control mechanisms were very effective in limiting its spread.[19] This is not to say that the *fear* of Ebola was not real, especially given its gruesome symptoms and high mortality rate, just that the likelihood of the disease spreading in an uncontrolled manner beyond West Africa was extremely low. Not least, transmission involved direct contact with bodily fluids of infected or recently deceased patients, while the contagious period coincided with symptoms being apparent rather than preceding them, meaning that people were generally aware that they were seriously ill when they were contagious. Both of these made control of the outbreak easier than with the 2009 PHEIC caused by the H1N1 ('swine flu') virus. Indeed, when the disease did spread from the three most infected states of Guinea, Liberia and Sierra Leone to Nigeria, action by the Nigerian government ensured that the outbreak was contained, with only 20 cases (one of which was unconfirmed) and eight deaths.[20]

The key element in the crisis narrative, however, is the sense of very large numbers of people suffering and dying from the disease. MSF's International President, Joanne Liu, provided a graphic example of this in her briefing to the UN:

> Six months into the worst Ebola epidemic in history…cases and deaths continue to surge. Riots are breaking out. Isolation centers are overwhelmed. Health workers on the front lines are becoming infected and dying in shocking numbers. Others have fled in fear, leaving people without care for even the most common illnesses. Entire health systems have crumbled. Ebola treatment centers are reduced to places where people go to die alone, where little more than palliative care is offered. It is impossible to keep up with the sheer number of infected people pouring into facilities. In Sierra Leone, bodies are rotting in the streets. Rather than building new Ebola care centers in Liberia, we are forced to build crematoria.[21]

With the WHO declaring a PHEIC in August, and CDC estimating over a million possible cases, this alone may provide the explanation for an understanding of the outbreak as a crisis. But making the case that the 2014–15 West African Ebola outbreak was a global crisis on the grounds of numbers of people who either caught the disease or died from it is problematic because, tragic though these numbers are, they do not come close to being among the highest causes of death from disease or other health-related causes in 2014. A decade previously HIV had become recognised as a global crisis, but the numbers of people dying from the disease in the early years of the millennium were not only over two million a year; this was repeated on a multi-year basis, with deaths still exceeding one million well into the second decade of the millennium. In contrast, the CDCs estimate of 1.4 million deaths was hedged with uncertainty – it assumed no interventions to prevent the spread of the disease, that case loads would continue to multiply in a similar manner as had occurred in previous weeks, and that underreporting would almost triple the number of actual cases. In contrast, its estimate of 8000 cases by the end of September (21,000 if underreporting was as serious as some believed) appeared an order of magnitude less serious.[22] In 2014 many more died of malaria than of Ebola without any sense of a global emergency, while 750,000 infants died of diarrhoeal disease with hardly any attention.[23] Nor does it explain why, when the WHO declared only the second PHEIC (on polio) in its history just weeks before the PHEIC on Ebola, the former received much less attention.[24]

This suggests that neither the declaration of a PHEIC nor the numbers of cases can fully explain why the West African Ebola outbreak became a global health crisis. This article therefore advances a different explanation. It does not deny the material basis of the outbreak, but suggests that it was 'made' a crisis because it could be tied into a narrative on global health which had been developing for the best part of two decades. It contrasts with previous analyses of the outbreak, which have largely focused on explaining how it became the largest outbreak of Ebola on record (for example because of high levels of poverty and the legacy of conflict),[25] or on the effectiveness (or otherwise) of the regional and international response.[26] It draws its theoretical inspiration from social constructivism and its key insight that the social world does not exist independent of observation, but rather is what we choose to make it, and that the ideas we use in observing and understanding the social world also shape that world.[27] This understanding of the social world also guides actions in establishing socially legitimate pathways of response. These should be distinguished from normatively determined ideas of what is 'right', but are rather products of the manner in which an issue is constructed leading to certain responses which accord with these understandings. The significance of ideational factors in constructing the social world does not mean that material factors are unimportant – in this article, for example, the numbers of people in West Africa who suffered and died from Ebola is a significant material factor in understanding how the disease was constructed as a crisis. Rather, material factors are given meaning and in turn (re)shape ideational constructions in a symbiotic, or mutually constitutive, manner.

The article draws on and contributes to a growing social constructivist literature in the study of global health politics.[28] Much of this literature has focused on how health issues have been framed around processes of securitisation but this article builds on the broader analysis of McInnes and Lee, which attempts a social constructivist reading of the manner in which health has become part of the study and practice of international relations.[29] Building on their analysis, it suggests that the manner in which health was constructed in the early years of the millennium was by way of a 'global health narrative'. Three key elements of this narrative – what may be broadly characterised as globalisation, securitisation and politicisation – not only shaped the way in which the West African Ebola outbreak could then be understood as a crisis, but also shaped the acceptable pathways of response.

The global health narrative

Over the past two decades the term 'global health' has become ubiquitous, replacing 'international health' almost entirely. The term is commonplace not only within scholarly circles but as part of key policy debates on the prioritisation, financing and delivery of health care services.[30] This development is often portrayed in rationalist terms – as a reflection of a profound shift in the ingredients that influence health policy. But it is also a concept that has contributed to that shift. In the creation and use of the term 'global health', a multiplicity of trends have been given a shared meaning which encourages us to see the world differently. Statements such as 'health is global',[31] therefore, are not simply a reflection of an external reality, but a call to reinterpret how we understand health in a particular way.

Central to the global health narrative is an emphasis on the perceived impact of globalisation.[32] This emphasis, however, is not simply a reaction to an exogenous reality. Rather, through the global health narrative a variety of developments is given both a shared identity as part of a single phenomenon and a shared meaning of transforming the world of health.

Most of this emphasis has focused on how disease vectors have changed, and in particular on the manner in which the increased frequency and rapidity of travel has allowed infectious diseases to spread quickly across state boundaries and continents.[33] But it also covers a much wider array of issues concerning epidemiology and the allocation and movement of health resources. These include issues such as the global market for pharmaceuticals (including patent protection), the mobility of health professionals, the management of information and disease surveillance, the privatised health care industry, increased access to food and drink with high fat, sugar or salt content produced by global companies, and the restructuring of health-related industries. Moreover, global communication technologies, especially the internet and social media, have allowed images and stories of health crises to be spread much further and more rapidly than before and to a much wider audience. This has not only fostered a spirit of shared humanity, giving normative power to charities such as MSF, but allowed fear of disease to be spread more easily. What is less frequently observed, however, is how globalisation has assisted in the standardisation of disease identification and responses. Kamradt-Scott, for example, demonstrates how the Western methodology of 'evidence-based medicine', using biostatistics and other quantifiable indices, has become the dominant frame in health and biomedical sciences.[34] Patricia Wald identifies the development of an 'outbreak narrative', which establishes a common understanding of and responses to disease outbreaks.[35] Starling et al note how the globalised system of vaccination and immunisation campaigns introduced by GAVI has often failed to take account of local weaknesses in public health systems, which compromised their introduction.[36] And HIV continues to be considered a single 'pandemic',[37] despite widely varying means of transmission between different regions (and even countries in the same region), meaning it is better understood as a series of epidemics. As a result, globalisation is not simply a narrative of changing health inputs, but one of responses as well.

The second element of the global health narrative is one of risk, specifically of the emergence of health risks with security implications.[38] In 1997 the US Institute of Medicine argued that exogenous health developments were a threat to US interests, while a decade later the WHO devoted the entirety of its annual *World Health Report* to 'global health security'.[39] Nor was interest limited to the health community: in January 2000, for example, the UN Security Council discussed for the first time the risk of a disease (HIV) to international peace and security and especially peacekeepers, and the US national security establishment co-opted public health in its bio-terrorism preparedness measures after 9/11 and the mailing of anthrax spores to members of the US Congress and media.[40] The nature of 'global health security' is contested, however. The language of security has been used in connection with traditional health issues, such as health promotion and laboratory safety, while at the same time being used to justify the inclusion of health issues in national security agendas. Moreover the level of analysis can be – and is sometimes simultaneously – global, national, community or individual (human).[41] Whether a health issue is fully 'securitised' or not may also be unclear, with different actors holding a variety of positions along a spectrum ranging from fully securitised to fully de-securitised.[42] From a more traditional national security perspective, however, attention has focused on a number of issues. These include the potential for health crises to lead to state failure, with wider consequences for regional stability and global security; the impact upon military forces and in particular peacekeepers; and the use of pathogens such as smallpox or anthrax as weapons of mass destruction, including their possible use for bio-terrorism. But the most common national security concern surrounds outbreaks of infectious disease.[43]

Specifically a subsidiary narrative has emerged whereby the apparent 'conquest' of infectious disease by the 1960s was overturned by the emergence of new (or new forms of existing) diseases. This was largely a product of changing social ecologies, including urbanisation and global travel, as well as climate change and deforestation, which allowed zoonotic diseases greater access to human populations. The potentially rapid spread of these new and re-emerging diseases, often possessing high morbidity and mortality rates (such as HIV, H5N1 and Ebola), for the first time in generations posed a risk to populations in both low-income and high-income countries because of increased and rapid travel. They threatened economic growth and regional stability, not least through worker absenteeism, migration, travel restrictions and reduced investment, at a time when economies were more interdependent than ever before.[44] And they risked state failure through a 'hollowing out' of state institutions, a lack of confidence in state authorities' capacity to manage the crisis, the stigma and alienation of infected communities and an exacerbation of pre-existing social inequalities.[45]

The final element of the global health narrative is perhaps the most obviously controversial. In bio-medical framings of health policy, political (value-based) interference has been resisted on the grounds that actions, from those of an individual clinician to global health initiatives, should be based on factually based (value-neutral) clinical evidence of health need. Politics is not only seen as unnecessary, but considered at best a hindrance and at worst potentially disastrous to rational decision making, in preventing an objective assessment, based on scientific evidence.[46] Similarly in a rights-based frame, political interference is seen as potentially undermining the rights of individuals to attain a basic level of health. This rights-based framing has influenced both the behaviour of health professionals (for example through the Hippocratic oath) and a range of international Declarations, including the 1978 Alma Ata Declaration on 'Heath for All'.[47] Since 2000, however, politics has been placed more explicitly within the arena of global health. In part this has been geared to how resources are used and mobilised and exemplified by the use of 'aid conditionalities', whereby aid resources are distributed only to organisations or authorities that comply with political agendas, such as good governance and pro-life policies.[48] But it has also been affected by a sense of the national interest – that health developments in low-income countries, including those in Africa, affect the interests of high-income countries. Particularly influential in this move was the WHO Commission on Macroeconomics and Health, which argued that the disease burden on the poor threatened the wealth of all.[49] Investment in the health needs of developing countries was required not simply for their economic growth and development strategies, but to avoid spill-over effects threatening regional or even global well-being. This had been presaged by the 1997 report from the US Institute of Medicine.[50] It was realised by a succession of initiatives in the first decade of the next century, many from the G8 either collectively (for example at the 2005 Gleneagles summit) or individually (for example PEPFAR in the USA), which, despite their humanitarian language, in operation also reflected national interests.[51]

For this article, however, a second dimension to the greater politicisation of health is important. At the same time as globalisation was creating a sense that the national interest might be affected by health developments elsewhere, so it was also understood as requiring changes to how decisions on health policy were made: if health was global, then collective solutions would be required for shared health problems. This became known as global health governance (GHG). Crucially GHG represented a move away from a sole focus on the technical competences of international institutions such as the WHO towards including questions of the increasingly complex relationships between the varied actors involved.[52] GHG became in the global health narrative not only a response to an increasingly globalised world, characterised by existing institutions acquiring new meanings and mandates, and the proliferation of new institutional arrangements; but also by an increased awareness that the global governance of health is not simply a technical or administrative matter but a political realm of cooperation and contestation.[53]

The key argument of this article is that this global health narrative – that health is now global, presenting a new range of security risks and requiring more obviously political forms of response – is not simply a rationalist account of a changing environment for health, but shapes both the understanding of global health and acceptable pathways of response. Specifically it shaped the understanding of the 2014–15 West African Ebola outbreak as a crisis and influenced the range of appropriate responses, not in a retrospective manner but as the outbreak developed. The next three sections therefore examine how each of the three key elements of this narrative shaped this understanding of the outbreak and the possibilities for action in response to it.

Ebola goes global

The 2014–15 outbreak of Ebola in West Africa was only the latest in a series of infectious disease outbreaks to have a global impact, following most notably on the heels of SARS in 2002–03 and H1N1 ('swine flu') in 2009. But it was far from the first outbreak of Ebola – indeed the US CDC identify 34 previous cases and outbreaks of the disease, as well as an outbreak in the Democratic Republic of Congo in August to November 2014, simultaneous to that in West Africa.[54] Nor was the outbreak spread evenly across the globe. The overwhelming numbers of cases was in the three geographically contiguous states of Guinea, Liberia and Sierra Leone (estimated in June 2015 at 27,352 with just 36 elsewhere, 29 of which were in other African states).[55] What, then, made the West African outbreak a global event, one where 'perceptions of Ebola virus disease [changed] from an exotic tropical disease to a priority for global health security'?[56]

One explanation of course is that the scale of the crisis passed a tipping point where it could no longer be considered as merely locally significant. The simple fact that more people died in this single outbreak than in all previous outbreaks of Ebola combined, that MSF – heavily engaged on the ground in West Africa – was describing the outbreak as being out of control, and that towards the end of September 2014 the US CDC was estimating a worst case of 1.4 million cases, cannot be ignored as factors influencing how the outbreak was seen and the reaction to it. The scale of suffering was certainly what appeared to underpin MSF's calls for concerted international action, including its head, Joanne Liu, appealing twice in person to the UN.[57] The problem with this argument, however, is that tipping points are not objectively set criteria where, after a preordained number of deaths in a set period, the international community starts to press the emergency response button.[58] Rather an outbreak has to fit into some idea of what constitutes a crisis in order for it to be described as such. This is not to suggest that mortality levels are not important but that what constitutes a sufficient number to call an outbreak a 'crisis' is socially constructed by the interplay between material factors (number of cases and deaths) and ideational ones (the global health narrative). A second explanation is that the outbreak met the understandings of a crisis established in the 2005 International Health Regulations, which in turn enabled the WHO to call a PHEIC in August 2014.[59] The problem with this is that, even if a PHEIC was necessary for establishing Ebola as a global health crisis, as the lack of a similar reaction to the PHEIC on polio in May 2014 demonstrated, this was not sufficient to generate the levels of attention and international action which Ebola received.

Instead, this article suggests that Ebola came to be understood as a global health crisis by linking it to the global health narrative that emphasised the shared risk from infectious disease. One of the features of the 2014–15 outbreak was the manner in which the growing numbers of deaths in West Africa in the first few months after its identification as Ebola in March 2014 generated comparatively little global attention and a poor international response.[60] The PHEIC was called five months after the WHO had first announced the outbreak and well into its second wave; the WHO published its 'roadmap' for international response in late August; the UN Security Council and General Assembly both met in early September; and UNMEER was established soon afterwards. This flurry of activity in August and September coincided with a growing awareness of the potential of the disease to spread beyond the three most affected countries. Cases began to appear in Nigeria from the end of July on, Western aid workers began to be med-evaced at a similar time, and cases of infection in the USA and Spain occurred in late September/early October. With the infections of health workers in the USA and Spain, in particular, public interest increased dramatically. An analysis of Twitter, for example, demonstrates how, when US CDC announced the first case of Ebola in the USA (Thomas Eric Duncan) and Spanish authorities confirmed that the nursing assistant Maria Teresa Romero Ramos had also caught the disease in Madrid, activity on the social media site concerning the disease increased exponentially.[61] As Margaret Chan observed, 'Fear and anxiety have spread well beyond West Africa to engulf the world'.[62] Consistent with the global health narrative, once the sense of shared risk was established, so too was the sense of a global crisis, *despite* the very small number of transmissions outside West Africa.

The global health narrative had also facilitated an accepted, globally applicable pathway of response to the risk of disease outbreaks based on three elements of surveillance, control (including an epidemiological understanding of the disease) and pharmacological interventions.[63] Despite the difficulties in applying each of these elements to West Africa and/or Ebola, the international response nevertheless relied upon them; when it failed the situation became a crisis not least *because* the globally accepted pathway of response had been seen to fail. The surveillance element of this response failed in part because the appearance of Ebola in West Africa was unprecedented and early cases were misdiagnosed, often as Lassa fever (another haemorrhagic fever endemic to the region).[64] But the system also failed because the disease surveillance infrastructure in the region was extremely weak (among other things there was a lack of available diagnostic kits) and because of failures at the WHO.[65]

The second element (control measures), was well established for Ebola and, based upon an understood epidemiology, had proven successful in previous outbreaks. Indeed, Margaret Chan commented during the 2014–15 outbreak that 'Experience tells us that Ebola outbreaks can be contained, even without a vaccine or cure',[66] suggesting a confidence in this approach. Such control measures included barrier nursing, the use of protective clothing by health workers, effective laboratory safety measures, disinfection, isolation and communication.[67] Nevertheless, these failed to contain the outbreak for much of the year. This was partly because of well-known weaknesses in the health systems in the region, which meant that there was no capacity to introduce these measures, and partly because of the difficulties in implementing them in local conditions, not least using protective gear in the heat and humidity.[68] But it was also a result of local customs and politics, which the standardised view of response failed to accommodate. The most heavily publicised of these was the local custom of washing the bodies of the dead, a practice which allowed the transmission of the virus. Although this practice was eventually curtailed, it was widely believed to have contributed to the early spread of the disease.[69] In addition to this, health workers were on occasion mistrusted, feared and avoided (not least as potential vectors for the disease, as well as because of long-standing mistrust of officialdom in some areas), while in some parts of the region the disease was seen as a product of witchcraft.[70] Joanne Liu also identified how 'in some cases, Ebola is being used as a political instrument, contributing to confusion and mistrust amongst communities'.[71] In a growing recognition that a standardised response was deficient and that greater cultural sensitivity was required, the WHO began calling for anthropologists to be deployed with its teams, both in West Africa and in subsequent large-scale health emergencies.[72]

Finally, pharmacological interventions failed for disease-specific reasons – there was no effective vaccine, or anti-viral, and even the transfusion of blood from patients who had recovered (Convalescent Whole Blood, or CWB therapy) was of uncertain effectiveness in a major outbreak, despite its apparent success in a small number of cases. Nevertheless, the power of the global health narrative was such that efforts were made to rush through untested vaccines and anti-virals, raising ethical questions over the risks involved as well as political unease over Africa being used as a 'laboratory' for Western pharmaceuticals.[73] What is also uncertain is whether, if any of the pharmacological interventions had been available, the countries in the region could have afforded to purchase them. International aid would almost certainly have been required, which would doubtless have led to further delays in treatment as financial authorisation was sought, while experience from the 2009 H1N1 pandemic suggests that fear in high-income states leads to pressure for them to stockpile anti-virals and vaccines even when the health risk is higher elsewhere. Therefore the globally accepted pathway of response to the risk of a disease outbreak failed for much of 2014, reinforcing the sense of crisis and reflected in statements from health leaders that the outbreak was 'out of control'.[74]

Ebola as a global health security risk

On 19 November 2014, when fear of Ebola in North America and Europe was at its height, the head of the US CDC Tom Frieden testified to Congress on US preparedness for public health threats. In his testimony he explicitly talked about Ebola as a threat to American lives and to national and global health security.[75] In so doing he was reflecting the manner in which security risks from disease outbreaks had been incorporated into the global health narrative. Specifically three concerns highlighted in this narrative – that disease outbreaks risked state failure, posed a risk to regional and global security, and threatened to spread beyond the region concerned creating fears for the lives of citizens elsewhere – were regularly identified in statements by key actors during the outbreak. As such they not only reflected an understanding of the outbreak as a global health crisis, but contributed through their speech acts to that understanding as well.

The risk of state failure was highlighted in UN Security Council Resolution 2177 in September 2014, which declared that 'the outbreak is undermining the stability of the most affected countries concerned and, unless contained, may lead to further instances of civil unrest, social tensions and a deterioration of the political and security climate'.[76] In her statement to the Security Council, WHO Director-General Margaret Chan drew attention to the economic instability caused by the outbreak, explicitly aligning herself with a World Bank report which had described the 'potentially catastrophic blow' to the region.[77] The next month she developed her concerns in a speech delivered in her name in the Philippines, arguing that 'I have never seen a health event threaten the very survival of societies and governments in already very poor countries. I have never seen an infectious disease contribute so strongly to potential state failure'.[78] Similarly the Korean Ambassador to the UN, Oh Joon, argued that the Ebola outbreak was a security issue because it was 'unravelling societies and threatening [the] gains' made through peace keeping,[79] while MSF's Joanne Liu warned in September 2014 of a collapse in state infrastructure.[80] These concerns were widespread, often picking up on what were identified as pre-existing vulnerabilities in the region resulting from past conflicts and weak economies. The WHO, for example, commented: 'The epidemic has had [a] broad impact on the socioeconomic stability of the region', before noting that all three countries 'were suffering economically, following years of civil war and unrest'.[81]

The UN Security Council also identified the second of the security concerns, the risk to regional and global security, stating in Resolution 2177 that 'the unprecedented extent of the Ebola outbreak in Africa constitutes a threat to international peace and security', although it was less explicit on how this was so.[82] Margaret Chan similarly argued that this was 'a threat to national security well beyond the outbreak zone'.[83] An October 2014 editorial in the *Lancet* was unequivocal in reporting a consensus that the outbreak was a 'clear threat to global health security',[84] while, in her statement to the UN, Liu referred somewhat vaguely to a 'transnational threat' from Ebola.[85] US President Obama appeared to draw a link between state failure and global security, stating in September 2014:

> if the outbreak is not stopped now, we could be looking at hundreds of thousands of people infected, with profound political and economic and security implications for all of us. So this is an epidemic that is not just a threat to regional security – it's a potential threat to global security if these countries break down, if their economies break down, if people panic. That has profound effects on all of us, even if we are not directly contracting the disease.[86]

The third concern, the fear of the disease spreading and threatening the lives of citizens in other countries, was reflected, for example, in comments made by the UK Chief Scientific Adviser, Sir Mark Walport, in July 2014 that 'deadly foreign diseases like Ebola are a "potential major threat to Britain"', a view also attributed to the British Prime Minister, David Cameron, after chairing a UK emergency COBRA meeting on the outbreak.[87] This view was similarly reflected in subsequent comments by David Heymann, chair of Public Health England, that 'as the Ebola virus crosses national borders, there is [a] clear understanding that the outbreaks in west [sic] Africa are a threat to *our* health security'.[88] Similarly Tom Frieden and three other colleagues from US CDC wrote 'the Ebola epidemic has shown how connected we are as a global community; we are only as safe as the most fragile states'.[89] Reaction to Frieden's November 2014 Congressional testimony suggested how this view resonated more widely outside public health circles.[90] Leaders were also at pains to emphasise the ability to control the disease should it spread to Europe or North America. In September 2014, when visiting CDC in Atlanta, President Obama commented, 'I want the American people to know that our experts, here at the CDC and across our government, agree that the chances of an Ebola outbreak here in the United States are extremely low'.[91] The UK Foreign Secretary, Philip Hammond, said 'it is not about the disease spreading in the UK because we have frankly different standards of infection control procedures that would make that most unlikely'.[92] Statements such as these, however, appeared to do little to allay the growing fear and sense of risk. Indeed, Margaret Chan felt moved to state the following month that 'in my long career in public health…I have never seen a health event strike such fear and terror, well beyond the affected countries'.[93] Data acquired from Twitter by *Time* indicated that 10.5 million tweets mentioning Ebola had been sent in 170 countries in the period 16 September to 6 October 2014 alone, with a dramatic spike at the very end of September and the beginning of October (when CDC announced the transmission of the virus in the USA for the first time).[94] Kim Yi Dionne drew an explicit link between this sense of fear and security: 'Fear of the Ebola virus and an out-of-control epidemic also make it easier for governments around the world to focus on security and military responses to public health solutions'.[95]

These three concerns were given legitimacy primarily by the credibility of the actors making the speech acts, but also by the modicum – however limited – of material evidence supporting them. Indeed, the very limited amount of material support for the claims suggests the power of the speech act in these circumstances. Not only did no state fail because of Ebola, but there had been no previous modern example of state failure because of a disease outbreak. This included the very heavy and long-term burden of HIV in sub-Saharan African states. Regional and global security does not seem to have been unduly affected, nor had it been during other recent major outbreaks of disease such as SARS, Middle East respiratory syndrome (MERS) and H1N1. And the outbreak was largely controlled, with only 36 cases outside the three most affected countries. Indeed, European and North American leaders emphasised their confidence in the ability to control an Ebola outbreak because of their public health infrastructure, while evidence from Nigeria during the outbreak demonstrated how effective control could be. This suggested difficulties in the outbreak spreading and at no point were cases of infection outside Africa anything other than isolated incidences, limited to health workers or those returning from working with aid agencies in West Africa. Nevertheless, the West African Ebola outbreak was successfully constructed as a security issue and generated feelings of fear and insecurity in countries far removed from the region, establishing the idea of the outbreak as a crisis.

Ebola and global health governance

The third element of the global health narrative includes ideas of how globalisation has created the need for effective collective action, not least in responding to health emergencies. However, the WHO complained that, during the outbreak, states failed to share information and exceeded recommended control measures, often without good reason and with potentially negative effects on global health more generally. In particular, travel restrictions were introduced in a number of states, despite uncertain – and potentially negative – consequences for global public health, in efforts to reassure the citizens of those states. The WHO commented that 'very few countries informed WHO that they were implementing additional measures significantly interfering with international traffic and when requested to justify their measures, few did so'.[96] Such states appeared to be privileging their national interests over the common good, a sentiment reflected in a *New York Times* op-ed that called on states to cease self-interested politicking at the WHO.[97] In a paradoxical twist, just as the failure to respond to the outbreak created the possibilities for greater global collaboration – what Kickbusch termed a 'cosmopolitan moment'[98] – so it revealed how states continued to privilege the national interest against exogenous threats.

These criticisms were largely ignored in the face of the apparent failure of the WHO, which led to calls for its reform, even replacement.[99] The slow and largely inadequate reaction to the 2014–15 West Africa Ebola outbreak revealed what Kickbusch describes as a 'structural global vulnerability',[100] while Gostin and Friedman commented that the West Africa Ebola outbreak had revealed a 'fragmented global health system' which was incapable of dealing with emergencies on this scale.[101] It demonstrated how the global response to health emergencies, including disease surveillance, was deficient – in the words of the *New York Times*, it had been a 'debacle' in which the WHO was the key culprit.[102] This point appeared to have been accepted by the WHO, when its Director-General reported to the WHO Executive Board that the outbreak had revealed 'some inadequacies' in the organisation.[103] The emergence of Ebola in West Africa in December 2013 was not identified by the WHO for three months, and even then it took until August before a PHEIC was called – some time after MSF had declared the spread of the disease to be 'out of control'.[104]

Despite the WHO declaring a PHEIC, the international response remained limited and slow to materialise. It was only on 28 August that the WHO produced its Ebola 'roadmap' to coordinate international efforts, followed on 18 September by the establishment of UNMEER.[105] Liu's call for action at the UN in the first week of September 2014 was followed two weeks later by her returning to the UN to complain publicly about continued inaction, arguing that 'the response remains totally, and lethally, inadequate'.[106] This was seven months after the outbreak had been identified, four months after the realisation that this was a more serious and complex outbreak of the disease than any previously encountered, and a month after the WHO had admitted that 'cases across the three worst countries were increasing at a rate that far outpaced the capacity of the traditional, core Ebola control package'.[107] These weaknesses in operational capacity were acknowledged when, in January 2015, the WHO proposed to its Executive Board a new capability to respond to large-scale health emergencies, a capability approved at the World Health Assembly (the WHO's governing body) in May 2015.[108] It was also seen in calls to revisit the International Health Regulations, the key international agreement enabling global surveillance of disease outbreaks.[109] The 2014–15 Ebola outbreak was therefore a crisis in terms of the global health narrative in a somewhat different sense: it was a crisis because it demonstrated the inadequacies of existing governance mechanisms and the need to urgently address capacities for collective action. If the global health narrative had established the need for new, collective action to meet global health challenges, then the 2014–15 outbreak was widely seen as demonstrating how the ability to respond was in crisis.

Conclusion

This article began from the basis that there was nothing 'natural' about the 2014–15 Ebola outbreak being considered a crisis; rather it was socially constructed as such. Specifically it suggested that the outbreak could be understood as a crisis because of the way in which it resonated with the global health narrative, which had been developing over the best part of two decades beforehand. This narrative consists of three themes which may be broadly characterised as globalisation, securitisation and politicisation. The outbreak tied into the narrative's theme of the impact of globalisation on health, through both ideas of shared risk and a globally accepted pathway of response which, when it failed, enhanced the sense of crisis. The outbreak was presented as a global health security risk through speech acts which claimed potential state failure, threats to regional and global security and that the spread of the disease threatened the well-being of citizens outside the region. And the poor response to the outbreak revealed weaknesses in global health governance exacerbating the sense of crisis, as well as the privileging of the national interest in response to exogenous threats. To suggest that the crisis was socially constructed is not, however, to deny the terrible suffering that occurred, especially in Guinea, Liberia and Sierra Leone during 2014. But it does serve to highlight the way in which the global health agenda is not an objective phenomenon. Rather it is one which is made and which reflects certain interests and understandings. Thus the 2014–15 outbreak was a global crisis which, for a short period of time, dominated headlines, fascinated social media and preoccupied decision makers. At the same time other diseases, with considerably higher annually recurring mortality rates, were largely ignored.

Disclosure statement

No potential conflict of interest was reported by the author.

Notes

1. Chan, "Report by the Director-General."
2. Although the first (retrospectively) identified case was in December 2013 and the epidemic continued into 2015, for convenience in this article the outbreak is referred to as '2014–15'. The article also uses 'West Africa', as this is where the first case was identified, where the outbreak was first detected and where the overwhelming majority of cases occurred, and it allows a differentiation from the separate Ebola outbreak over the summer of 2014 in the DRC.
3. WHO, "Ebola Situation Report."
4. Determination made by comparing WHO, "Current Context and Challenges," paragraph 19 for the 2014–15 West Africa outbreak with CDC, "Outbreaks Chronology" for previous outbreaks and cases.
5. WHO, "Key Events."
6. MSF, "Ebola in West Africa"; and WHO, "Current Context and Challenges."
7. "Reform after the Ebola Debacle." See also Frieden, "Joanne Liu"; House of Commons International Development Committee, *Responses to the Ebola Crisis*; Park, "WHO announces Changes"; Petherick, "Ebola in West Africa"; and Beaubien, "Critics."
8. WHO, "Current Context and Challenges."
9. Comments reported in WHO, "UN Senior Leaders."

10. UN Security Council, *Resolution 2177*.
11. Ban Ki-moon, "Statement."
12. CDC, "Estimating the Future Number of Cases."
13. Duncan contracted Ebola in Liberia before travelling to the USA, where he fell ill from the disease.
14. WHO, "Current Context and Challenges," paragraph 8. See also Holehouse, "David Cameron rounds on European Leaders"; and Dionne, "Obama's Ebola Failure."
15. "#BBCtrending."
16. See, for example, UN, "With Spread of Ebola outpacing Respose"; Liu, "United Nations Special Briefing"; Liu, "Ebola UN Speech"; Gostin et al., "The Ebola Epidemic"; and Oxfam, "More Military, more Medics."
17. Despite the PHEIC supposedly being criteria-based, rumours persist that political pressure was exerted to avoid calling one over the West African Ebola outbreak. See, for example, "Political Considerations"; and Gostin, "The Future of the World Health Organization."
18. As we have seen with HIV/AIDS, where the risk is arguably higher since it is a long-wave event. See Barnett and Whiteside, "The Jaipur Paradigm"; and McInnes and Rushton, "HIV, AIDS and Security."
19. Chan, "Ebola Virus Disease." See also the comments of WHO head of global health security, Keiji Fukuda, reported in "WHO."
20. The source of this information is a senior Nigerian Ministry of Health official.
21. Liu, "United Nations Special Briefing."
22. CDC, "Estimating the Future Number of Cases."
23. See WHO, "Top 10 Causes of Death." Interestingly Margaret Chan alluded to this discrepancy between the attention paid to Ebola and the greater number of deaths from other causes in an October 2014 speech – in other words, at the height of concern over Ebola. Chan, "WHO Director-General's Speech."
24. WHO, "WHO Statement."
25. For example, WHO, "Ebola Virus Disease"; Rowden, "West Africa's Financial Immune Deficiency"; Fauci, "Ebola"; Chan, "Ebola Virus Disease"; and MSF, "International Response to West Africa Ebola."
26. Compare, for example, WHO's somewhat self-congratulatory assessments with the more acerbic pieces which appeared in the press. WHO, "Current Context and Challenges"; WHO "Highlight of Efforts"; "Reform after the Ebola Debacle"; and "Lack of Leadership."
27. Onuf, *A World of our Making*.
28. Examples include Davies et al., *Disease Diplomacy*; Shiffman, "A Social Explanation"; Labonte and Gagnon, "Framing Health and Foreign Policy"; and McInnes and Lee, *Framing Global Health Governance*.
29. McInnes and Lee, *Global Health and International Relations*.
30. See, for example, "Oslo Ministerial Declaration"; Garrett, "The Challenge of Global Health"; Davies, *The Global Politics of Health*; MacFarlane et al., "In the Name of Global Health"; and Beaglehole and Bonita, "What is Global Health?"
31. Department of Health, *Health is Global*.
32. Lee, *Globalization and Health*; and McInnes and Lee, *Global Health*, 6–22.
33. For example, Brown and Chalk, *The Global Threat*; Department of Health, *Health is Global*; Prescott, "SARS"; Ingram, "The New Geopolitics"; and Institute of Medicine, *America's Vital Interest*. See also Tatem et al., "Global Transport Networks" for a discussion of how transport has affected disease vectors.
34. Kamradt-Scott, "Evidence-based Medicine." See also Jennings, "Chinese Medicine."
35. Wald, *Contagious Cultures*.
36. Starling et al., *New Products*, esp. 51–52.
37. See, for example, Elbe, *Virus Alert*; and Simms, "Sub-Saharan Africa's HIV Pandemic."
38. McInnes and Lee, *Global Health and International Relations*, 130–157.
39. Institute of Medicine, *America's Vital Interest*; and WHO, *The World Health Report 2007*.

40. UN, "Security Council holds Debate"; Department of Homeland Security, "Office of Health Affairs"; McInnes and Rushton, "HIV, AIDS and Security"; and Elbe, *Virus Alert*. Elbe subsequently argued that not only had ideas of security affected health concerns, but that the reverse had also occurred. Elbe, *Security and Global Health*.

41. See Rushton and Youde, *Handbook of Global Health Security* for a thorough review of global health and security issues.

42. See McInnes and Rushton, "HIV, AIDS and Security."

43. Enemark, "Is Pandemic Flu?"; Enemark, *Disease and Security*; and Rushton and Youde, *Handbook of Global Health Security*, esp. 83–150.

44. A US National Intelligence Committee Report on the 2002–03 SARS epidemic concluded that it caused a 'significant, if temporary, slowing of economic growth in East Asia and Canada', although initial estimates of a $100 billion cost were almost certainly exaggerated. NIC, *Strategic Implications of Global Health*, 23.

45. The most thorough examination of this is with respect to HIV. See, for example, International Crisis Group, *HIV/AIDS as a Security Issue*.

46. Kamradt-Scott, "Evidence-based Medicine," S112; and Kristiansen and Mooney, *Evidence-based Medicine*.

47. See, for example, WHO, "The Right to Health."

48. See, for example, Burchardt, "Faith-based Humanitarianism"; Ingram, "HIV/ AIDS'; and Ingram "Governmentality and Security."

49. WHO, *Macroeconomics and Health*.

50. Institute of Medicine, *America's Vital Interest in Global Health*.

51. Ingram, "HIV/AIDS"; and Ingram, "Governmentality and Security."

52. See, for example, Harman, *Global Health Governance*; Youde, *Global Health Governance*; and Davies, *The Global Politics of Health*, 31–61.

53. For a discussion and analysis of this, see McInnes and Lee, *Framing Global Health Governance*.

54. CDC, "Outbreaks Chronology."

55. CDC, "2014 Ebola Outbreak."

56. Arwady et al., "Evolution of Ebola Virus Disease," 578.

57. Liu, "UN Special Briefing"; and Liu, "Ebola UN Speech."

58. This analysis is influenced by Finnemore and Sikkink's work on norm entrepreneurship in international institutions, as used by Davies et al. in their study of norms and global health security. For both sets of authors, norms 'cascade' once a tipping point has been reached but the identification of the tipping point is left vague. Davies et al., *Disease Diplomacy*, esp. 46.

59. A PHEIC has to meet two criteria: that an outbreak in one state poses a risk of spreading to others; and that it is potentially sufficiently serious to warrant a coordinated international response. See WHO, "PHEIC Procedures." These are of course sufficiently imprecise as to warrant interpretation and the WHO Director-General (who calls the PHEIC) is required to establish a committee of experts to advise on this. They are also amenable to different interpretations of whether an outbreak has met these criteria or not.

60. See, for example, the pleas of MSF for action throughout the summer of 2014. MSF, "Ebola in West Africa"; MSF, "Ebola: Official MSF Response"; and MSF, "International Response to West Africa Ebola."

61. srogers [sic], "Two Months in #Ebola on Twitter," Accessed May 25, 2015. https://srogers. cartodb.com/viz/98cb3c42-4d7b-11e4-b811-0e4fddd5de28/public_map. However, the often ephemeral nature of social media was demonstrated when, in October 2014, the proposed euthanisation of Ramos' dog Excalibur became the second most trending story on Twitter. It is believed that this is the only occasion that incidents relating to Ebola reached this level of social media activity.

62. Chan, "Ebola Virus Disease."

63. Wald, *Contagious Cultures*.

64. WHO, "Current Context and Challenges"; and Feldmann, "Ebola."

65. WHO, "Current Context and Challenges"; Fidler, "The Ebola Outbreak"; and Stocking, *Report*.

66. Chan, "Ebola Virus Disease."

67. Dixon and Schafer, "Ebola Viral Disease Outbreak"; and Briand et al., "The International Ebola Emergency."
68. Rowden, "West Africa's Financial Immune Deficiency"; and MSF, "Ebola: Pushed to the Limit."
69. WHO, "Ebola Virus Disease," 2; Chan, "Ebola Virus Disease"; and Frieden et al., "Ebola 2014."
70. Briand et al., "The International Ebola Emergency."
71. Liu, "Speech by MSF International President."
72. WHO, "Ensuring WHO's Capacity," 5.
73. WHO, "Fast Tracking"; WHO, "Ebola Virus Disease"; Gutfraind and Meyers, "Evaluating Large-scale Blood Transfusion Therapy"; Easton and Leppard, "Experimental Drugs"; and Tappero et al., "Global Health Security Agenda."
74. MSF, "Ebola in West Africa."
75. Frieden, "Preparedness and Response."
76. UN Security Council, *Resolution 2177*.
77. Chan, quoted in UN, "Spread of Ebola."
78. Chan, "WHO Director-General's Speech."
79. Oh Joon, quoted in UN, "With the Spread of Ebola outpacing Response."
80. Liu, "UN Special Briefing."
81. WHO, "Current Context and Challenges." See also Maron, "Ebola now poses a Threat"; MSF, "International Response to West Africa Ebola"; and Chen and Takemi, "Ebola."
82. UN Security Council, *Resolution 2177*.
83. Key elements of Chan's statement are reproduced in UN, "With the Spread of Ebola outpacing Response."
84. "Ebola: What Lessons?". See also Maron, "Ebola now poses a Threat."
85. Liu, "UN Special Briefing."
86. Obama, "Remarks."
87. Knapton, "Ebola Outbreak"; and Watts, "Ebola." So-called COBRA meetings are *ad hoc* emergency committees, chaired either by the UK prime minister or another senior minister. The name comes from the meeting room used – Cabinet Office Briefing Room A.
88. Heymann, "The True Scope of Health Security" (emphasis added).
89. Tappero et al., "Global Health Security Agenda."
90. For example, Winfield Burns, "The CDC's Tom Frieden"; and Dionne, "Obama's Ebola Failure." See also Basch et al., "Coverage of the Ebola Virus Disease."
91. Obama, "Remarks."
92. Quoted in "Ebola: NHS can deal with Threat." See also "Ebola Outbreak."
93. Chan, "WHO Director-General's Speech."
94. Luckerson, "Watch how Word of Ebola." See also "#BBCtrending."
95. Dionne, "Obama's Ebola Failure."
96. WHO, "IHR and Ebola," paragraph 10. See also WHO, "Current Context and Challenges," paragraph 13; and "WHO, "IHR and Ebola," paragraphs 8, 9.
97. "Reform after the Ebola Debacle."
98. Kickbusch, "Global Health Security."
99. See for example Stocking, *Report*; Beaubien, "Critics"; and Gostin, "The Future of the World Health Organization."
100. Kickbusch, "Global Health Security."
101. Gostin and Friedman, "A Retrospective and Prospective Analysis," 1903.
102. "Reform after the Ebola Debacle." See also Stocking, *Report*.
103. Chan, "Report of the Director-General."
104. The comment is from MSF's head of operations, Bart Janssens. MSF, "Ebola in West Africa."
105. WHO, *Ebola Response Roadmap*; UNMEER, *UN Mission*; and Ban Ki-moon, "Statement by the Secretary-General."
106. Liu, "Ebola UN Speech."
107. See, for example, WHO, "Current Context and Challenges," para 6.
108. WHO, "Ensuring WHO's Capacity"; and WHO, "WHO Response."
109. WHO, "IHR and Ebola"; WHO, "Ensuring WHO's Capacity"; and Katz and Dowell, "Revising the International Health Regulations." See also Gostin, "The Future of the World Health Organization."

Bibliography

Arwady, M. Allison, Luke Bawo, Jennifer C. Hunter, Moses Massaquoi, Almea Matanock, Bernice Dahn, Patrick Ayscue, et al. "Evolution of Ebola Virus Disease from Exotic Infection to Global Health Priority, Liberia, Mid-2014." *Emeegin infectious Diseases* 21 (2015). http://wwwnc.cdc.gov/eid/article/21/4/14-1940_article

"#BBCtrending: How Panic about Ebola is spreading faster than the Virus." *BBC News*, October 14, 2014. http://www.bbc.co.uk/news/blogs-trending-29618224.

Ban Ki-moon. "Statement by the Secretary-General on the Establishment of the United Nations Mission for Ebola Emergency Response (UNMEER)." Accessed June 10, 2015. http://www.un.org/sg/statements/index.asp?nid=8006.

Barnett, Tony, and Alan Whiteside. "The Jaipur Paradigm: A Conceptual Framework for Understanding Social Susceptibility and Vulnerability to HIV." *South African Medical Journal* 90 (2000): 1098–1101.

Basch, Corey H., Charles E. Basch, and Irwin Redlener. "Coverage of the Ebola Virus Disease Epidemic in three widely circulated United States Newspapers: Implications for Preparedness and Prevention." *Health Promotion Perspectives* 4, no. 2 (2014): 247–251.

Beaglehole, Robert, and R. Bonita. "What is Global Health?" *Global Health Action* 3 (2010): 5142.

Beaubien, Jason. "Critics say Ebola Crisis was WHO's Big Failure. Will Reform Follow?" US National Public Radio (npr), February 6, 2015. http://www.npr.org/sections/goatsandsoda/2015/02/06/384223023/critics-says-ebola-crisis-was-whos-big-failure-will-reform-follow.

Briand, Sylvie, Eric Bertherat, Paul Cox, Pierre Formenty, Marie-Paule Kieny, Joel K. Myhre, Cathy Roth, et al. "The International Ebola Emergency." *New England Journal of Medicine* 371, no. 13 (2014): 1180–1183.

Brown, Jennifer, and Peter Chalk. *The Global Threat of New and Re-emerging Infectious Diseases*. Santa Monica, CA: RAND, 2003.

Burchard, Marian. "Faith-based Humanitarianism: Organizational Change and Everyday Meanings in South Africa." *Sociology of Religion* 74, no. 1 (2013): 30–55.

Centers for Disease Control and Prevention (CDC). "Estimating the Future Number of Cases in the Ebola Epidemic – Liberia and Sierra Leone, 2014–2015." November 2014 update. http://www.cdc.gov/vhf/ebola/outbreaks/2014-west-africa/qa-mmwr-estimating-future-cases.html.

CDC. "Outbreaks Chronology – Ebola Virus Disease." March 4, 2015 update. http://www.cdc.gov/vhf/ebola/outbreaks/history/chronology.html.

CDC. "2014 Ebola Outbreak in West Africa: Case Counts." Accessed Juen 23, 2015. http://www.cdc.gov/vhf/ebola/outbreaks/2014-west-africa/case-counts.html.

Chan, Margaret. "Ebola Virus Disease in West Africa – No Early End to the Outbreak." *New England Journal of Medicine* 371, no. 13 (2014): 1183–1185.

Chan, Margaret. "Report by the Director-General to the Special Session of the Executive Board on Ebola." January 25, 2015. http://www.who.int/dg/speeches/2015/executive-board-ebola/en/.

Chan, Margaret. "WHO Director-General's Speech to the Regional Committee for the Western Pacific." October 13, 2014. http://who.int/dg/speeches/2014/regional-committee-western-pacific/en/.

Chen, Lincoln, and Keizo Takemi. "Ebola: Lessons in Human Security." *Lancet* 385, issue 9980 (2015). http://www.thelancet.com/journals/lancet/article/PIIS0140-6736(15)60858-3/fulltext.

Davies, Sara E. *The Global Politics of Health*. Cambridge: Polity, 2011.

Davies, Sara E., Adam Kamradt-Scott, and Simon Rushton. *Disease Diplomacy*. Baltimore, MD: Johns Hopkins University Press, 2015.

Department of Health. *Health is Global*. London: HMSO, 2008.

Department of Homeland Security. "Office of Health Affairs." http://www.dhs.gov/office-health-affairs.

Dionne, Kim Yi. "Obama's Ebola Failure." *Foreign Affairs*, September 15, 2014. https://www.foreignaffairs.com/articles/africa/2014-09-15/obamas-ebola-failure.

Dixon, Meredith G., and Ilana J. Schafer. "Ebola Virus Disease Outbreak – West Africa 2014." *Morbidity and Mortality Weekly Report* 63, no. 25 (2014): 548–551.

Easton, Andrew, and Keith Leppard. "Experimental Drugs were used for HIV, but Ebola is a riskier Bet." *The Conversation*, August 18, 2014. http://theconversation.com/experimental-drugs-were-used-for-hiv-but-ebola-is-a-riskier-bet-30578.

"Ebola: NHS can deal with Threat to UK, says Hammond." *BBC News*, July 30, 2014. http://www.bbc.co.uk/news/uk-28558783.

"Ebola Outbreak: Britain has Expertise to Cope, say Ministers." *Guardian*, July 30, 2014. http://www.theguardian.com/society/2014/jul/30/ebola-outbreak-uk-ministers-emergecny-cobra-meeting.

"Ebola: "What Lessons for the International Health Regulations?" *Lancet* October 8, 2014. http://www.thelancet.com/journals/lancet/article/PIIS0140-6736(14)61697-4/fulltext.

Elbe, Stefan. *Virus Alert: Security, Governmentality and the AIDS Pandemic*. New York: Columbia University Press, 2009.

Elbe, Stefan. *Security and Global Health: Toward the Medicalization of Insecurity*. Cambridge: Polity, 2010.

Enemark, Christian. *Disease and Security*. Abingdon: Routledge, 2007.

Enemark, Christian. "Is Pandemic Flu a Security Threat?" *Survival* 51, no. 1 (2009): 191–214.

Fauci, Anthony S. "Ebola – Underscoring the Global Disparities in Health Care Resources." *New England Journal of Medicine* 371, no. 12 (2014): 1084–1086.

Feldmann, Heinz. "Ebola – A Growing Threat?" *New England Journal of Medicine* 371, no. 15 (2014): 1375–1378.

Fidler, David P. "The Ebola Outbreak and the Future of Global Health Security." *Lancet* 385, issue 9980 (2015). http://www.thelancet.com/journals/lancet/article/PIIS0140-6736(15)60858-3/fulltext.

Frieden, Tom, Inger Damon, Beth P. Bell, Thomas Kenyon, and Stuart Nichol. "Ebola 2014 – New Challenges, New Global Response and Responsibility." *New England Journal of Medicine* 371, no. 13 (2014): 1177–1180.

Frieden, Tom. "Joanne Liu." *Time*, 100 Leaders, April 16, 2015. http://time.com/3822834/joanne-liu-2015-time-100/.

Frieden, Tom. "Preparedness and Response to Public Health Threats: How Ready are We?" *Testimony before the Senate Committee on Homeland Security and Governmental Affairs*, November 19, 2014. http://www.cdc.gov/washington/testimony/2014/t20141119.htmlast.

Garrett, L. "The Challenge of Global Health." *Foreign Affairs*, January/February 2007. https://www.foreignaffairs.org/articles/2007-01-01/challenge-global-health.

Gostin, Lawrence O. "The Future of the World Health Organization." *Milbank Quarterly* 93, no. 3 (2015): 475–479. http://www.milbank.org/the-milbank-quarterly/search-archives/article/4046/the-future-of-the-world-health-organization-lessons-learned-from-ebola.

Gostin, Lawrence O., and Eric A. Friedman. "A Retrospective and Prospective Analysis of the West African Ebola Virus Disease Epidemic: Robust National Health Systems at the Foundation and an Empowered WHO at the Apex." *Lancet* 385, issue 9980 (2015): 1902–1909.

Gostin, Lawrence O., Daniel Lucey, and Alexandra Phelan. "The Ebola Epidemic: A Global Health Emergency." *Journal of the American Medical Association* 312, no. 11 (2014): 1095–1096.

Gutfraind, Alexander, and Lauren Ancel Meyers. "Evaluating Large-scale Blood Transfusion Therapy for the Current Ebola Epidemic in Liberia." *Journal of Infectious Diseases* 211, no. 8 (2015): 1262–1267.

Harman, Sophie. *Global Health Governance*. Abingdon: Routledge, 2011.

Heymann, David. "The True Scope of Health Security." *Lancet* 385, issue 9980 (2015). http://www.thelancet.com/journals/lancet/article/PIIS0140-6736(15)60858-3/fulltext.

House of Commons International Development Committee. *Responses to the Ebola Crisis*. Eighth Report of Session 2014–15. http://www.publications.parliament.uk/pa/cm201415/cmselect/cmintdev/876/876.pdf.

Holehouse, Matthew. "David Cameron rounds on European Leaders who spend less Fighting Ebola than Ikea." *Daily Telegraph*, October 23, 2014. http://www.telegraph.co.uk/news/worldnews/ebola/11183784/David-Cameron-rounds-on-European-leaders-who-spend-less-fighting-Ebola-than-Ikea.html.

Ingram, Alan. "The New Geopolitics of Disease: Between Global Health and Global Security." *Geopolitics* 10, no. 3 (2005): 522–545.

Ingram, Alan. "HIV/AIDS, Security and the Geopolitics of US–Nigerian Relations." *Review of International Political Economy* 14, no. 3 (2007): 510–534.

Ingram, Alan. "Governmentality and Security in the US President's Emergency plan for AIDS Relief (PEPFAR)." *Geoforum* 21, no. 4 (2010): 607–616.

Institute of Medicine. *America's Vital Interest in Global Health*. Washington, DC: National Academies Press, 1997.

International Crisis Group (ICG). *HIV/AIDS as a Security Issue*. Brussels: ICG, 2001.

Jennings, Michael. "Chinese Medicine and Medical Pluralism in Dar-es-Salaam." *International Relations* 19, no. 4 (2005): 457–473.

Kamradt-Scott, Adam. "Evidence-based Medicine and the Governance of Pandemic Influenza." *Global Public Health* 7, Supplement 2 (2012): S111–126.

Katz, Rebecca, and Scott F. Dowell. "Revising the International Health Regulations: Call for a 2017 Review Conference." *Lancet Global Health*, published online May 8, 2015. http://www.thelancet.com/journals/langlo/article/PIIS2214-109X(15)00025-X/fulltext.

Kickbusch, Ilona. "Global Health Security: A Cosmopolitan Moment." *G7G20*. Accessed June 22, 2015. http://www.g7g20.com/articles/ilona-kickbusch-global-health-security-a-cosmopolitan-moment.

Knapton, Sarah. "Ebola Outbreak: Deadly Foreign Diseases are 'Potential Major Threat', says Chief Scientist." *Daily Telegraph*, July 30, 2014. http://www.telegraph.co.uk/news/science/science-news/10998514/Ebola-outbreak-deadly-foreign-diseases-are-potential-major-threat-says-Chief-Scientist.html.

Kristiansen, I. S., and G. Mooney. *Evidence-based Medicine in its Place*. Abingdon: Routledge, 2004.

Labonte, Ron, and Michelle Gagnon. "Framing Health and Foreign Policy." *Globalization and Health* 6, no. 14 (2010): http://www.globalizationandhealth.com/content/6/1/14.

"Lack of Leadership hurts Ebola Fight in West Africa: MSF." *Reuters*, August 21, 2014. http://uk.reuters.com/article/2014/08/21/us-health-ebola-msf-idUKKBN0GL24P20140821.

Lee, Kelley. *Globalization and Health: An Introduction*. Basingstoke: Macmillan, 2003.

Liu, Joanne. "Ebola UN Speech: 'The Response remains totally, and lethally, Inadequate.'" September 16, 2014. http://www.msf.org.uk/article/ebola-un-speech-response-remains-totally-and-lethally-inadequate.

Liu, Joanne. "Speech by MSF International President Joanne Liu to the EU High Level Meeting on Ebola." March 3, 2015. http://www.msf.org/article/speech-msf-international-president-joanne-liu-eu-high-level-meeting-ebola-–-3-march-2015.

Liu, Joanne. "United Nations Special Briefing." September 2, 2014. http://www.msf.org.uk/article/msf-international-president-united-nations-special-briefing-ebola.

Luckerson, Victor. "Watch how Word of Ebola exploded in America." *Time*, October 7, 2014. http://time.com/3478452/ebola-twitter/.

Macfarlane, Sarah B., Marian Jacobs, and Ephata E. Kaaya. "In the Name of Global Health: Trends in Academic Institutions." *Journal of Public Health Policy* 29, no. 4 (2008): 383–401.

Maron, Dina Fine. "Ebola now poses a Threat to National Security in West Africa." *Scientific American*, September 2, 2014. http://www.scientificamerican.com/article/ebola-now-poses-a-threat-to-national-security-in-west-africa/.

McInnes, Colin, and Kelley Lee, eds. *Framing Global Health Governance. Special Supplement of Global Public Health* 7, SS2 (2012).

McInnes, Colin, and Kelley Lee. *Global Health and International Relations*. Cambridge: Polity, 2012.

McInnes, Colin, and Simon Rushton. "HIV, AIDS and Security: Where are we Now?" *International Affairs* 86, no. 1 (2010): 225–245.

Médecins Sans Frontières (MSF). "Ebola: Official MSF Response to WHO declaring Epidemic an 'Extraordinary Event.'" August 8, 2014. http://www.msf.org.uk/article/ebola-official-msf-response-who-declaring-epidemic-extraordinary-event.

MSF. "Ebola in West Africa: Epidemic requires Massive Deployment of Resources." June 21, 2014. http://www.msf.org/article/ebola-west-africa-epidemic-requires-massive-deployment-resources.

MSF. "Ebola: Pushed to the Limit and Beyond – MSF Report." March 23, 2015. http://www.msf.org.uk/article/ebola-pushed-to-the-limit-and-beyond-msf-report.

MSF. "International Response to West Africa Ebola Epidemic dangerously Inadequate." August 15, 2014. http://www.msf.org/article/international-response-west-africa-ebola-epidemic-dangerously-inadequate.

National Intelligence Council (NIC). *Strategic Implications of Global Health*. 2008. http://www.dni.gov/nic/NIC_specialproducts.html.

Obama, Barack. "Remarks by the President on the Ebola Outbreak." Press release, September 16, 2014. https://www.whitehouse.gov/the-press-office/2014/09/16/remarks-president-ebola-outbreak.

Onuf, Nicholas. *A World of our Making: Rules and Rule in Social Theory and International Relations*. Columbia, SC: University of South Carolina Press, 1989.

"Oslo Ministerial Declaration – Global Health: A Pressing Foreign Policy Issue of our Time." *Lancet* 369, no. 9570 (2007): 1373–1378.

Oxfam. "More Military, more Medics and more Money needed to prevent Definitive Humanitarian Disaster of our Generation." Press release, October 18, 2014. https://www.oxfam.org/en/pressroom/pressreleases/2014-10-18/ebola-more-military-medics-money-needed.

Park, Madison. "WHO announces Changes after Widespread Ebola Criticism." CNN online. Accessed May 18, 2015. http://edition.cnn.com/2015/05/18/health/who-ebola-reform/.

Petherick, Anna. "Ebola in West Africa: Learning the Lessons." *Lancet*, published online February 10, 2015. http://ebola.thelancet.com/pb/assets/raw/Lancet/pdfs/S0140673615600757.pdf.

"Political Considerations delayed WHO Ebola Response, Emails Show." Associated Press. Accessed September 3, 2015. http://www.cbsnews.com/news/political-considerations-delayed-who-ebola-response-emails-show/.

Prescott, Elizabeth. "SARS: A Warning." *Survival* 45, no. 3 (2003): 207–226.

"Reform after the Ebola Debacle." *New York Times*, February 10, 2015. http://www.nytimes.com/2015/02/10/opinion/reform-after-the-ebola-debacle.html?_r=0.

Rowden, Rick. "West Africa's Financial Immune Deficiency." *Foreign Policy*, October 30, 2014. http://foreignpolicy.com/2014/10/30/west-africas-financial-immune-deficiency/.

Rushton, Simon, and Jeremy Youde. *Handbook of Global Health Security*. Basingstoke: Palgrave, 2014.

Shiffman, Jeremy. "A Social Explanation for the Rise and Fall of Global Health Issues." *Bulletin of the World Health Organization* 87, no. 8 (2009): 608–613.

Simms, Chris. "Sub-Saharan Africa's HIV Pandemic." *American Psychologist* 69, no. 1 (2014): 94–95.

Starling, Mary, Ruairi Brugha, and Gill Walt. *New Products into Old Systems*. London: Save the Children, 2002.

Stocking, Barbara. *Report of the Ebola Interim Assessment Panel*. Geneva: WHO, 2015.

Tappero, Jordan W., Matthew J. Thomas, Thomas A. Kenyon, and Thomas R. Frieden. "Global Health Security Agenda: Building Resilient Public Health Systems to stop Infectious Disease Threats." *Lancet* 385, issue 9980 (2015). http://www.thelancet.com/journals/lancet/article/PIIS0140-6736(15)60858-3/fulltext.

Tatem, A. J., D. J. Rogers, and S. I. Hay. "Global Transport Networks and Infectious Disease Spread." *Advances in Parasitology* 62 (2006): 293–343. http://www.ncbi.nlm.nih.gov/pmc/articles/PMC3145127/.

UN. "Security Council holds Debate on Impact of AIDS on Peace and Security in Africa." Press Release 6781, January 10, 2000. http://www.un.org/press/en/2000/20000110.sc6781.doc.html.

UN. "With Spread of Ebola outpacing Response, Security Council adopts Resolution 2177 (2014) urging Immediate Action, End to Isolation of Affected States." Media Release SC11566, September 18, 2014. http://www.un.org/press/en/2014/sc11566.doc.htm.

UN Security Council. *Resolution 2177*. September 18, 2014. http://www.un.org/en/ga/search/view_doc.asp?symbol=S/RES/2177%20(2014).

UNMEER. *UN Mission for Ebola Emergency Response*. Website. https://ebolaresponse.un.org/un-mission-ebola-emergency-response-unmeer.

Wald, Priscilla. *Contagious Cultures: Cultures, Carriers and the Outbreak Narrative*. Durham, NC: Duke University Press, 2007.

Watts, Joseph. "Ebola: David Cameron considers Outbreak as a 'Serious Threat' in the UK." *London Evening Standard*, July 30, 2014. http://www.standard.co.uk/news/health/philip-hammond-calls-cobra-meeting-over-ebola-amid-fears-it-could-spread-to-uk-9637146.html.

"WHO: Ebola 'an International Emergency'." *BBC News*, August 8, 2014. http://www.bbc.co.uk/news/world-africa-28702356.

WHO. "Current Context and Challenges: Stopping the Epidemic, and Preparedness in Non-affected Countries and Regions." Paper for WHO Executive Board Special Session on Ebola EBSS/3/2. http://apps.who.int/gb/e/e_ebss3.html.

WHO. *Ebola Response Roadmap*. Geneva: WHO, 2014. http://apps.who.int/iris/bitstream/10665/131596/1/EbolaResponseRoadmap.pdf?ua=1.

WHO. "Ebola Situation Report – 3 June 2015." http://apps.who.int/ebola/ebola-situation-reports.

WHO. "Ebola Virus Disease." Factsheet 103, April 2015 update. http://www.who.int/mediacentre/factsheets/fs103/en/.

WHO. "Ensuring WHO's Capacity to prepare for and respond to future Large-scale and Sustained Outbreaks and Emergencies." Paper for WHO Executive Board Special Session on Ebola EBSS/3/3. http://apps.who.int/gb/e/e_ebss3.html.

WHO. "Fast-tracking the Development and Prospective Roll-out of Vaccines, Therapies and Diagnostics in Response to Ebola Virus Disease." Paper for WHO Executive Board Special Session on Ebola EBSS/3/INF1. http://apps.who.int/gb/e/e_ebss3.html.

WHO. "Highlight of Efforts made to date towards preparing Non-affected Countries and Regions to respond to Potential Importation of EVD." Paper for WHO Executive Board Special Session on Ebola EBSS/3/INF3. http://apps.who.int/gb/e/e_ebss3.html.

WHO. "IHR and Ebola." Paper for WHO Executive Board Special Session on Ebola EBSS/3/INF4. http://apps.who.int/gb/e/e_ebss3.html.

WHO. "Key Events in the WHO Response to the Ebola Outbreak." Accessed June 10, 2015. http://www.who.int/csr/disease/ebola/one-year-report/who-response/en/.

WHO. *Macroeconomics and Health: Investing in Health for Economic Development*. Report of the Commission on Macroeconomics and Health. Geneva: WHO, 2001.

WHO. "PHEIC Procedures." Accessed October 1, 2015. http://www.who.int/ihr/procedures/pheic/en/.

WHO. "The Right to Health." Fact Sheet 323, 2007 update. http://www.who.int/mediacentre/factsheets/fs323/en/index.html.

WHO. "Top 10 Causes of Death." Fact Sheet 310, 2014 update. http://www.who.int/mediacentre/factsheets/fs310/en/.

WHO. "UN Senior Leaders outline Needs for Global Ebola Response." http://www.who.int/mediacentre/news/releases/2014/ebola-response-needs/en/.

WHO. "WHO Statement on the Meeting of the International Health Regulations Emergency Committee concerning the International Spread of Wild Poliovirus." May 5, 2014. http://www.who.int/mediacentre/news/statements/2014/polio-20140505/en/.

WHO. *The World Health Report 2007 – A Safer Future: Global Public Health Security in the 21st Century*. Geneva: WHO, 2007.

Winfield Burns, Alison. "The CDC's Tom Frieden and Ebola Virus Disease." *Huffington Post*, October 17, 2014. http://www.huffingtonpost.com/alison-winfield-burns/the-cdcs-tom-frieden-and-_b_6000342.html.

Youde, Jeremy. *Global Health Governance*. Cambridge: Polity, 2012.

WHO's to blame? The World Health Organization and the 2014 Ebola outbreak in West Africa

Adam Kamradt-Scott

Centre for International Security Studies, Department of Government and International Relations, University of Sydney, Australia

ABSTRACT
Since 2001 the World Health Organization (WHO) has been actively promoting its credentials for managing 'global health security'. However, the organisation's initial response to the 2014 Ebola outbreak in West Africa has attracted significant criticism, even prompting calls for its dissolution and the creation of a new global health agency. Drawing on principal–agent theory and insights from previous disease outbreaks, this article examines what went wrong, the extent to which the organisation can be held to account, and what this means for the WHO's global health security mandate.

Introduction

Since May 2001 the secretariat of the World Health Organization (WHO) has promoted its ability to manage global health security, which it subsequently defined as 'the activities required, both proactive and reactive, to minimize vulnerability to acute public health events that endanger the collective health of populations living across geographical regions and international boundaries'.[1] Yet, whereas the organisation's response to the 2003 Severe Acute Respiratory Syndrome (SARS) outbreak was seen as efficient, competent and effective, the WHO's management of the 2009 H1N1 pandemic and of the 2014 outbreak of Ebola Virus Disease (EVD) in West Africa has been perceived as inept, dysfunctional, even shambolic. Indeed, so poorly has the organisation's handling of these global health crises been viewed that each public health emergency of international concern (PHEIC) has spurred several independent external reviews of the organisation's performance. Every review has subsequently concluded that there is an urgent need to reform the organisation.

These events are understandably disconcerting, and on the surface would suggest that the WHO has been shirking its delegated responsibilities, exhibiting a type of dysfunctional behaviour often attributed to international organisations (IOs).[2] But has it? This article interrogates the WHO's management of the 2014 EVD outbreak from March to September 2014 in an attempt to evaluate whether the IO's initial response to the crisis was appropriate and reasonable, and whether the criticisms that have emerged are justified. To accomplish this task the article explores, first, the WHO's constitutional obligations and customary practice in managing global health security before, second, comparing the organisation's handling of the 2014 EVD epidemic with its handling of previous outbreaks. What this analysis reveals is that, while mistakes were clearly made, criticisms that the secretariat was remiss in its initial response are somewhat misguided when taking account of previous outbreaks and of the IO's customary practice. Moreover, the investigation reveals that there are far more fundamental issues at stake which – if left unaddressed – will continue to impede the WHO's ability to fulfil its delegated responsibilities. The article then concludes by considering what this event signifies for the future of the WHO and global health security.

WHO's evolving authority to control and eradicate disease outbreaks

The WHO was created in 1948 with the overall objective of improving the health of all populations worldwide. Within this, the containment and eradication of infectious diseases was considered to be the IO's primary task, and the organisation was imbued with considerable authority and autonomy to pursue this goal.[3] The priority attached to this specific function reflected the postwar world-view, which regarded good health as a precondition for international peace and security.[4] Health was essential for security; and as infectious diseases were recognised to adversely affect not only the health of populations but also the global economy, by disrupting international trade, great weight was attached to preventing their spread. The WHO, which had been established to serve as the 'directing and coordinating authority' in all international health matters,[5] was thus tasked with seeking to eliminate infectious diseases wherever they arose.

To give effect to this mandate, and in a classic example of principal–agent (PA) delegation,[6] several specific powers were conferred upon the organisation. These notably included the authority to: (1) adopt regulations pertaining to sanitary and quarantine measures that – if two-thirds of member states agree – are automatically binding on all governments; (2) designate disease and public health-related nomenclatures; and (3) pass emergency powers that, once enacted, allow the director-general to use every available resource at the organisation's disposal to respond to any event requiring 'immediate action'.[7] The WHO's member states also ensured that the organisation soon exercised this new found authority, adopting the International Sanitary Regulations in 1951 and launching the first global eradication programme targeting malaria in 1958.

Over time and based on a number of eradication initiatives the organisation developed a standard approach to managing disease outbreaks, one characterised by collating epidemic intelligence and issuing policy advice. Importantly, however, following the prominent failure of the malaria eradication programme, the secretariat fastidiously refrained from even the appearance of instructing governments on the precise measures they should take to eradicate or control diseases. Instead the WHO secretariat consistently demurred, proffering advice derived from expert consensus and coordinating efforts only where it had been explicitly invited to do so. This standard, or classical, approach to disease eradication typified the WHO secretariat's efforts throughout the remainder of the 20th century, and demonstrated that the IO had developed a customary practice towards fulfilling its obligations.[8]

Perhaps more significantly member states were broadly content with the WHO's classical approach, and robustly resisted any perceived IO autonomy or mission creep. This was most clearly exemplified by the WHO director-general Marcolino Candau's decision in 1970 to report an outbreak of cholera underway in Guinea, despite the fact that the Guinean government had not officially notified the secretariat of the event. Although the director-general maintained that he took this action 'in order to fulfil the Organization's obligations under Article 2 of the WHO Constitution,'[9] member states reacted swiftly in condemning his breach of the now renamed and updated 1969 International Health (formerly Sanitary) Regulations (IHR), which required government notification before publicly disseminating any alert.[10] This one incident had a notable impact on the secretariat – including on the publicly chastised director-general – for it revealed very clearly that governments would not tolerate infringement of their sovereignty.

In 2003 the emergence of a novel pathogen in the form of SARS aided the WHO secretariat in establishing a new approach to global health security. By the end of the 20th century, confronted by the emergence of new diseases like HIV/AIDS, the resurgence of new and resistant forms of disease such as multi-drug-resistant tuberculosis and the threat of biological weapons, governments increasingly appreciated that the WHO's former methods of coordinating disease outbreaks were no longer fit for purpose. The IHR, which formed an integral part of the IO's delegation contract with member states, were identified to be in urgent need of reform. Even so, several delays were encountered,[11] and before the IHR revisions could be completed the SARS-associated coronavirus spread internationally to cause over 700 deaths and economic damage of over US$30 billion.[12] Among governments the SARS experience became widely regarded as a timely 'wake-up call'; thus the WHO secretariat was encouraged to redouble its efforts to finalise the IHR revisions.

The updated IHR framework was adopted by the 58th Worldl Health Assembly (WHA) in 2005, and officially entered into force in June 2007. Under the terms of the IHR 2005 member states tasked themselves with developing national disease surveillance and response capacities to prevent the international spread of disease, while instructing the WHO to provide technical support to those countries struggling to meet these requirements. In addition, new powers were conferred upon the secretariat to utilise non-government sources of information to detect disease outbreaks, and to 'name and shame' countries that refused assistance or attempted to cover up public health risks.

At the same time, however, member states also ensured new checks and balances were placed on the WHO to prevent a repeat of what some viewed as unmitigated autonomy by the secretariat throughout the SARS epidemic, particularly with regard to issuing travel advisories that might cause economic damage. These new measures included, among others, the explicit requirement for the director-general to convene an emergency committee for expert advice before declaring a PHEIC or recommending measures (such as travel advisories). While the director-general may select specific individuals to serve on an emergency committee, s/he may only choose from a roster of experts nominated by member states. This conceivably opens the committee to political interference; and although the director-general is only obligated to consider the committee's advice, it is nevertheless difficult to envisage a situation in which the director-general would dismiss such advice without having his or her own legitimacy publicly questioned. Thus, while in many respects the WHO secretariat's authority to eradicate diseases was refreshed for the conditions of a highly interconnected, globalised world, the organisation's principals also guaranteed that there were limits to the secretariat's autonomy that prevented their agent from becoming too independent or powerful.

In 2009 the revised IHR 2005 framework was put to its inaugural test with the emergence of a novel strain of influenza A(H1N1), which achieved effective human-to-human transmission, sparking the first pandemic of the 21st century. This event also proved to be a critical test of the WHO secretariat, one that many commentators subsequently concluded it failed. Indeed, the organisation's handling of the crisis sparked considerable controversy, resulting in at least three independent investigations. Although all three reviews had ultimately concluded by 2011 that the organisation's integrity had not been compromised, they nevertheless each recommended a series of measures designed to strengthen both member states' and the WHO secretariat's capacities for managing the next PHEIC more effectively. Regrettably, by 2014 when the West African EVD outbreak was identified, only limited progress had been made in implementing the measures and many of the recommendations remained unaddressed.

WHO responds to the 2014 EVD outbreak in West Africa

An outbreak of EVD was officially declared to be underway in Guinea on 23 March 2014.[13] By this time, however, the virus had already been circulating undetected for some three months and, as a result, had spread across border regions into neighbouring Liberia and Sierra Leone. Initially suspected to be Lassa Fever, within hours of confirming that the etiological agent was Ebola, the WHO secretariat in Geneva mobilised a response team via the Global Outbreak Alert and Response Network (GOARN) to deploy to Guinea to assist local health authorities. The secretariat also alerted Liberian and Sierra Leonean health officials to commence surveillance. On 27 March 2014 both Liberia and Sierra Leone confirmed that they had identified a small number of suspected EVD cases;[14] and within 72 hours laboratory testing verified that cases had indeed appeared in Liberia.[15] The GOARN team, which had arrived in Guinea on 28 March 2014, immediately began an assessment of local conditions and then presented these findings at a press conference in Geneva on 8 April 2014. At the briefing it was noted by WHO officials that the outbreak underway in Guinea was 'one of the most challenging Ebola outbreaks that we have ever faced'.[16] Yet, even as the weeks progressed and additional suspected cases were reported in Liberia, Sierra Leone and Mali,[17] significant concerns were not raised by the secretariat in Geneva until late June 2014.

Having said this, it would be erroneous to suggest – as some have – that the WHO secretariat did nothing. Throughout April 2014, for instance, the organisation continued to mobilise technical support and resources to assist the affected countries. As a result, by 7 May 2014 some 113 technical experts had been deployed to assist the health authorities in Guinea (88), Liberia (23), Sierra Leone (1) and the WHO African regional office (AFRO).[18] Moreover, the expertise deployed represented a wide array of skill sets, including coordination, surveillance and epidemiology, infection prevention and control, clinical case management, anthropology, logistics, laboratory services, risk communication, social mobilisation, finance, health informatics, and resource mobilisation. These were drawn from partner organisations and recruited via the WHO's surge capacity mechanisms. Thus, while the WHO's response was extensively criticised by Médecins Sans Frontières (MSF) for its perceived lack of action throughout this period,[19] given that the number of suspected cases and deaths were consistent with the size of previous EVD outbreaks in other parts of Africa,[20] it would be improper to suggest that the WHO secretariat had been negligent.

Indeed, it seems only reasonable that, when evaluating the WHO secretariat's initial reaction to the 2014 EVD outbreak, the IO's actions are also compared against previous outbreaks. In this regard it is important to note that in the immediate decade preceding the 2014 epidemic, the WHO had received reports of a total of nine EVD outbreaks – four in the Democratic Republic of Congo (DRC), four in Uganda and one outbreak of Ebola Reston Virus in the Philippines.[21] Critically, however, with the exception of the 2007 DRC outbreak, which even necessitated deployment of UN peacekeepers to provide logistical support as a result of the size of the outbreak,[22] the WHO secretariat had previously sent very limited numbers of personnel to countries affected by Ebola. In fact, from all the available evidence it appears that the WHO secretariat has, on average, only ever dispatched between two and five technical experts for each EVD outbreak over the previous 10 years.[23]

That the WHO secretariat has only ever deployed very modest numbers of technical experts is understandable when recalling that the IO was never intended to be a 'first responder' agency, but rather the 'directing and coordinating authority' in international health. Its primary task has always been to coordinate, only assisting governments upon request. In this respect the IO's 'arm's length' approach to fulfilling its delegated functions is not a modern phenomenon, as Frank Gutteridge's observations in 1963 demonstrate: 'Although it possesses…wider scope and powers than its predecessors, the World Health Organization remains without any direct authority over its Members. Thus it may advise, assist, co-ordinate and recommend, but it is not enabled to legislate or execute.'[24] Even after SARS acutely demonstrated the need for a new approach, governments have consistently resisted attempts to expand the IO's staffing levels to one that might enable the secretariat to adopt a more operational role. As a result, since its failed malaria eradication programme the WHO has never retained large numbers of staff that can be deployed in emergencies.[25] Consistent with the organisation's customary practice, the WHO secretariat's response to previous EVD outbreaks has thus been to draw on networks such as GOARN to gather the requisite expertise to assist national health authorities to lead any operational response.

Given, therefore, that in previous EVD outbreaks the number of personnel mobilised by the WHO has consistently been between two and five persons, the fact that the secretariat had deployed 113 experts to West Africa within six weeks of the outbreak being confirmed suggests that the IO's initial response was at least reasonable and arguably defensible. However, confusion over the outbreak was then further compounded in mid-May 2014, when all epidemiological indicators suggested that the EVD outbreak, which was primarily still concentrated in Guinea,[26] might be nearing its end. This perception was reinforced at the 67th WHA in May 2014 when the Guinean Minister for Health reported that the outbreak in his country was 'yielding very encouraging results' and was now essentially under control.[27] In these circumstances it can be appreciated that the secretariat in Geneva believed it had acted appropriately and proportionately to the Ebola crisis. Of course, in hindsight it is now clear that the sense of security was misplaced, for immediately after the 67th WHA Sierra Leone notified the WHO of 16 either suspected or confirmed EVD cases that proved to be the first of thousands.[28]

By mid-June 2014 a very different epidemiological picture was emerging, and it was at this juncture the flaws in the WHO secretariat's management of the crisis especially materialised. Between 28 May and 10 June 2014, for instance, Guinea and Sierra Leone recorded some 150 new infections, bringing the cumulative total to 440 suspected or confirmed EVD cases. The rise in cases so alarmed some officials in AFRO that they contacted the secretariat in Geneva recommending a PHEIC be declared, but the response they received discouraged invoking the IHR 2005, suggesting a declaration of that nature would only damage relations with the affected countries.[29] By 17 June the cumulative number of cases throughout the region had risen again, to 528 suspected or confirmed cases, with Liberia reporting nine new suspected cases and five deaths – the first since April earlier that year.[30] Reacting to this news the AFRO convened a high-level meeting on 23 June 2014 in Conakry with the Guinean president, the US ambassador to Guinea, WHO officials, and representatives from the Centers for Disease Control and Prevention (CDC), while in Geneva the GOARN steering committee met to review the situation.[31] The conclusion these meetings drew was that the WHO needed to take greater control of the response. Thus on 27 June 2014 the WHO director-general was sent a report that outlined the case for more 'forceful leadership'.[32]

By late July 2014, however, beyond a series of additional meetings little further effort had been expended. The director-general, who purportedly assumed personal responsibility for managing the crisis in late June, convened yet another high-level meeting of officials in early July in Ghana, where additional commitments were made from partners that included airlines, mining companies and the African Development Bank to support the outbreak response. Yet, in terms of practical measures, no further steps were taken. This was despite the fact that across the region EVD infections had effectively doubled to almost 1000 suspected or confirmed cases.[33] Somewhat inevitably, therefore, at the same time as a conference was being held in the third week of July to identify the technical and human resources required to contain the virus's spread, a Liberian man who had contracted EVD boarded a plane for Nigeria, where he subsequently initiated a local outbreak.[34] This event understandably alarmed health authorities around the world, prompting the director-general, finally, to invoke the IHR and assemble an emergency committee to review the epidemiological situation and determine whether the conditions for a PHEIC had been reached.

The IHR emergency committee met for the first time via teleconference over two days on 7–8 August 2014 and conveyed to the director-general their assessment that the declaration of a PHEIC was justified. Yet, again, despite the fact that a PHEIC was declared that same day,[35] and almost 1800 EVD cases had now been reported,[36] few additional measures were implemented to assist those countries affected. On 27 August 2014 the WHO secretariat in Geneva released its 'Ebola Roadmap', which outlined various strategies and targets to contain the virus.[37] But by this stage public criticisms of the organisation's response, combined with anxiety about the risk of the virus spreading internationally, had grown to such an extent that plans had already been drawn up to elevate the crisis to the peak UN body – the UN Security Council – while advance teams of foreign military personnel arrived in Liberia and Sierra Leone to begin assessing how international civil–military cooperation might support such efforts.[38]

At the beginning of September 2014 several organisations, including MSF and the WHO, as well as representatives from the countries worst affected by the outbreak, were invited to New York to brief the UN and world leaders on the Ebola crisis. In an explicit attempt to highlight the severity of the emergency MSF issued an unprecedented call for urgent military intervention, declaring the response to date 'lethally inadequate',[39] while Liberia's defence minister opined that the virus was 'spreading like wild fire and devouring everything in its path'.[40] In response, the UN Security Council was convened on 15 September 2014 and passed resolution UNSC 2176 authorising the extension of the UN mission to Liberia (UNMIL) by an initial three months (with provision for further extensions) to provide additional support in containing the virus.[41] This announcement was followed the next day by US President Barack Obama declaring his country's commitment to deploy 3000 military personnel to support affected countries; just two days later on 18 September the UN Security Council passed resolution UNSC 2177 that declared the outbreak a 'threat to international peace and security'.[42] On the basis of these resolutions Secretary-General Ban Ki-Moon obtained authorisation from the UN General Assembly the following day to create the UN's first-ever public health mission – the United Nations Mission for Ebola Emergency Response (UNMEER) – and tasked the entity with coordinating the international humanitarian response in West Africa.[43]

So what went wrong and why?

The official launch of UNMEER has been interpreted by many as a stunning admission of the WHO's failure to respond adequately to the EVD crisis.[44] In October 2014 this perception was reinforced when the unauthorised release of a draft internal review of the WHO's handling of the Ebola outbreak confirmed what many had already suspected: that 'A perfect storm' had been 'brewing, ready to burst open in full force' but that the WHO secretariat had 'failed to see some fairly plain writing on the wall'.[45] Subsequent international media reports exposed the fact that, despite dire warnings of a growing humanitarian crisis and responder agencies being overwhelmed, senior officials within WHO had resisted calls to invoke the IHR 2005, suggesting such steps would not only be unhelpful but potentially viewed as a 'hostile act'.[46] As time has progressed, a series of scholarly analyses has added to the litany of critiques calling for the WHO to undergo significant reforms in the wake of the EVD outbreak. World leaders called for the establishment of entirely new global health institutions to prevent a repeat of similar crises in the future and an independent panel established by the WHO director-general released an interim report noting that the IO's response was 'surprising' and that it was 'still unclear…why early warnings, approximately from May through to July 2014, did not result in an effective and adequate response'.[47]

In light of such assessments, elements of the WHO secretariat, including the director-general, periodically attempted to defend the organisation. As early as 3 September 2014, for example, Assistant Director-General for Health Security, Keiji Fukuda, emphasised to international media that WHO did not have 'enough health workers, doctors, nurses, drivers, and contact tracers' to manage the high numbers of EVD cases.[48] The following day the director-general emphasised in an interview with a *New York Times* reporter that: 'First and foremost people need to understand WHO. WHO is the UN specialized agency for health. And we are not the first responder. You know, the government has first priority to take care of their people and provide health care.'[49] Ensuing reports produced by the secretariat have also noted the large number of other humanitarian crises that preceded or were concurrent with the EVD outbreak, pointing to their limited capacity to respond to all emergencies with equal attention.[50]

Even so, the WHO secretariat has acknowledged on several occasions that mistakes were made. For instance, on 4 October 2014 Richard Brennan, director of the IO's emergency risk management department, admitted: 'In retrospect, we could have responded faster. Some of the criticism is appropriate.'[51] This was followed on 25 January 2015 by the special session of the Executive Board to review the Ebola response, where the director-general agreed that the organisation had been 'too slow to see what was unfolding before us', and that the response had revealed several administrative, managerial and technical infrastructure shortcomings.[52]

At the 68th WHA in May 2015 the director-general went on to outline a series of reforms to address identified failings, including merging departments to create a single programme for responding to health emergencies, helping establish a global emergency health workforce and a $100 million contingency fund, and expanding the organisation's existing capabilities in emergency management and response.[53]

Importantly, however, while the majority of attention to date has focused on fixing certain aspects of the WHO secretariat, there are several far more fundamental structural factors that contributed to the IO's inadequate EVD response that are being overlooked. These notably include various financial, cultural, political and design constraints which, in virtually every instance, can be directly traced to the IO's principal–agent relationship with its member states. For instance, in the immediate 12-month period before the EVD outbreak in one department central to the WHO's emergency response capacity the number of staff had been reduced from 90 to 36 persons.[54] These staffing reductions were admittedly instituted by the secretariat, but they were executed in response to a 51% spending cut by member states in 2013 to the WHO's 'outbreak and crisis response' budget for 2014–15.[55] In making these staffing reductions the secretariat in Geneva had anticipated that the IO's regional offices, which possess far more autonomy over their finances, would mitigate some of these reductions by increasing their own capacity but, as one senior WHO official observed, 'this didn't happen.'[56] Faced with such reductions it is likely that any organisation would struggle, but the EVD outbreak placed demands on the organisation that, according to the director-general, were 'more than 10 times greater than ever experienced in the almost 70-year history.'[57] Worse still, the EVD crisis occurred at a time when the IO was responding to at least three other significant humanitarian emergencies in Syria, South Sudan and the Central African Republic.[58] The collective decision by member states to reduce the IO's crisis response budget was thus not only ill-timed, but it directly compromised the secretariat's ability to respond to the EVD outbreak.

That said, from the narrative above it is apparent that the internal culture of the WHO secretariat also contributed to shortcomings in the organisation's response. Yet, even here, much of this can be attributed to former conduct of the IO's principals. As mentioned earlier, between March and June 2014 the governments of Liberia, Sierra Leone and Guinea repeatedly downplayed the extent of their respective outbreaks. As early as March 2014, for instance, rumours emerged of large numbers of deaths suspected to be EVD-related occurring in Monrovia,[59] yet by the end of April the government – whether through negligence or obfuscation – had only ever reported one suspected case within the entire county of Montserrado.[60] Further, as noted above, the Guinean Minister for Health emphasised at the 67th WHA that his country was seeing tremendous progress in containing the outbreak, with five out of the six foci areas of the epidemic effectively now controlled.[61] This attempt at obfuscation reportedly even persisted to the extent that, when Liberia's president, Ellen Johnson-Sirleaf, later did call for international assistance, the leaders of neighbouring Guinea and Sierra Leone criticised her for doing so.[62] When the AFRO and specifically its regional director also failed to counter these views,[63] it can perhaps be appreciated why the secretariat in Geneva did not adopt an emergency mind-set.

Nevertheless, the WHO secretariat's unwillingness to challenge or gainsay official reports emerging from the affected countries is arguably one of the most damning indictments of the IO's performance. The secretariat's error is made particularly acute when considering the historical record of governments' attempts to conceal disease-related events as a result of concerns that these may lead to trade and travel sanctions – a practice that, ironically, member states had hoped would be addressed when they commissioned the IHR to be revised. It is thus perplexing that the organisation failed to contest the affected countries' official reports when the poor state of their healthcare systems, and, in particular, the absence of any comprehensive disease surveillance, were well known.

At the same time, whenever the WHO secretariat has publicly challenged governments' official positions or pushed hard to intervene in an event, member states have often responded negatively. It is a pattern of behaviour witnessed many times over, extending from events such as the 1970 cholera outbreak in Guinea that resulted in diplomatic rebukes, to the 2003 SARS outbreak, which culminated in the imposition of new control mechanisms to limit the IO's autonomy. Throughout the IHR negotiations, for example, while many governments initially welcomed the secretariat's rebuke of the Chinese for attempting to cover up the true nature of their SARS outbreak, they subsequently rejected draft proposals to allow the WHO equivalent autonomy to intervene in public health emergencies, emphasising instead the need to protect state sovereignty.[64] Similarly, in 2009 when the WHO secretariat publicly questioned Russia's decision to ban pork imports over alleged concerns about influenza transmission, Russian bureaucrats reacted by stating: 'Health officials should stick to their own business and not promote the world pork trade'.[65] These events underscore the precarious position in which the WHO secretariat frequently finds itself. For member states, as the IO's principals, preserve various means to reprimand the secretariat, ranging from immediately ceasing voluntary contributions (which make up the majority of the WHO's budget – see below) to more substantive measures such as altering the IO's design, function and autonomy – a fact the IO remains acutely aware of.

This same dynamic also underlines the broader political challenge confronting the WHO. It must be recalled, for instance, that the 2014 EVD outbreak occurred in an environment in which the secretariat had been extensively accused of 'crying wolf' over its response to the 2009 H1N1 influenza pandemic.[66] These criticisms essentially revolved around the perception that the pandemic did not turn out to be as severe as first predicted. In this context, when it is recalled how member states reacted in the wake of SARS, the multiple investigations into the WHO's handling of H1N1, and that the organisation's normative reputation remains one of the IO's most powerful tools,[67] it can be appreciated why the secretariat might have approached the EVD outbreak cautiously, only escalating its discourse and activities when it was apparent that the virus's spread remained uncontrolled. Of course, in hindsight it is also easy to criticise the WHO secretariat for the fact that it judged the situation poorly. Yet, given the above set of circumstances, the difficult line the IO must constantly tread between its principals' sovereignty, public health and significant economic interests when facing crises characterised by pervasive uncertainty, mistruths and obfuscation can at least be understood.

Lastly, in reviewing the WHO's actions it is clear that structural factors related to the IO's design additionally contributed – and arguably exacerbated – its ineffectual response. This was most clearly exemplified in the first months of the response by the disjointed approach taken by the secretariat in Geneva and its regional office, AFRO. As revealed in a leaked internal memo dated 25 March 2014, the AFRO had convened an emergency teleconference the previous day, where the high number of suspected cases and deaths in Guinea and the 'high possibility of cross-border transmission' were noted with concern.[68] In response, the AFRO secretariat advocated that the regional director declare an 'internal WHO Grade

2 emergency' and establish a *regional* emergency support team to coordinate technical and operational support. This action plan was approved the same day.[69] Yet by 5 May 2014, whereas the WHO secretariat in Geneva had deployed almost 90 staff to Guinea, only 20 were sent to Liberia, one was dispatched to Sierra Leone and four were sent to the regional office.[70] This suggests that information and decisions taken at the regional level were not sufficiently communicated to the central office or, if they were, were not acted upon. Sending the bulk of personnel to Guinea also suggests that the Geneva-based secretariat lacked sufficient insight into how the outbreak might unfold and spread to affect neighbouring states, which is rather odd given that the outbreak was known to have started in a region close to international borders and that the poor surveillance capacity of all three countries was well documented. At the same time the AFRO ignored its own standard operating procedures (SOPs) for disease outbreaks which, astonishingly, were released in the very same month the outbreak was detected and which advocated the mobilisation and deployment of expertise within 72 hours of official notification.[71]

These events underscore yet again the disjointed nature of the WHO's division into seven organisations (six regional offices and central headquarters) that have long been identified as impeding its effectiveness. Importantly, however, the regional offices, which are separate and largely autonomous from the central headquarters in Geneva, are a result of disagreement over the incorporation of the Pan American Sanitary (later Health) Bureau that dates back to 1946.[72] Yet, while the regional structure has consistently been identified as a problem in multiple reviews of the IO's functioning for perpetuating a raft of inefficiencies, duplication of services, poor health outcomes and unhelpful infighting,[73] governments have resisted calls to significantly reform this element of the WHO's design. Accordingly, it raises the question: are the reforms now being proposed going to address the various structural issues that inhibited the WHO's response to Ebola?

So what happens now?

As revealed at the 68th WHA in May 2015, the WHO director-general is proceeding with a series of proposed reforms designed to prevent a repeat of the organisation's EVD mistakes and strengthen the IO's global health security and emergency response capacities. Among the recommended changes are establishing a global emergency health workforce and a $100 million replenishable contingency fund that the WHO secretariat can immediately draw upon whenever a PHEIC arises to mobilise resources and personnel. These measures, combined with internal restructuring efforts to streamline and augment the WHO secretariat's emergency response capacity, will arguably go some way to enhancing the IO's overall ability to respond to health emergencies when they arise. In the longer term, however, it remains doubtful that the international community will see any substantive change in the way the organisation responds to future health crises; ultimately, the responsibility for this rests with the IO's principals.

In January 2015, for instance, the WHO director-general observed at the special session of the Executive Board on Ebola that the IHR 2005 clearly needed 'more teeth' if the world was ever to 'reach true health security'.[74] Yet, although the independent expert panel established in the aftermath of the 2009 H1N1 pandemic also identified this precise issue, viewing it as fundamental to several of the recommendations it produced,[75] practical proposals for how the IHR 2005 framework might be further strengthened have been few or politically naive.[76] In fact, in many respects the exact opposite has now occurred, with member states agreeing to extend the deadline for those countries yet to develop the core capacities to 2019 – seven years beyond the original target date.[77] Given that the deadline has now been extended once, political pressure on non-compliant governments has been lifted, raising the prospect that these core capacities will never be achieved.

Even more disconcerting is the fact that on two distinct occasions now countries have ignored WHO recommendations and imposed various trade and travel sanctions that contravene the spirit and purpose of the IHR 2005. Throughout the 2009 H1N1 influenza pandemic and again in the 2014 EVD outbreak roughly 40 governments implemented policies and measures that the IO explicitly advised against, purportedly on the basis of wanting to protect themselves from the risk the diseases would spread to their respective territories.[78] Disappointingly, in both contexts the WHO secretariat under Margaret Chan's leadership selected not to exercise its ability to 'name and shame' these governments; given that no other provision exists within the IHR 2005 to penalise countries that contravene the framework, these governments have eluded reprimand. Crucially, however, preventing such behaviour was one of the fundamental reasons why the IHR revision process was instigated in the first place. These developments thus signal a disturbing trend whereby governments can act with impunity, without fear of retribution, while simultaneously undermining a framework intended to strengthen global health security.

Further, and as noted above, the budgetary restrictions and efficiency savings imposed on the WHO directly contributed to the organisation's poor EVD response. It had been hoped at the beginning of the 68th WHA that member states would reconsider their long-held opposition to increasing their assessed contributions, which have remained unchanged since the 1980s,[79] thereby allowing the IO greater flexibility and autonomy to reallocate funds to respond to health emergencies. To that end the director-general had put forward a suggestion ahead of the meeting to increase member states' assessed contributions by 5%, which would in turn raise the organisation's overall operational budget by 8%.[80] Even before the meeting commenced, however, Chan was forced to drop the proposed 5% increase in order to secure broader consensus on raising the overall budget ceiling.[81] By the time the WHA concluded, a budget increase had been approved but with any additional funds to be donated on a voluntarily basis only.[82] Such a concession does not augur well for the WHO, however, as it fails to provide any surety of financial sustainability and evades entirely the need for the organisation to have greater autonomy around its finances to redeploy them, as the founders intended, for events demanding 'immediate action'.

Alongside the financial circumstances, the second major structural issue that has remained unaddressed in the wake of the EVD crisis is the WHO's division into seven effectively distinct entities. As noted above, the disjuncture between the AFRO and the WHO secretariat in Geneva contributed to delays in how the IO responded throughout the first six months of the EVD outbreak. Yet, while the regional director, Dr Luis Gomes Sambo, was replaced in January 2015,[83] the wider structural arrangements have been left untouched. In fact, rather than member states taking up the challenge to reform this system, the director-general has been left to try and integrate services designed to streamline the organisation into 'one WHO'.[84] Previous attempts by directors general at such realignment have conspicuously failed, however.[85] Until member states are prepared to collectively intervene and reshape the IO's organisational design the international community is unlikely to see any significant progress in this area.

In the meantime, addressing the cultural factors and the broader political environment in which the WHO secretariat operates entails a far more complex set of problems which, regrettably, are intimately tied to member state behaviour. To see lasting change here, governments would – collectively – have to regulate themselves and be prepared not only to sacrifice a degree of state sovereignty to facilitate a more interventionist role by the IO when PHEICs arise, but also to accept a greater level of uncertainty and avoid knee-jerk reactions when events do not play out as anticipated. Put another way, it would require the IO's principals to collectively agree to relinquish some of their control over their agent, allowing it greater scope and autonomy to act in the interests of global health security. Unfortunately, the prospects of such a fundamental transformation in the PA relationship between the WHO and its member states are currently very remote.

Conclusion

It would be easy, as a number of media commentators and scholars have already done, to blame the WHO for its perceived failure in responding to the Ebola outbreak. Yet, as is often the case in international relations, the picture is rarely, if ever, so clear-cut. As this article has sought to highlight, there are several examples of where the WHO's dysfunction can be clearly and directly attributed to the organisation's customary practices and internal culture. It can be expected that in the coming months, as the various independent investigations, including the UN high-level panel, hand down their findings, much more attention will be paid to the WHO's overall response and, while the above factors are not the only examples of where the IO failed in its delegated duty, they arguably represent some of the most serious, given the IO's global health security mandate.

Equally, however, any reasonable evaluation of the WHO's actions must also take into account the various structural constraints upon the secretariat that contributed to the IO's slow response. The budget cuts and efficiency savings instituted by governments as part of the WHO reform process are part of this, but some culpability must also be accepted by member states for their past opposition to the IO assuming a more proactive, interventionist role. The fact that governments have now finally acted on a four-year-old proposal to establish a $100 million contingency fund, as well as instructing the director-general to form and coordinate a global emergency health workforce, will arguably serve to strengthen global health security capacities to some extent. But for the people of West Africa, these reforms come too little too late to save the thousands of lives that have been lost as a result of EVD. It also remains decidedly unclear how willing governments are to address some of the wider, more important reforms such as the organisation's design and financial arrangements.

Within this mix the governments of West Africa must also accept some responsibility for not calling for assistance earlier. Indeed, the fact that Liberia's president attracted criticism from the leaders of Guinea and Sierra Leone even after it had become apparent that the virus was wreaking widespread havoc is a damning critique of the political leadership throughout this crisis. Attempts at subterfuge are not uncommon in disease outbreaks. But the EVD crisis once again highlights the desperate need for governments to develop sufficient capacity to detect and verify disease outbreaks, to be open and willing to share that information and, if necessary, call for assistance, whenever a public health crisis with international transmission potential arises. Disappointingly the 2014 EVD outbreak has shown that this lesson is yet to be learned, which raises the question of what it will take and how many lives will be lost before it is.

Intergovernmental organisations are, by design, answerable to their member states and, as much as it is tempting to single out agencies for their perceived and actual failings, it must also be appreciated that they are ultimately the creations of governments. These governments are also organisations' principals, and possess the ultimate authority over how their agents execute their duties. Accordingly, governments also bear the bulk of responsibility for when IOs – such as the WHO in the context of the Ebola outbreak – fail. It is also the case that, if these organisations are to ever improve, governments must take the lead in reforming them. Time and again, however, it seems such political leadership is intentionally absent.

Disclosure statement

No potential conflict of interest was reported by the author.

Funding

I would like to acknowledge the University of Sydney HMR+ Implementation grant and the Marie Bashir Institute for Infectious Diseases and Biosecurity, which provided funding for the fieldwork.

Acknowledgements

I would like to thank the two anonymous reviewers for their helpful suggestions.

Notes

1. WHO, *The World Health Report 2007*, ix.
2. Barnett and Finnemore, *Rules for the World*; and Hawkins et al., "Delegation under Anarchy," 3–38.
3. Kamradt-Scott, *Managing Global Health Security*.
4. Shimkin, "The World Health Organization," 281–283.
5. WHO, "Constitution," Article 2.
6. Kassim and Menon, "The Principal–Agent Approach," 121–139.
7. WHO, "Constitution," Articles 21, 28.
8. Kamradt-Scott, *Managing Global Health Security*, 45–78.
9. WHO, "Cholera," 377.
10. Weir and Mykhalovskiy, *Global Public Health Vigilance*, 75; and Fidler, *SARS, Governance and the Globalization of Disease*, 64–65.

11. Davies et al., *Disease Diplomacy*.
12. WHO, *The World Health Report 2007*, 40.
13. WHO, "Ebola Virus Disease in Guinea, 23 March 2014."
14. WHO, "Ebola Virus Disease in Guinea – Update, 27 March 2014."
15. WHO, "Ebola Virus Disease in Guinea – Update, 30 March 2014"; and WHO, "Ebola Virus Disease in Liberia, 30 March 2014."
16. WHO, "Key Events."
17. AFRO, "Ebola Virus Disease, West Africa (Situation as of 7 April 2014)."
18. AFRO, "Ebola Virus Disease, West Africa (Situation as of 7 May 2014)."
19. Hussain, "Ebola Response of MSF."
20. As of May 7, 2014 the number of confirmed EVD cases in Guinea was 235, including 157 deaths. These numbers were consistent with former outbreaks in locations like Uganda. See CDC, "Ebola Outbreaks 2000–2014."
21. WHO, "Ebola Virus Disease: Disease Outbreak News"; and CDC, "Outbreaks Chronology."
22. WHO, "Ebola Haemorrhagic Fever."
23. This number is derived from systematically reviewing photographic evidence and secretariat reports from WHO teams deployed to EVD outbreaks between 2005 and 2012. However, this excludes the 2007 outbreak in the DRC, which entailed WHO deploying country teams, the African Regional Office and staff from headquarters. See WHO, "Ebola Virus Disease: Disease Outbreak News."
24. Gutteridge, "The World Health Organization," 6–7.
25. Kamradt-Scott, *Managing Global Health Security*, 46–54.
26. By May 15, 2014 only 12 EVD cases and 11 deaths had been recorded. WHO, "Ebola Virus Disease, West Africa – Update, 12 May 2014."
27. WHO, "Key Events."
28. WHO, "Ebola Virus Disease, West Africa – Update, 28 May 2014."
29. "Bungling Ebola."
30. AFRO, "Ebola Virus Disease, West Africa (Situation as of 17 June 2014)."
31. WHO, "Key Events."
32. Ibid.
33. WHO, "Ebola Virus Disease, West Africa – Update, 15 July 2014."
34. WHO, "Ebola Virus Disease, West Africa – Update, 27 July 2014"; and WHO, "Ebola Virus Disease, West Africa – Update, 8 August 2014."
35. WHO, "8 August 2014 Press Briefing."
36. AFRO, "Ebola Virus Disease, West Africa (Situation as of 8 August 2014)."
37. WHO, *Ebola Response Roadmap*.
38. Interview with US military official, Monrovia, Liberia, March 25, 2015.
39. MSF, "Press Release."
40. Nichols, "Ebola seriously threatens Liberia's National Existence."
41. UN Security Council, S/RES/2176.
42. UN Security Council, S/RES/2177.
43. UN General Assembly, *Resolution 69/1*.
44. Sengupta, "Effort on Ebola hurt WHO Chief."
45. Cheng, "UN: We botched Response."
46. WHO, "BRIEFING NOTE"; and "Bungling Ebola."
47. WHO, "2014 Ebola Virus Disease Outbreak." A68/25, 3–4.
48. WHO, "Key Events."
49. Fink, "WHO Leader describes the Agency's Ebola Operations."
50. WHO, "WHO Response."
51. Sun et al., "Out of Control."
52. Chan, "Report by the Director-General."
53. WHO, "Address by Dr. Margaret Chan."
54. Interview with senior WHO official, Geneva, May 27, 2015.
55. Butler, "Agency gets a Grip on Budget," 18–19.

56. Interview with senior WHO official, Geneva, May 27, 2015.
57. WHO, "Address by Dr, Margaret Chan."
58. WHO, "WHO Response," 1.
59. Sengupta, "Effort on Ebola hurt WHO Chief."
60. WHO, "Ebola Virus Disease, West Africa – Update, 14 April 2014"; and WHO, "Ebola Virus Disease, West Africa – Update, 25 April 2014."
61. WHO, "Key Events."
62. Interview with UN official, Monrovia, March 25, 2015.
63. The AFRO regional director did not visit all three affected countries until July 21, 2014. AFRO, "Ebola Virus Disease, West Africa – Update 23 July 2014."
64. Kamradt-Scott, *Managing Global Health Security*, 134–135.
65. Budrys, "Russia says extends Pork Import Ban"; and Davies et al., *Disease Diplomacy*, 108.
66. Dumiak, "Push needed for Pandemic Planning," 800–801; and Carney and Bennett, "Framing Pandemic Management," 136–147.
67. Burci and Vignes, *World Health Organization*.
68. Cheng and Satter, "Emails."
69. AFRO, "AFRO-MEMORANDUM."
70. AFRO, "Ebola Virus Disease, West Africa (Situation as of 5 May 2014)."
71. AFRO, *Standard Operating Procedures*.
72. WHO, *The First Ten Years*; and Lee, *The World Health Organization*.
73. Godlee, "The World Health Organization," 1424–1428; WHO, "Looking Ahead"; and Burci and Vignes, *World Health Organization*, 121.
74. Chan, "Report by the Director-General," 4.
75. WHO, "Implementation of the International Health Regulations (2005): Report of the Review Committee."
76. Moon et al., "Will Ebola change the game?," 2204–2221.
77. WHO, "Decisions and List of Resolutions."
78. Davies et al., *Disease Diplomacy*; and WHO, "Implementation of the International Health Regulations (2005): Responding to Public Health Emergencies," 3.
79. Legge, "Future of WHO hangs in the Balance," e6877.
80. Lei Ravelo, "To accommodate Reforms."
81. Interview with senior WHO official, Geneva, May 20, 2015.
82. Garrett, "The Ebola Review."
83. AFRO, "WHO Executive Board appoints Dr. Matshidiso Moeti."
84. Chan, "Report by the Director-General," 4.
85. Notably the reforms attempted by Dr. Gro H. Brundtland between 1998 and 2003. See Yamey, "Have the latest Reforms reversed WHO's Decline?," 1107–1112; and Lerer and Matzopoulos, "'The Worst of Both Worlds,'" 415–438.

Bibliography

AFRO. Standard Operating Procedures for Coordinating Public Health Event Preparedness and Response in the WHO African Region. Brazzaville: AFRO, 2014. http://www.afro.who.int/en/clusters-a-programmes/dpc/epidemic-a-pandemic-alert-and-response.html.

AFRO. "AFRO-MEMORANDUM." http://www.documentcloud.org/documents/1689998-afro-memorandum-march-2014.html.

AFRO. "Ebola Virus Disease, West Africa (Situation as of 7 April 2014)." http://www.afro.who.int/en/clusters-a-programmes/dpc/epidemic-a-pandemic-alert-and-response/outbreak-news/4087-ebola-virus-disease-west-africa-7-april-2014.html.

AFRO. "Ebola Virus Disease, West Africa (Situation as of 5 May 2014)." http://www.afro.who.int/en/clusters-a-programmes/dpc/epidemic-a-pandemic-alert-and-response/outbreak-news/4131-ebola-virus-disease-west-africa-5-may-2014.html.

AFRO. "Ebola Virus Disease, West Africa (Situation as of 7 May 2014)." http://www.afro.who.int/en/clusters-a-programmes/dpc/epidemic-a-pandemic-alert-and-response/outbreak-news/4133-ebola-virus-disease-west-africa-situation-as-of-7-may-2014.html.

AFRO. "Ebola Virus Disease, West Africa (Situation as of 17 June 2014)." http://www.afro.who.int/en/clusters-a-programmes/dpc/epidemic-a-pandemic-alert-and-response/outbreak-news/4166-ebola-virus-disease-west-africa-17-june-2014.html.

AFRO. "Ebola Virus Disease, West Africa – Update 23 July 2014." http://www.afro.who.int/en/clusters-a-programmes/dpc/epidemic-a-pandemic-alert-and-response/outbreak-news/4230-ebola-virus-disease-west-africa-23-july-2014.html.

AFRO. "Ebola Virus Disease, West Africa (Situation as of 8 August 2014)." http://www.afro.who.int/en/clusters-a-programmes/dpc/epidemic-a-pandemic-alert-and-response/outbreak-news/4241-ebola-virus-disease-west-africa-8-august-2014.html.

AFRO. "WHO Executive Board appoints Dr. Matshidiso Moeti as new Regional Director for Africa." http://www.afro.who.int/en/media-centre/pressreleases/item/7319-who-executive-board-appoints-dr-matshidiso-moeti-as-new-regional-director-for-africa.html.

Barnett, Michael, and Martha Finnemore. *Rules for the World: International Organizations in Global Politics*. London: Cornell University Press, 2004.

Budrys, Alexsandras. "Russia says extends Pork Import Ban to Canada, Spain." Reuters, May 4, 2009. http://www.reuters.com/article/2009/05/04/us-flu-russia-idUSTRE5431PB20090504.

"Bungling Ebola – Documents." Associated Press. Accessed 20 June 2015. http://interactives.ap.org/specials/interactives/_documents/who-ebola/.

Burci, Gian-Luca, and Claude Vignes. *World Health Organization*. The Hague: Kluwer, 2004.

Butler, Declan. "Agency gets a Grip on Budget." *Nature* 498 (2013): 18–19.

Carney, Terry, and Belinda Bennett. "Framing Pandemic Management: New Governance, Science or Culture?" *Health Sociology Review* 23, no. 2 (2014): 136–147.

Centers for Disease Control and Prevention (CDC). "Ebola Outbreaks 2000–2014." Accessed September 9, 2015. http://www.cdc.gov/vhf/ebola/outbreaks/history/summaries.html.

CDC. "Outbreaks Chronology: Ebola Virus Disease." Accessed September 8, 2015. http://www.cdc.gov/vhf/ebola/outbreaks/history/chronology.html.

Chan, Margaret. "Report by the Director-General to the Special Session of the Executive Board on Ebola. Geneva, Switzerland, 25 January 2015." apps.who.int/gb/Statements/PDF/ReportbytheDirector-General.pdf.

Cheng, Maria. "UN: We botched Response to the Ebola Outbreak." Associated Press, October 17, 2014. http://www.bigstory.ap.org/article/6fd22fbcca0c47318cb178596d57dc7a/un-we-botched-response-ebola-outbreak.

Cheng, Maria, and Raphael Satter. 2015. "Emails: UN Health Agency resisted Declaring Ebola Emergency." *New York Times*, March 20. http://www.nytimes.com/aponline/2015/03/20/world/ap-un-who-bungling-ebola.html?_r=0.

Davies, Sara, Adam Kamradt-Scott, and Simon Rushton. *Disease Diplomacy: International Norms and Global Health Security*. Baltimore, MD: Johns Hopkins University Press, 2015.

Dumiak, Michael. "Push needed for Pandemic Planning." *Bulletin of the World Health Organization* 90, no. 11 (2012): 800–801.

Fidler, David. *SARS, Governance and the Globalization of Disease*. Basingstoke: Palgrave Macmillan, 2004.

Fink, Sheri. 2014. "WHO Leader describes the Agency's Ebola Operations." *New York Times*, September 4. http://www.nytimes.com/2014/09/04/world/africa/who-leader-describes-the-agencys-ebola-operations.html.

Garrett, Laurie. "The Ebola Review, Part I." *Foreign Policy*, June 6, 2015. http://foreignpolicy.com/2015/06/06/ebola-review-world-health-organization-g-7-merkel/.

Godlee, Fiona. "The World Health Organization: WHO in Crisis." *British Medical Journal* 309, no. 6966 (1994): 1424–1428.

Gutteridge, Frank. "The World Health Organization: Its Scope and Achievements." *Temple Law Quarterly* 37, no. 1 (1963): 1–14.

Hawkins, David, David Lake, Daniel Nielson, and Michael Tierney. "Delegation under Anarchy: States, International Organizations, and Principal-Agent Theory." In *Delegation and Agency in International*

Organizations, edited by David Hawkins, David Lake, Daniel Nielson and Michael Tierney, 3–38. Cambridge: Cambridge University Press, 2006.

Hussain, Misha. "Ebola Response of MSF and 'Boiling Frog' WHO under Scrutiny." Reuters.com, August 21, 2014. http://uk.reuters.com/article/2014/08/21/us-foundation-health-ebola-response-idUKKBN0GL1TT20140821.

Kamradt-Scott, Adam. *Managing Global Health Security: The World Health Organization and Disease Outbreak Control*. London: Palgrave, 2015.

Kassim, Hussein, and Anand Menon. ""The Principal-Agent Approach and the Study of the European Union: Promise Unfulfilled?" *Journal of European Public Policy* 10, no. 1 (2003): 121–139.

Lee, Kelley. *The World Health Organization (WHO)*. London: Routledge, 2009.

Lei Ravelo, Jenny. "To accommodate Reforms, Chan proposes 5 percent Increase in WHO Contributions." Devex.com, May 19, 2015. https://www.devex.com/news/to-accommodate-reforms-chan-proposes-5-percent-increase-in-who-contributions-86179.

Legge, David. "Future of WHO hangs in the Balance." *British Medical Journal* 345 (2012): e6877.

Lerer, Leonard, and Richard Matzopoulos. "'The Worst of Both Worlds': The Management Reform of the World Health Organization." *International Journal of Health Services* 31, no. 2 (2001): 415–438.

Moon, Surie, Muhammad Pate, Ashish Jha, Chelsea Clinton, Sophie Delaunay, Valnora Edwin, Mosoka Fallah, et al. "Will Ebola change the game? Ten essential reforms before the next pandemic. The report of the Harvard-LSHTM Independent Panel on the Global Response to Ebola." *Lancet* 386, no. 10009 (2015): 2204–2221.

MSF. "Press Release: Global Bio-disaster Response urgently needed in Ebola Fight, 2 September 2014." http://www.doctorswithoutborders.org/news-stories/press-release/global-bio-disaster-response-urgently-needed-ebola-fight.

Nichols, Michelle. "Ebola seriously threatens Liberia's National Existence – Minister." Reuters.com, September 10, 2014. http://af.reuters.com/article/topNews/idAFKBN0H50IM20140910.

Sengupta, Somini. 2015. "Effort on Ebola hurt WHO Chief." New York Times, January 6. http://www.nytimes.com/2015/01/07/world/leader-of-world-health-organization-defends-ebola-response.html?_r=0.

Shimkin, Michael. "The World Health Organization." *Science* 104, no. 2700 (1946): 281–283.

Sun, Lena, Brady Dennis, Lenny Bernstein, and Joel Achenbach. 2014. "Out of Control: How the World's Health Organizations failed to stop the Ebola Disaster." *Washington Post*, October 4. http://www.washingtonpost.com/sf/national/2014/10/04/how-ebola-sped-out-of-control/.

UN General Assembly. *Resolution 69/1: Measures to contain and combat the recent Ebola Outbreak in West Africa*. A/RES/69.1. Accessed September 9, 2015. http://www.un.org/en/ga/search/view_doc.asp?symbol=A/RES/69/1.

UN Security Council. S/RES/2176(2014). Accessed June 20, 2015. http://www.un.org/en/ga/search/view_doc.asp?symbol=S/RES/2176%20%282014%29.

UN Security Council. S/REST/2177(2014). Accessed September 9, 2015. http://www.un.org/en/ga/search/view_doc.asp?symbol=S/RES/2177%20%282014%29.

Weir, Lorna, and Eric Mykhalovskiy. *Global Public Health Vigilance: Creating a World on Alert*. London: Routledge, 2012.

WHO. "8 August 2014 Press Briefing on Ebola Outbreak in West Africa by Dr. Margaret Chan, Director-General, and Dr. Keiji Fukuda, Assistant Director-General for Health Security, WHO." Accessed September 11, 2015. http://www.who.int/mediacentre/multimedia/ebola_briefing/en/index1.html.

WHO. "2014 Ebola Virus Disease Outbreak and Follow-up to the Special Session of the Executive Board on Ebola: Ebola Interim Assessment Panel – Report by the Secretariat." A68/25. Geneva, 2015: 1–12.

WHO. "Address by Dr. Margaret Chan, Director-General, to the Sixty-eighth World Health Assembly." A68/3. Geneva. apps.who.int/gb/ebwha/pdf_files/WHA68/A68_3-en.pdf.

WHO. "BRIEFING NOTE TO THE DIRECTOR-GENERAL." Accessed June 20, 2015. http://www.documentcloud.org/documents/1690004-briefing-to-who-dg-on-ebola-in-guinea-june-2014.html.

WHO. "Cholera." Weekly Epidemiological Record 45, no. 36 (1970): 377.

WHO. "Constitution." In Basic Documents. 45th ed. Geneva: WHO, 2005.

WHO. "Decisions and List of Resolutions." A68/DIV./3. Geneva, 2015.

WHO. *The First Ten Years of the World Health Organization*. Geneva: WHO, 1958.

WHO. "Ebola Haemorrhagic Fever in the Democratic Republic of Congo – Update 2." 20 September 2007. http://www.who.int/csr/don/2007_09_20/en/.

WHO. "Ebola Virus Disease: Disease Outbreak News." Accessed September 8, 2015. http://www.who.int/csr/don/archive/disease/ebola/en/.

WHO. "Ebola Virus Disease in Guinea." 23 March 2014. http://www.who.int/csr/don/2014_03_23_ebola/en/.

WHO. "Ebola Virus Disease in Guinea – Update." 27 March 2014. http://www.who.int/csr/don/2014_03_27_ebola/en/.

WHO. "Ebola Virus Disease in Guinea - Update." 30 March 2014. http://www.who.int/csr/don/2014_03_30_ebola/en/.

WHO. "Ebola Virus Disease in Liberia." 30 March 2014. http://www.who.int/csr/don/2014_03_30_ebola_lbr/en/.

WHO. "Ebola Virus Disease, West Africa – Update." 14 April 2014. http://www.who.int/csr/don/2014_04_14_ebola/en/.

WHO. "Ebola Virus Disease, West Africa – Update." 25 April 2014. http://www.who.int/csr/don/2014_04_25_ebola/en/.

WHO. "Ebola Virus Disease, West Africa – Update." 12 May 2014. http://www.who.int/csr/don/2014_05_12_ebola/en/.

WHO. "Ebola Virus Disease, West Africa – Update." 28 May 2014. Accessed 20 June 2015. http://www.who.int/csr/don/2014_05_28_ebola/en/.

WHO. "Ebola Virus Disease, West Africa – Update." 15 July 2014." http://www.who.int/csr/don/2014_07_15_ebola/en/.

WHO. "Ebola Virus Disease, West Africa – Update." 27 July 2014. http://www.who.int/csr/don/2014_07_27_ebola/en/.

WHO. "Ebola Virus Disease, West Africa – Update." 8 August 2014. http://www.who.int/csr/don/2014_08_08_ebola/en/.

WHO. *Ebola Response Roadmap*. Geneva: WHO, 2014. http://www.who.int/csr/resources/publications/ebola/response-roadmap/en/.

WHO. "Implementation of the International Health Regulations (2005): Report of the Review Committee on the Functioning of the International Health Regulations (2005) in Relation to Pandemic (H1N1) 2009." A64/10. Geneva, 2011. apps.who.int/gb/ebwha/pdf_files/WHA64/A64_10-en.pdf.

WHO. "Implementation of the International Health Regulations (2005): Responding to Public Health Emergencies: Report by the Director-General." A68/22. Geneva, 2015.

WHO. "Key Events in the WHO Response to the Ebola Outbreak." January 2015. http://www.who.int/csr/disease/ebola/one-year-report/who-response/en/.

WHO. "Looking ahead for WHO after a Year of Change: Statement by the Director-General to the Fifty-second World Health Assembly." A52/3. Geneva, 1999.

WHO. "WHO Response in Severe, Large-scale Emergencies: Report of the Director-General." A68/23. Geneva: WHO.

WHO. *The World Health Report 2007: A Safer Future – Global Public Health Security in the 21st Century*. Geneva: WHO, 2007.

Yamey, Gavin. "Have the Latest Reforms reversed WHO's Decline?" *British Medical Journal* 325, no. 7372 (2002): 1107–1112.

Public health emergencies: a new peacekeeping mission? Insights from UNMIL's role in the Liberia Ebola outbreak

Sara E. Davies[a] and Simon Rushton[b]

[a]Centre for Governance and Public Policy, Griffith University, Nathan, Australia; [b]Department of Politics, University of Sheffield, UK

ABSTRACT

The UN Security Council meeting on 18 September 2014 represented a major turning-point in the international response to the Ebola outbreak then underway in West Africa. However, in the light of widespread criticism over the tardiness of the international response, it can be argued that the UN, and particularly the Security Council, failed to make best use of a potential resource it already had on the ground in Liberia: the United Nations Mission in Liberia (UNMIL). This article examines whether UNMIL could have done more to contribute to the emergency response and attempts to draw some lessons from this experience for potential peacekeeper involvement in future public health emergencies. UNMIL could have done more than it did within the terms of its mandate, although it may well have been hampered by factors such as its own capacities, the views of Troop Contributing Countries and the approach taken by the Liberian government. This case can inform broader discussions over the provision of medical and other forms of humanitarian assistance by peacekeeping missions, such as the danger of politicising humanitarian aid and peacekeepers doing more harm than good. Finally, we warn that a reliance on peacekeepers to deliver health services during 'normal' times could foster a dangerous culture of dependency, hampering emergency responses if the need arises.

Introduction

On 23 March 2014 the World Health Organization (WHO) reported on its Disease Outbreak News website that the Guinean government had informed it of a virulent form of Ebola Virus Disease (EVD) affecting the southeastern region of the country, with a case fatality rate of 59% (29 deaths out of 49 cases).[1] The same day, Médecins Sans Frontières (MSF) released a statement reporting that it had launched an emergency response in collaboration with the Guinean Ministry of Health.[2] Seven days later, on 30 March, the Liberian Ministry of Health reported its first two confirmed cases of EVD to WHO, followed by Sierra Leone in late May. From that point on there were near daily reports of new EVD cases in Guinea, Liberia and Sierra Leone. In early August the spread of the disease into Nigeria, and the repatriation of two infected health workers to the USA, provided the catalyst for the Director-General of the WHO to convene an Emergency Committee under the International Health Regulations and formally declare the outbreak a Public Health Emergency of International Concern (PHEIC).[3]

Although assistance to the region gradually began to increase following the declaration of a PHEIC, the meeting of the UN Security Council on 18 September represented a major turning-point in the international response. At that meeting the Security Council passed Resolution 2177 (2014), determining that the 'unprecedented extent of the Ebola outbreak in Africa constitutes a threat to international peace and security'.[4] The operative clauses of that Resolution called on a range of actors to do more. They included the governments of Sierra Leone, Liberia and Guinea; the African Union; the Economic Community of West African States (ECOWAS); the EU; WHO; the United Nations Humanitarian Air Service (UNHAS); and other UN member states. The Resolution also called on governments in the region to lift border restrictions that had been imposed as a result of the outbreak. At the same time the Council welcomed 'the intention of the Secretary-General to convene a high-level meeting on the margins of the sixty-ninth United Nations General Assembly to urge an exceptional and vigorous response to the Ebola outbreak',[5] signalling its approval of the creation of the United Nations Mission for Ebola Emergency Response (UNMEER).[6]

While the Security Council even discussing a health issue was unusual (although not unique – it has periodically discussed HIV/AIDS since 2000), the 2014–15 Ebola outbreak was the first example of the Security Council taking on a major leadership role in response to a public health emergency. Certainly, however, the Council had a longstanding interest in West Africa. Indeed, long before the creation of UNMEER, the Council had a mission present in one of the most severely affected countries: the United Nations Mission in Liberia (UNMIL). At the time Ebola struck, UNMIL was in its 'drawdown' phase, designed to deliver 'a successful transition of complete security responsibility' to the Liberian government in 2016.[7] UNMIL was not a mission designed to deal with a major public health emergency and it was only present in one of the three most affected countries. However, the drawdown continued through the crucial early months of the outbreak (and in August the Secretary-General recommended that it continue as planned[8]), despite the fact that 'the mission in Liberia sent increasingly dire cables [to WHO] about the virus, calling for help from [WHO Executive-Director] Dr Chan and others about what to do'.[9]

Given the widespread criticism over the tardiness of the international response (a PHEIC was not declared until 8 August and UNMEER was only established in September, almost six months after the first cases were detected, by which time there had been over 5000 confirmed, probable or suspected cases and 2622 deaths[10]), there is a case to be made that the UN, and particularly the Security Council, failed to make best use of the potential resource it had in UNMIL during the early stage of the outbreak. Michael R Snyder, for example, wrote (before the Security Council's first Ebola meeting):

> [UNMIL's] mandate includes the provision of humanitarian assistance and, crucially, the protection of civilians. In the past, this mostly meant protection against armed groups; however, UNMIL now needs to interpret this language to mean supporting the government in its effort to protect the population against a deadly pathogen.[11]

The delay in mounting a coordinated response on the part of the UN, particularly between the WHO and the Department of Peacekeeping Operations, could be seen as all the more puzzling given there appeared to be a precedent: the UN's Mission in the Democratic Republic of Congo (MONUC) had played a role in providing logistical support and communications capabilities during an EVD outbreak in the Democratic Republic of Congo seven years earlier.[12]

In this article we examine the question of whether UNMIL could and should have done more with the assets it already had deployed in Liberia to contribute to the emergency response. In particular, given the concerns that the UN mission had about the capacity of the Liberian government to respond to the crisis, we consider the effect of the mission drawdown as security and health personnel crises unfolded around the country at the height of the outbreak. The broader question underlying the analysis of this case is whether, given the recent emphasis on civilian protection in peacekeeping mandates and the Security Council's apparently expanding role in global disease response, public health emergencies could and should become a 'new peacekeeping mission'.

We begin by briefly outlining the context of the outbreak in Liberia before looking at whether UNMIL had the necessary authorisation and capacity to play a greater role than it did. In the final section of the paper we shift the focus to look at question of appropriateness, drawing out some lessons from the Liberian Ebola case to shed light on the issue of whether or not peacekeepers should be used to address future public health emergencies in the developing countries in which they are often deployed.

We find that UNMIL could have done more than it did within the terms of its mandate, although, even if it had chosen to do so, it may well have been hampered by a number of factors, including its own capacities, the view of the Troop Contributing Countries (TCCs) involved, and the approach taken by the Liberian government. Despite these limitations, continuing the drawdown process and largely confining UNMIL troops to their barracks during the first months of the outbreak reduced the overall response capacity available in Liberia – and included the effective withdrawal of vital health services that the mission had previously provided. More generally we suggest that this case can inform broader discussions over the provision of medical and other forms of humanitarian assistance by peacekeeping missions, including those around the dangers of politicising humanitarian aid and of peacekeepers doing more harm than good.[13] Overall we argue that peacekeeping missions may have a minor supporting role to play but are not a reliable mechanism for responding to public health emergencies. It is important that the lessons learned from Liberia's EVD outbreak do not lead them to be seen as a reliable mechanism , even if the Security Council continues to carve out a role for Itself as a leader In the field of 'global health security'.

Finally, we suggest that UNMIL's pre-Ebola practices may contain some valuable lessons about the desirability of peacekeeping missions providing medical services to civilian populations, even outside of public health emergencies. While such activities can be understood in both humanitarian and strategic terms (as a response to manifest need and as a way of building positive relations with host communities), there is a danger of fostering dependency, unwittingly undermining the development of the sustainable domestic health systems that will be crucial to the response to any future public health crisis.

UNMIL and the Ebola outbreak in Liberia

The first EVD cases in Liberia were confirmed in Lofa county on 30 March 2014. On 2 April an infected individual from Lofa travelled to the capital Monrovia, unknowingly bringing the disease to a major urban centre.[14] From that point onwards infections increased exponentially. When the WHO declared Ebola a PHEIC on 8 August, there had been 294 deaths in the country as a result of the disease.[15] By the time the Security Council met on 18 September this had increased to 1459. Liberia was officially declared Ebola-free on 9 May 2015, by which stage the death toll stood at 4716.[16] A few further cases were diagnosed in June and July, before the country was once again declared officially Ebola-free on 3 September 2015.[17]

Originally created as a multidimensional peacekeeping operation to monitor the August 2003 ceasefire agreement that brought an end to Liberia's civil war, at the time the Ebola outbreak began UNMIL was in the second phase of its drawdown plan.[18] From a peak of 15,520 troops in 2006, by June 2014 and the start of Liberia's EVD outbreak the number had been reduced to just over 4500.[19] The potential impact of Ebola on these mission personnel quickly attracted attention, especially from TCCs. Several expressed concern for the safety of their personnel, and the Philippines announced on 23 August that it was withdrawing its 115 troops from the mission – despite assurances from Secretary-General Ban Ki-moon that the threat posed to them was limited:

> All United Nations personnel in Liberia have been educated about the appropriate preventive measures that would minimize the risk of contracting Ebola, which is not airborne and requires direct contact with the bodily fluids of a symptomatic infected person or the deceased. I am therefore confident that United Nations personnel may continue their important work in Liberia.[20]

Nevertheless, the emergence of Ebola in areas where UNMIL units were stationed led to the mission's general advice to its units to close UNMIL facilities to public access.[21] All personnel were restricted to essential movement only, and an isolation centre was created to screen personnel for possible infection.[22] Despite these measures, the mission did suffer from infections. The first death of an UNMIL staff member from EVD came on 25 September; the second on 13 October.

At the end of August the Secretary General reversed his recommendation from two weeks earlier and recommended a rollover of UNMIL's mandate for three months 'to monitor the human rights situation and better facilitate humanitarian assistance during the crisis by helping maintain the necessary security conditions'.[23] In a series of meetings in September 2014 the Security Council discussed the situation in Liberia, focusing largely on the efforts of the Department for Peacekeeping Operations (DPKO) to keep UNMIL peacekeepers safe from the outbreak – although Karin Landgren, Head of UNMIL, also briefed the Council on the situation in Liberia more generally and reported that UNMIL 'had turned its full focus on Ebola since late July and was working in four areas: security and rule of law, logistics, communications and outreach and coordination at the central and country level'. Even once they got underway, however, these types of activity were in the vast majority of cases 'supportive' and indirect: donating vehicles, providing medical training to local health workers and providing public communication on Ebola prevention via UNMIL radio and community outreach.[24] The mission did not play an active role in treating Ebola patients (other than its own personnel) and (despite its security provision role) explicitly distanced itself from involvement in the Liberian government's disease containment-related security operations, such as the isolation of the West Point district of Monrovia, which led to violent clashes between the public and the Liberian security forces.[25]

These decisions to play only a supporting role were in many ways understandable, not least because of the need to keep concerned TCCs in the mission and a desire to avoid associating the mission with the (inappropriate in the view of many) militarised response of the Liberian government.[26] Nevertheless, these decisions had considerable impact, given

UNMIL's previous practice in delivering both health and security services, which we discuss in the following section. Effectively returning mission personnel to their barracks once EVD had emerged did not, therefore, represent merely a failure to step up and provide direct assistance, but in fact led to the effective withdrawal of assistance (both security and medical) that had previously been provided. [27] This was despite the fact that the weaknesses of the Liberian health system were well-known (one of the reasons UNMIL was so active in its medical outreach activities), and that in 2014 the mission's progress report expressed concerns about the political and security practices of the Liberian government. The relationship between these weaknesses and the Ebola response was not examined in depth in the August report.[28] Indeed, it was not until the Security Council session in early September that the head of UNMIL, Karin Landgren, openly doubted the effectiveness of the Liberian government's response.[29]

These choices may be interpreted – and indeed were by some – as a missed opportunity to make a fuller contribution in the crucial early months of the outbreak. But they also raise more general questions about the role of peacekeeping missions in public health emergencies. The idea that UNMIL could and should have done more rests on a series of underlying assumptions: that peacekeeping missions (in particular in this case UNMIL) are authorised to play a greater role; that they are capable of doing so safely and effectively; and that they are an appropriate mechanism for carrying out such tasks. In the following sections of this paper we discuss the issues of authorisation and capacity, before turning to a discussion of the appropriateness of peacekeeping forces as a mechanism for addressing public health emergencies in the developing countries in which they are most often deployed.

Authorisation

The first assumption that we examine is that UNMIL was authorised to play a more active role in responding to Ebola than it did. This is not uncontroversial – and such a role could entail various things, from providing security to allow humanitarian aid agencies to work to more direct forms of medical assistance such as treatment by UNMIL's medical staff.

The mandate is always the starting point for examining issues of peacekeeping authorisation, with the mandate for each mission being specified in the relevant resolution(s) of the UN Security Council. The original UNMIL mandate, as set out by the Security Council, acting under Chapter VII of the UN Charter, in Resolution 1509 (2003) outlined a 19-point mandate, the most important clauses of which charged UNMIL with the tasks of observing and monitoring the ceasefire; assisting with the development and operation of cantonment sites; developing and implementing a Disarmament, Demobilisation, Rehabilitation and Reintegration (DDRR) action plan; and providing security services at key institutions.[30]

Resolution 2116 (2013), the authorising resolution in force at the beginning of the Ebola outbreak, reaffirmed that 'UNMIL's primary tasks are to continue to support the Government in order to solidify peace and stability in Liberia and to protect civilians'.[31] Civilian protection was thus a part of the mandate, although this did not include an explicit requirement to deliver medical aid or other forms of humanitarian assistance. Indeed, the mandate was clear that UNMIL's mission was to play a *facilitating* rather than a direct humanitarian assistance role:

> (k) to facilitate the provision of humanitarian assistance, including by helping to establish the necessary security conditions.

As discussed in the previous section, in September 2014 the Security Council passed Resolution 2176, which expressed 'grave concern about the extent of the outbreak of the Ebola virus', and extended UNMIL's mandate to December 2014 (in the process deferring the planned drawdown). In that Resolution the Council noted that it was

> expressing deep appreciation for and commending the continued contribution and commitment of United Nations personnel, especially the troop- and police-contributing countries of the United Nations Mission in Liberia (UNMIL), to assist in consolidating peace and stability in Liberia, and the efforts of the Special Representative of the Secretary-General.[32]

That was followed on 15 December 2014 by Resolution 2190 (2014), which repeated the sentiments of the September resolution and updated UNMIL's mandate. The humanitarian assistance mandate given to the mission remained very similar to that of 2003:

> (b)(i) to facilitate the provision of humanitarian assistance, including in collaboration with the Government of Liberia, and those supporting it, and by helping to establish the necessary security conditions.[33]

What can be said, therefore, is that, notwithstanding the overall civilian protection mandate, there is nothing in UNMIL's mandate – even as renewed during the Ebola outbreak – that tasked it with directly providing humanitarian assistance, although it was given a role in facilitating the provision of such assistance by other parties by helping to establish the necessary security conditions.

In addition to each mission's mandate, the DPKO has also produced a range of other guidance and information relevant to peacekeeper provision of humanitarian (including medical) assistance, perhaps the most notable of which is the 2008 *Principles and Guidelines to Peacekeeping Operations* (commonly known as the 'Capstone Doctrine'), which provides generic guidance on the roles and responsibilities of peacekeepers serving in UN missions.[34] *Principles and Guidelines* includes material concerning the organisation, management and support of missions and states clearly that the 'core business' of peacekeepers is to stabilise the situation and provide a secure environment for civilians and humanitarian actors.[35] When it comes to playing a more direct role in the delivery of humanitarian assistance, meanwhile, the document notes that responsibility:

> rests primarily with the relevant civilian United Nations specialized agencies, funds and programmes, as well as the range of independent, international and local NGOs which are usually active alongside a United Nations peacekeeping operation. The primary role of United Nations peacekeeping operations with regard to the provision of humanitarian assistance is to provide a secure and stable environment within which humanitarian actors may carry out their activities.[36]

Could it nevertheless have been argued that UNMIL was authorised to play a more direct role in delivering medical aid during the EVD outbreak, even without a specific request from the Security Council? In our view it possibly could. There are two particular areas where we find official endorsement of a role for peacekeepers in the direct delivery of humanitarian medical aid (rather than solely as facilitators of humanitarian access): Civil Military Cooperation (Cimic), which includes health care delivery and services (sometimes referred to as Quick Impact Projects' – QIPs),[37] and cases of extreme emergency.

First, the DPKO does recommend that in some circumstances missions should engage in QIPs, designed to benefit the population through small-scale infrastructure and/or public communication projects, which may include a health or medical component, although it emphasises that these are 'not a substitute for humanitarian and/or development assistance'.[38] As we discuss below, UNMIL has a long track-record of engaging in such projects in the health field, with medical outreach and related activities being undertaken by a number of different national contingents over the history of the mission. The impetus for such activities frequently comes from the contingents on the ground rather than from New York. The UN's Department of Field Support (DFS), responsible for the day-to-day management of peace-keeping operations, states that all civil assistance, including health care delivery, should be 'coordinated with other humanitarian entities and subject to review by the UN-CIMIC and the mission approval process'.[39]

The other set of circumstances in which peacekeepers are authorised to play an explicit humanitarian role is in cases of extreme emergency. Office for the Coordination of Humanitarian Affairs (OCHA) provides guidance on the relationship between civilian and mili-tary actors during complex emergencies, as well as mission specific guidance.[40] The priority in both cases is to ensure that conflict is avoided between military and humanitarian actors and that the principles of neutrality and impartiality of humanitarian aid provision are respected (and are seen to be respected). In terms of coordination these guidelines seek to forward the broader UN integration policy to 'Deliver as One', while at the same time ensuring that peacekeepers maintain primary responsibility for a mission's political and security objectives, as humanitarian agencies lead the response in that sector. The intention is to see these roles blend only in situations where an emergency is so great as to require it, for example where 'only the use of military assets can meet a critical humanitarian need', and even then only as a 'last resort'.[41] The DPKO has similarly made reference to 'emergency response periods' in which there is a potential need for humanitarian assistance to be provided directly by a peacekeeping mission rather than by specialised humanitarian agencies. In such cases the only objective is to save lives, ensure protection, and meet basic, urgent needs. The DPKO goes on to note that in these situations, 'it is important to keep longer-term objectives in mind and begin planning for the more comprehensive humanitarian programmes that will be possible in a more stable environment'.[42]

It would surely be the case that the Ebola outbreak in Liberia, as it developed through 2014, would qualify as such an 'emergency', justifying UNMIL playing a greater role without compromising the terms of its mandate, and without the mission contravening more gen-eral UN guidelines and principles. Particularly in the early stages of the outbreak the acute shortage of trained medical personnel reduced any danger of problematic overlap with the activities of humanitarian aid agencies. That UNMIL did not use the developing emergency as a basis to justify doing more suggests that issues of capacity and competence were the primary limitation. Certainly that is the implication to be derived from the comments of the Under-Secretary-General for UN Peacekeeping Operations, Hervé Ladsous, when he stated that 'a peacekeeping mission is not a public health operation [as] this is not what we are trained for'.[43]

Capacity and competence

As is the case with all peacekeeping operations, UNMIL was deployed with its own medical services, whose primary role was (and is) to provide healthcare services to mission staff (both military and civilian) during their deployment.[44] Yet it is clear from UNMIL's public communications that, before Ebola, assisting with logistics and even in the direct delivery of medical services to local populations in the mission area, and not just to mission personnel, was a significant part of its daily work – and also an important aspect of the 'public face' of the mission.

Indeed, the extent to which the outer provinces of Liberia in particular were dependent upon the presence and assistance of UNMIL is striking. UNMIL has provided the only supply chain for moving essential logistical equipment, as well as personnel from the Liberian National Police force and medical staff to the outer provinces. In the (six-month) rainy season 'roads become impassable and cannot sustain major logistics movements...There are no in-country commercial alternatives to the UNMIL military engineering units that keep critical supply lines open; there are also serious shortfalls in the national medical system.' UNMIL – despite the drawdown – was still required to 'support civilian personnel, including police [and presumably medical staff], deployed throughout the country'.[45] This situation has resulted in two dependencies – a reliance on UNMIL to facilitate access to Liberian medical staff in the outer provinces or, failing that, reliance on UNMIL itself to provide medical assistance to Liberian citizens.

The mission's publication, UNMIL Today, frequently included reports of troops' involvement in providing medical services to civilian populations – in particular (but not only) to women and children. Examples include reports of medical outreach initiatives in Bensonville, near Monrovia, where more than 300 patients were treated by Nigerian UNMIL medical personnel (reported June 2009);[46] a paediatric de-worming programme along the Zorzor–Voinjama road (carried out by Bangladeshi troops and reported in November 2009);[47] a weekly 'meet the doctor' organised by the Bangladeshi battalion at Camp Charlie in Ganta which, at the time of the report in July 2010, was claimed to have treated over 1350 patients;[48] a Pakistani Battalion-run clinic providing medical assistance to the blind and visually impaired in Tubmanburg, Bomi County (reported July 2010);[49] and an outreach programme, again run by troops from Pakistan, in Careysburg, Montserrado County, where over 500 received treatment (reported August 2010).[50] The UNMIL Facebook page – which was launched in 2011 – has similarly featured regular reports of medical outreach activities. These have included treating 900 residents of Plumkor Community in Brewerville, Montserrado County;[51] offering training to medical staff in a Liberian hospital;[52] a Christmas–time medical outreach day at Virginia Christian Academy near River View, Monrovia;[53] and countless other examples of outreach days in communities, including to students at the Darussalam International Islamic Mission,[54] inmates at Monrovia Central Prison,[55] and the Hotel Africa community.[56]

Of course, neither UNMIL's important role in providing logistical capabilities to the Liberian health sector nor the medical outreach initiatives (most of which were for limited periods of time and involved relatively small numbers of UNMIL personnel) meant that the mission was in a position (either in terms of manpower or equipment) to play a major part in responding to a public health emergency on the scale of Ebola. But they do indicate that it may have been able to play a greater part than it did, and it remains striking that the first reaction was for battalions to return to barracks – and also, as we noted above, that the vast majority of existing medical outreach activities ceased once the Ebola outbreak had begun.

One obvious lesson here is that the views and demands of TCCs were a key capacity constraint on the mission. The withdrawal of the Philippines contingent and the reluctance of other TCCs to see their troops put 'in harm's way' in a rapidly developing health crisis certainly limited the extent to which peacekeepers could play a more active role. But, even without these constraints, there were good reasons to question whether the UNMIL medical services could have effectively (and safely) made a significant contribution to controlling Ebola in public health terms (as opposed to the mission making a greater potential logistical and security contribution if it had not continued drawdown – a point to which we return below).

For one thing, there had over a number of years been serious criticisms of the quality and safety of UNMIL's medical services. In 2009 the UN's Office of Internal Oversight Services' (OIOS) audit of UNMIL identified failures in the quality of medical care being provided in this mission to both troops and civilian populations.[57] Among other things, it found a lack of standard operating procedures to guide TCC's provision of medical care; no professional support and training available to upgrade medical personnel skills; inadequate hygiene in TCC clinics; and failures to comply with WHO guidelines on the disposal of medical waste. During the audit the OIOS also found that peacekeepers were providing medical treatment to local populations, despite their clinics not meeting basic medical standards for hygiene and waste management. All this means that there must be caution in the presumption that UNMIL's medical services were well-placed to assist with an infectious disease outbreak as deadly and virulent as EVD. Indeed, as noted by the OIOS audit, one of the major health concerns surrounding UN peacekeeping is the potential for peacekeepers to be 'vectors' of disease – to spread infection through the local community.[58] As well as the obvious negative health impact on affected civilians, such events can have other damaging effects, including straining relations between a mission and the host community.

Where UNMIL may have been better-placed to play a more active role earlier than it did is in relation to logistical support (continuing or augmenting its previous role), and in assisting the Liberian government with the spread of information about the virus throughout the provinces. However, the drawdown had a significant detrimental effect on UNMIL's provincial presence. As we noted above, UNMIL was one of the few international actors with a strong logistical capability in the provinces before the outbreak, and it was noted during the Ebola crisis that the peacekeeping mission in Liberia had the comparative advantage over other UN agencies in terms of its geographic reach and political leverage.[59] But by the time of the Security Council session on 9 September 2014 it was reported that UNMIL had completed drawdown from four provinces and was now only present in seven of 15 provinces. Improving the limited capacity to provide rapid response in the outer provinces was later noted by WHO as vital to containing the outbreak.[60]

The lack of international coordination in responding to the Ebola outbreak also hampered UNMIL's response to the emergency in Liberia. For example, in late July the UN had asked the US Centers for Disease Control (CDC) not to publicly release projected end-of-year Ebola cases, in part because UNMIL had reported that the situation was tense on the ground. This advice was not followed and UNMIL – still in drawdown mode at the time – had to prepare quickly for a security response to riots and shootings in Monrovia.[61] The delay in WHO Headquarters convening an emergency committee to declare Ebola a PHEIC also impaired the ability of UNMIL to raise the alarm. Technically UNMIL could not request support to mount an emergency response action to the outbreak without prior action from WHO, the body authorised to declare a health emergency. If WHO Headquarters had acted sooner, there is the possibility that the UNMIL Head of Mission may have had a greater opportunity to do more earlier on.

In relation to assisting with security (a task which would on the face of it seem to explicitly fit within the 'facilitating humanitarian access' provisions of the mission's mandate), one of the difficulties faced by the mission was the controversial nature of some of the Liberian government's own responses. Those responses became increasingly militarised over time

– with one of the most high-profile incidents being the attempt to forcibly quarantine the West Point district of Monrovia, an attempt that culminated in clashes between the public and the security services.[62] Not only was UNMIL not involved in such operations, it was at pains to distance itself from them.[63] This dimension of the Ebola response highlights the difficult choices that peacekeeping missions such as UNMIL face when dealing with complex emergencies within their mission areas. In the next part of this paper we go on to unpack some of these issues, considering the question of whether or not, where present on the ground, peacekeeping missions are appropriate bodies for responding to rapidly developing public health emergencies.

Peacekeepers: a role in responding to health emergencies?

In the previous section we argued that UNMIL could have done more within the terms of its mandate, although the types of contribution it was in a position to make was limited by a range of factors, including the views of the TCCs involved, the resources and competences of the mission, problems of inter-agency coordination, and the actions of the host government. But, aside from these issues, what can we say about the appropriate role of peacekeepers in responding to the Ebola outbreak and to future public health emergencies?

It is clearly not the case – and nobody would try to argue – that peacekeepers are ideally suited to responding to major disease outbreaks. The question, rather, is whether, in the absence of other agencies better-placed to take on the burden of the task, it is appropriate for peacekeepers that are already on the ground to play a role as emergency 'first responders'.

It was noted in the Introduction to a recent special issue of *Third World Quarterly* on the 'local turn' in peace building that critics often point to the 'shallowness of interventions that serve the intervener better than the targets of intervention. Practices remain as they were, and peace building in post-conflict contexts remains volatile'.[64] Liberia, even before the Ebola outbreak, was a country struggling to live up to the liberal peace ideal. The dependence we described above on external agencies, including UNMIL, for local healthcare service delivery – a problem identified long before EVD – points to a collective failure by the national government and international donors to build domestic health system capacities.[65] As was widely noted, the Ebola outbreak graphically illustrated the weaknesses of the health infrastructure in Liberia (as well as the other two most-affected countries). Liberia had resided near the bottom of all the league tables for health indicators and health system development for many years before the outbreak. In terms of life expectancy it ranked 166th in the world.[66] On the league table of physicians per 1000 people it did even worse, being ranked 194th in the world (jointly with Sierra Leone, at 0.03 physicians per 1000 people).[67] The Ebola outbreak (and certainly its scale) was to a great extent the product of a decade and more of failure to transition Liberia to an effective state.

Yet, taking the Liberian health system as it was in 2014, what can the UNMIL experience reveal about the suitability of peacekeeping missions as first responders to major public health crises? If the Security Council continues to play a leading role in international responses to such events, it may be tempted to view the peacekeeping forces which it has stationed around the world as a potential tool – as might the Secretary-General, given his recommendation of extending the UNMIL mandate to enable it to assist in the response. In this section we raise two doubts about the appropriateness of peacekeeping forces playing a significant role in responding (especially in a medical capacity) to health emergencies. While there were opportunities for UNMIL to have done more, as we have discussed above, there are dangers (and the potential for dangerous precedents) that must be acknowledged before advocating that peacekeepers should be in the front line of responding to health emergencies. In this section we discuss, first, the danger of humanitarian aid becoming politicised and, second, the potential that even well-intentioned actions could do more harm than good.

Politicisation

One of the potential downsides of the engagement of military forces (even those serving in blue helmets) in delivering aid is that it can undermine the perceived neutrality of humanitarian assistance. This fact is well-recognised by the UN itself. In discussing QIPs, *Principles and Guidelines* recommends that missions should consult with humanitarian actors and:

> be aware that humanitarian actors may have concerns about the characterization of QIPs, or Civil Military Coordination (CIMIC) projects, 'hearts and minds' activities, or other security or recovery projects as being of a humanitarian nature, when they see these as primarily serving political, security or reconstruction priorities.[68]

A clear expression of this fear from the humanitarian aid community's side was seen in 1997, when Cornelio Sommaruga, then President of the International Committee of the Red Cross (ICRC), argued that the separation of peacekeeping duties from the provision of humanitarian assistance was essential:

> UN military missions are an essential component of successful conflict management; in certain anarchic situations they may prove indispensable in securing respect for international humanitarian law and thus restoring the necessary security environment for the conduct of humanitarian activities. That being said, peacekeeping, and especially peace-enforcement operations, should be clearly distinct in character from humanitarian activities. Military forces should not be directly involved in humanitarian action, as this would associate humanitarian organizations, in the minds of the authorities and the population, with political or military objectives which go beyond humanitarian concerns.[69]

Similar concerns were apparent in the 2011 WHO Global Health Cluster's position paper on civil–military roles and responsibilities. That report noted that neither the Inter-Agency Standing Committee (IASC) nor the Security Council has adequately addressed the division of responsibilities that reflect the multidisciplinary UN mission environment. The concern, as voiced by the WHO was that:

> This blending of strategies and tactics serves to undermine the international humanitarian community's core humanitarian principles. The integrated mission concept developed by the UN follows a similar trend. Although there are significant attempts to protect the humanitarian space within integrated missions, the concept foresees the integration of different agencies and components into an overall political/strategic crisis management framework. This can blur the lines between the UN's different political and humanitarian branches, with predictably negative results.[70]

While protection of humanitarian space was not a major problem in the case of Liberia (although the mission was reluctant to associate itself with the government's controversial security operations for fear of politicisation), the transfer of responsibility *was* proving a problem, particularly to local government structures outside Monrovia.[71] In this respect, of course, Liberia was not typical of all peacekeeping missions: this was a relatively stable country in the midst of a drawdown of the UN presence, without the kinds of antagonism that other peacekeeping missions may face. In the Liberia case, indeed, the widespread acceptance of UNMIL's presence was itself part of the problem, creating a worrying dependence on the mission for access outside of Monrovia at a time when it was continuing with drawdown, despite the developing humanitarian emergency. Yet in other cases peacekeeping missions are more controversial, and their engagement in delivering humanitarian assistance could pose risks to perceptions of aid neutrality.

Doing more harm than good

A second danger relates to Lasdous' comment that 'this is not what we are trained for', and relates to the possibility that peacekeeping missions attempting to provide assistance in cases of a major public health emergency could unwittingly end up doing more harm than good. We have already mentioned the findings of the OIOS audit of UNMIL's medical services that there were worrying failures – including in hygiene standards in facilities used to provide treatment to the civilian population. Although steps were taken to address these issues in the intervening years, the high standards of infection control required in the treatment of infectious diseases such as Ebola point to the potential dangers of under-equipped and ill-prepared interventions – however well-intentioned. The experience of the UNMIH mission in Haiti, which was accused of having been responsible for a serious cholera outbreak following the 2010 earthquake,[72] serves as a warning about the importance of infection control, and the possible implications of peacekeeping missions failing to maintain strict standards in this respect.

In terms of the potential for logistical and security assistance to do more harm than good the risks are perhaps more limited – but are not entirely absent. Even if there is a mandate provision to respond to a health emergency, the Security Council remains dependent on TCCs to provide it with the personnel and other resources that it needs. This posed a problem in the Ebola outbreak, with TCCs being extremely wary of exposing their troops to risk of infection and it would probably similarly arise in future situations. Difficult relationships and policy disagreements with host governments can also pose problems – clearly a factor in UNMIL's desire to disassociate itself from some of the security operations of the Liberian government. Even though (indeed precisely because) they are humanitarian emergencies, major outbreak events can be deeply politicised, with governments often opting to take unpopular and authoritarian actions in the name of disease control. There are clearly risks in the UN becoming associated with such actions, not least given its position of support for human rights around the world. Engagement in such controversial activities could create new complications both for the mission itself and for the UN family as a whole.

Conclusions

This discussion leads us to two final observations on the role of UNMIL in the Liberian Ebola outbreak, and more generally on the potential role of peacekeeping missions in responding to public health emergencies in the developing world.

First, there may have been opportunities for UNMIL to play a greater role than it did – especially early in the outbreak – but it could never have been an optimal response mechanism for a number of reasons. While the mission probably did have scope under its mandate to justify a bigger role (especially, for example, in logistics and support in the provinces), it suffered a number of limitations, including the willingness of TCCs to allow their personnel to play this role and the effects that drawdown had already begun to have. The actions of the Liberian government also arguably made it more politically difficult for UNMIL to play a more significant role in providing the security conditions under which the humanitarian response could operate effectively. What is more, there are important questions to be asked about the competence and capacity of some TCCs' medical services when confronting a deadly infectious disease threat. At the very least, however, we would argue that the drawdown should have been halted at an earlier stage in the outbreak, a decision that may have allowed UNMIL to contribute more to the developing international effort.

Second, there are broader questions raised by the Liberia case about the provision of medical assistance to civilians by peacekeeping missions. While we would accept that there is a case for mission medics to play a role in emergency situations such as the Ebola outbreak, the desirability of such a role in 'normal' times is more debateable. Indeed, in this case the reliance on external actors, including UNMIL, to 'prop up' a failing national health system by delivering services seems to have been one of the underlying causes of the country's failure to develop a sustainable national health system. Greater attention needs to be paid to peacekeeper involvement in such activities, and to how transitions can be made to national 'ownership', shifting health care delivery from blue helmets to local authorities. Ebola, coupled with the UNMIL drawdown, revealed the over-dependence of national service provision on external support – including that provided by what was always designed to be a temporary peacekeeping mission. This is a moral hazard for peacekeepers, and is one that all humanitarian actors feed into, but the consequences may not become tragically apparent until a country is thrown into the perfect storm of health insecurity, as happened with in Ebola outbreak.

Disclosure statement

No potential conflict of interest was reported by the authors.

Acknowledgement

We are grateful to Vanessa Newby for her invaluable research assistance in the preparation of this article. Dr Sara Davies is the recipient of an Australian Research Council Future Fellowship (project number FT130101040).

Notes

1. WHO, "Ebola Virus Disease in Guinea."
2. MSF, "Ebola Epidemic Declared."
3. Enserik. "WHO declares Ebola Emergency."
4. UN Security Council, S/RES/ 2177, 1.
5. UN Security Council, S/RES/ 2177, 3.
6. UN General Assembly, A/RES/69/1. UNMEER was based in Ghana and initially led by Assistant Secretary General for Field Support, Anthony Banbury. Banbury had already been appointed 'Ebola Crisis Manager' by the Secretary General on September 8. UN General Assembly and Security Council, A/69/389-S/2014/679.
7. UN Security Council, S/RES/2066.
8. UN Secretary General, Twenty-eighth Progress Report'. S/2014/598 .
9. Sengupta, "Effort on Ebola." Chan's office, according to Sengupta, claimed that it had no record of receiving the cables.
10. WHO, "Ebola Response Roadmap."
11. Snyder, "What Role for Peacekeepers?"
12. WHO, "Ebola Haemorrhagic Fever."
13. For further discussion of these issues see Davies & Rushton, *Healing or Harming?*
14. WHO, "Liberia."
15. WHO AFRO, "Ebola Virus Disease."
16. WHO, "Ebola Situation Report – 6 May."
17. WHO, "Ebola Transmission in Liberia Over."
18. UN Security Council, S/RES/2066.
19. UN Secretary General, "Twenty-eighth Progress Report," 14.
20. Quoted in Lynch, "Ban says UN Troops are Safe."
21. Menkor, "Ebola Fear closes UNMIL."
22. Snyder, "What Role for UN Peacekeepers?"
23. "Citing Ebola Outbreak's Profound Toll."
24. Wesee, "Liberia."
25. "Citing Ebola Outbreak's Profound Toll."
26. Landgren, "Combatting Ebola".
27. "Liberia."
28. UN Security Council, "Twenty-eighth Progress Report," 5, 11.
29. UN Security Council, "7260th Meeting."
30. UN Security Council, S/RES/1509.
31. UN Security Council, S/RES/2116.
32. UN Security Council, S/RES/2176.
33. UN Security Council, S/RES/2190.
34. UN DPKO, *Principles and Guidelines*.
35. Ibid., Figure 2, 23–24.
36. UN DPKO, *United Nations Peacekeeping Operations*, 30.
37. UN DPKO, *Civil–Military Coordination*. Indeed, QIPs were rolled out to support country health teams when government funds were inexplicably held up in reaching the province. See UN Security Council, "7260th Meeting," 5.
38. UN DPKO, *Principles and Guidelines*, 30.
39. UN DPKO, *Civil–Military Coordination*.
40. OCHA, *Humanitarian Civil–Military Coordination*.
41. OCHA, "Civil–Military Guidelines," xi.
42. UN Peacekeeping Operations, *Handbook on Multidimensional Peacekeeping*, 175 .
43. "Ebola."
44. UN DPKO, *Medical Support Manual*, para.1.01.
45. UN Secretary General, S/2014.598, 6, 15.
46. UNMIL, "Medical Outreach in Gurmoshor."

47. UNMIL, "Banengr-12 Deworming Exercise."
48. UNMIL, "Meet the Doctor."
49. UNMIL, "PakEng-13 helps Blind."
50. UNMIL, "PakEngr-14 in Medical Outreach."
51. UNMIL, Facebook page, July 19, 2012.
52. UNMIL, Facebook page, July 25, 2012.
53. UNMIL, Facebook page, December 17, 2012.
54. UNMIL, Facebook page, June 6, 2013.
55. UNMIL, Facebook page, October 9, 2013.
56. UNMIL, Facebook page, December 26, 2013.
57. UN OIOS, "Audit of the Provision."
58. For further discussion of this issue, see Davies & Rushton, *Healing or Harming?*
59. UN Security Council "Twenty-eighth Progress Report," 10; and UN Security Council, "Letter dated 28 August 2014," 2.
60. WHO, "Liberia."
61. Karin Landgren, quoted in "Combating Ebola in Liberia," 2–3.
62. Onishi. "Clashes Erupt."
63. In a letter to the Security Council on August 28, 2014, Secretary-General Ban reported: 'Though it has not, and will not, enforce the Government-imposed isolation of affected areas, UNMIL will continue to facilitate the provision of humanitarian assistance, including by helping to provide the necessary security conditions, in accordance with Security Council resolution 1509 (2003)'. UN Security Council, "Letter dated 28 August 2014," 2.
64. Hughes et al., "The Struggle versus the Song," 823.
65. Downie, *The Road to Recovery*; and Petit et al., "Implementing a Basic Package."
66. WHO, "Life Expectancy by Country."
67. "Physicians per 1000 People."
68. UN DPKO, *United Nations Peacekeeping Operations*, 30.
69. Sommaruga, "Humanitarian Action."
70. WHO, "Civil–Military Coordination," 11–12.
71. UN Security Council, "Twenty-eighth Progress Report," 8. See also Leonardsson and Rudd, "The 'Local Turn'."
72. For a full discussion of this case see Davies & Rushton, *Healing or Harming?*

Bibliography

"Citing Ebola Outbreak's Profound Toll on Liberia, Top Official tells Security Council Plaque must be stopped in its Tracks." UN News. September 9, 2014. http://www.un.org/press/en/2014/sc11553. doc.htm.

Davies, S., and Rushton, S. *Healing or Harming? United Nations Peacekeeping and Health*. Providing for Peacekeeping No.9. (New York: International Peace Institute, March 2015). Available at: http://www. ipinst.org/2015/03/healing-or-harming-united-nations-peacekeeping-and-health

Downie, Richard. *The Road to Recovery: Rebuilding Liberia's Health System*. Washington, DC: Center for International Strategic Studies. August 2012. http://csis.org/files/publication/120822_Downie_ RoadtoRecovery_web.pdf.

"Ebola: UN will 'stay the Course' in Liberia, Peacekeeping Chief Says." UN News Centre, September 11, 2014. http://www.un.org/apps/news/story.asp?NewsID=48693#.VXZSwc-qpBc.

Enserik, Martin. "WHO declares Escalating Ebola Outbreak an International Emergency." *Nature*, August 8, 2014. http://news.sciencemag.org/africa/2014/08/who-declares-escalating-ebola-outbreak-international-emergency.

Hughes, Caroline, Joakim Öjendal, and Isabell Schierenbeck. "The Struggle versus the Song – The Local Turn in Peace Building: An Introduction." *Third World Quarterly* 36, no. 5 (2015): 817–824.

Landgren, K. 'Combating Ebola in Liberia: The Role of the International Community'. Speech delivered at Chatham House, London, November 10, 2014. https://www.chathamhouse.org/sites/files/ chathamhouse/field/field_document/20141110EbolaLiberia.pdf

Leonardsson, H., and Rudd, G. "The 'Local Turn' in Peace Building: A Literature Review of Effective and Emancipatory Local Peace Building." *Third World Quarterly* 36, no. 5 (2015): 825–839.

"Liberia: Samukai outlines Effects of Ebola – Wants Support to lift Travel Ban and Statement to the UNSC by Defence Minister Brownie Samukai." All Africa, September 11, 2014. http://allafrica.com/stories/201409111254.html.

Lynch, C. "Ban says UN Troops are Safe, needed to quash Ebola Unrest." *Foreign Policy: The Cable*, September 2, 2014. http://thecable.foreignpolicy.com/posts/2014/09/02/ban_says_un_troops_are_safe_needed_to_quash_ebola_unrest.

Menkor, I. F. 2014. "Ebola Fear closes UNMIL Facilities in Nimba 'Indefinitely.'" *Liberian Observer*, July 16. http://www.liberianobserver.com/security/ebola-fear-closes-unmil-facilities-nimba-%E2%80%98indefinitely%E2%80%99

MSF. "Ebola Epidemic declared in Guinea: MSF launches Emergency Response." March 23, 2014. http://www.doctorswithoutborders.org/news-stories/field-news/ebola-epidemic-declared-guinea-msf-launches-emergency-response.

"Physicians per 1000 People." Nationmaster, 2015. http://www.nationmaster.com/country-info/stats/Health/Physicians/Per-1,000-people.

OCHA. *Humanitarian Civil–Military Coordination.* 2014. http://www.unocha.org/what-we-do/coordination-tools/UN-CMCoord/publications.

OCHA. *Civil–Military Guidelines and Reference for Complex Humanitarian Emergencies.* Geneva: United Nations, 2005. https://docs.unocha.org/sites/dms/Documents/ENGLISH%20VERSION%20Guidelines%20for%20Complex%20Emergencies.pdf.

Onishi, Norimitsu. 2014. "Clashes erupt as Liberia sets an Ebola Quarantine." *New York Times*, August 21. http://www.nytimes.com/2014/08/21/world/africa/ebola-outbreak-liberia-quarantine.html?_r=0.

Petit, Dörte, Egbert Sondorp, Susannah Mayhew, Maria Roura, and Bayard Roberts. "Implementing a Basic Package of Health Services in Post-conflict Liberia: Perceptions of Key Stakeholders." *Social Science and Medicine* 78 (2013): 42–49.

Sengupta, Somini. 2015. "Effort on Ebola hurt UN Chief." *New York Times*, January 6. http://www.nytimes.com/2015/01/07/world/leader-of-world-health-organization-defends-ebola-response.html?_r=0.

Snyder, M. R. 2014. "What Role for UN Peacekeepers in tackling Ebola?" *IPI Global Observatory*, September 8. http://theglobalobservatory.org/2014/09/role-un-peacekeepers-unmil-tackling-ebola/.

Sommaruga, Cornelio. "Humanitarian Action and Peace-keeping Operations." *International Review of the Red Cross*, no. 317 (1997). http://www.icrc.org/eng/resources/documents/misc/57jnj7.htm.

UN DPKO. *Civil–Military Coordination in UN Integrated Peacekeeping Missions.* New York: United Nations, 2010. https://docs.unocha.org/sites/dms/Documents/DPKO%20UN-CIMIC%20(2010).pdf.

UN DPKO. *Medical Support Manual for United Nations Peacekeeping Operations.* 2nd ed. New York: United Nations, 1999. http://reliefweb.int/sites/reliefweb.int/files/resources/D196C0B0FF3A637BC1256DD4004983B9-dpko-medical-1999.pdf.

UN DPKO. *Handbook on United Nations Multidimensional Peacekeeping Operations.* New York: United Nations, 2003. http://www.unrol.org/files/Handbook%20on%20Multi-Dimensional%20Peacekeeping.pdf

UNDPKO. *United Nations Peacekeeping Operations: Principles and Guidelines.* New York: United Nations, 2008.

UN General Assembly. A/RES/69/1. New York, September 19, 2014.

UN General Assembly and UN Security Council. Identical letters dated 17 September 2014 from Secretary-General addressed to the President of the General Assembly and the President of the Security Council. A/69/389-S/2014/679. New York, 2014.

UNMIL. "Banengr-12 in Deworming Exercise." *UNMIL Today* 9, no. 6 (2009). http://reliefweb.int/sites/reliefweb.int/files/resources/8CC159C1AD21E8894925768700185A05-Full_Report.pdf.

UNMIL. "Medical Outreach in Gurmoshor." *UNMIL Today* 6, no. 1 (2009). http://reliefweb.int/sites/reliefweb.int/files/resources/EE2C0DBB1ACB36EF4925761F001AD414-Full_Report.pdf.

UNIMIL. "Meet the Doctor." *UNMIL Today* 7, no. 2 (2010). http://reliefweb.int/sites/reliefweb.int/files/resources/A73FCCFE15906B2C4925777B0004A60F-Full_Report.pdf.

UNIMIL. "PakEng-13 helps the Blind." *UNMIL Today* 7, no. 2 (2010). http://reliefweb.int/sites/reliefweb.int/files/resources/A73FCCFE15906B2C4925777B0004A60F-Full_Report.pdf.

UNMIL. "PakEngr-14 in Medical Outreach." *UNMIL Today* 7, no. 3 (2010). http://reliefweb.int/sites/reliefweb.int/files/resources/C7B9AAE1AD84B98649257799000CE8DA-Full_Report.pdf.

UN OIOS. "Audit of the Provision of Medical Services in UNMIL." Assignment No. AP2008/626/08. April 8, 2009. http://usun.state.gov/documents/organization/140720.pdf.

UN Security Council. "Twenty-eighth Progress Report of the Secretary-General on the United Nations Mission in Liberia." S/2014/598. New York, August 15, 2014.

UN Security Council. "Letter dated 28 August 2014 from the Secretary-General addressed to the President of the Security Council." S/2014/644. New York, September 2, 2014. http://www.un.org/ga/search/view_doc.asp?symbol=S/2014/644.

UN Security Council. "7260th Meeting of the Security Council, 9 September 2014." S/PV.7260. New York, 2014.

UN Security Council, S/RES/1509. New York, NY, September 19, 2003.

UN Security Council. S/RES/2066. New York, September 17, 2012.

UN Security Council. S/RES/2116. New York, NY, September 19, 2013.

UN Security Council. S/RES/2176. New York, September 15, 2014.

UN Security Council. S/RES/2177. New York, September 18, 2014.

UN Security Council, S/RES/2190. New York, December 15, 2014.

Wesee, B.P. "Liberia: UNMIL, UN commit to Ebola Fight." All Africa, July 24, 2014. http://allafrica.com/stories/201407241090.html.

World Health Organization (WHO). "Civil–Military Coordination during Humanitarian Health Action." Global Health Cluster. February 2011. http://www.who.int/hac/global_health_cluster/about/policy_strategy/ghc_position_paper_civil_military_coord_2_feb2011.pdf?ua=1.

WHO. "Ebola Haemorrhagic Fever in the Democratic Republic of the Congo – Update 2." Emergency Preparedness and Response, September 20, 2007. http://www.who.int/csr/don/2007_09_20/en/.

WHO. "Ebola Response Roadmap Situation Report: 18 September 2014." http://apps.who.int/iris/bitstream/10665/133833/1/roadmapsitrep4_eng.pdf?ua=1.

WHO. "Ebola Situation Report: 6 May 2015." http://apps.who.int/ebola/en/current-situation/ebola-situation-report-6-may-2015.

WHO. "Ebola Transmission in Liberia Over. Nation enters 90-day Intensive Surveillance Period." September 3, 2015. http://www.who.int/mediacentre/news/statements/2015/ebola-transmission-over-liberia/en/.

WHO. "Ebola Virus Disease in Guinea." March 23, 2014. http://www.who.int/csr/don/2014_03_23_ebola/en/.

WHO. "Liberia: A Country – and its Capital – are overwhelmed with Ebola Cases." January 2015. http://www.who.int/csr/disease/ebola/one-year-report/liberia/en/.

WHO. "Life Expectancy by Country." Global Health Observatory Data Repository, 2015. http://apps.who.int/gho/data/node.main.688?lang=en.

WHO AFRO. "Ebola Virus Disease, West Africa – Update 8 August 2014." http://www.afro.who.int/en/clusters-a-programmes/dpc/epidemic-a-pandemic-alert-and-response/outbreak-news/4241-ebola-virus-disease-west-africa-8-august-2014.html.

Ebola respons-ibility: moving from shared to multiple responsibilities

Clare Wenham

London School of Hygiene & Tropical Medicine, UK

ABSTRACT

Combating threats of infectious diseases has been increasingly framed as a global shared responsibility for a multi-actor framework of states, international organisations and nongovernmental actors. However, the outbreak of Ebola Virus Disease (EVD) has shown that this governance framework has not been able to limit the spread of this virus, despite the normative and legislative changes to global disease control. By unbundling the concept of responsibility, this article will assess how global shared responsibility may have failed because accountability does not fall on any one state or stakeholder, highlighting an inherent weakness in the global disease governance regime. The paper concludes that a move towards multiple responsibilities may prove a more effective mechanism for ensuring global health security.

Introduction

'There is no one to take responsibility, absolutely no one, since the beginning of the [EVD] crisis', claimed a Médecins Sans Frontières (MSF) advisor (*New York Times*, September 3, 2014), summarising the unprecedented scale of the West African outbreak. This paper seeks to question this assumption of responsibility for disease control. It suggests that the framing of a global shared responsibility for disease threats, which has developed in the post-SARS era, is inherently flawed if no one actor is able to be held accountable for any one part of it. This empirical study of EVD offers an alternative reframing, as multiple accountabilities may prove more fruitful for understanding failures in this health crisis. The paper suggests three sets of actors that contributed to the chaotic response to the global health threat: the E3 states (Sierra Leone, Liberia and Guinea), the World Health Organization (WHO) and Western states. As such, instead of relying on a global shared responsibility for disease control, the paper suggests global health should seek a new framework for governance of infectious disease, with more clearly defined responsibilities for individual actors, based on established accountability chains.

The EVD outbreak

EVD is a relatively rare disease, yet the 2014–05 crisis represents the largest and most complex outbreak on record, witnessing over 28,000 cases and over 11,000 deaths. This amounts to more cases than all previous outbreaks of EVD combined, since the 'discovery' of the disease in 1976.[1] These previous outbreaks were successfully controlled through rapid diagnosis, effective treatment of infected individuals, isolation of patients, contact tracing of all potential infections, safe burials and effective community mobilisation. This EVD outbreak, however, is paradoxical: from a public health perspective the pathogen is readily controllable and yet for much of 2014 it was out of control.[2] Consequently the global health community has sought to understand what or who may be responsible for the unprecedented scale of the outbreak.

One plausible analysis by Piot suggests that a series of delays and an uncoordinated response created a 'perfect storm' for the outbreak to spread rapidly through the population.[3] One such delay was the time-lag between the episode emerging in rural Guinea in December 2013 and its being reported to the WHO on 22 March 2014. Further factors contributing to Piot's perfect storm narrative include: the spread within a dense urban area, highly mobile populations, porous international borders, the pathogen's appearance in a previously uninfected location, the lack of health system capacity, and mistrust within West African governments.[4] This paper works within this perfect storm narrative and seeks to suggest a further contributing factor: the failure of global shared responsibility in global disease governance.

Global shared responsibility

The framing of an issue is vital to understanding the ensuing response. The outbreaks of SARS (2003), H5N1 (2005), H1N1 (2009) and Middle East Respiratory Syndrome Coronavirus (MERS-CoV) (2012–15) highlighted global mutual vulnerabilities to infectious disease, leading to disease being framed as a collective security threat.[5] This collective security suggests that the responsibility for protection from the threat (of disease) is held collectively rather than by individual members of the community. Such an understanding can be seen through the favouring of a dynamic global disease governance arrangement championing global shared responsibility for disease control. The framework of global disease governance involves many actors, each maintaining an important position in a multi-actor mosaic. This includes states, international organisations (such as WHO, the UN, World Bank etc), NGOs (ranging from large charities such as MSF down to grassroots initiatives, such as those seen in the EVD crisis offering community awareness about the risks of the disease), the private sector, public–private partnerships and many more besides. Although this produces a series of complex interactions between the stakeholders, one point of convergence appears to be their mutual understanding of global shared responsibility.

International organisations have started to use the language of global shared responsibility for global health. The WHO website suggests that 'in the 21st century, health is a shared responsibility, involving…collective defence against transnational threats'. The UN has also used the language of shared responsibility for addressing major global threats, in particular in the Millennium Declaration, which states that there is a 'shared responsibility for managing…threats to international peace and security',[6] and in calling a key report *A More*

Secure World: Our Shared Responsibility, which explicitly recognised that 'no state, no matter how powerful can by its own efforts alone make itself invulnerable to today's threats...we all share responsibility for each other's security'.[7]

Academic scholars have similarly used this framing of global shared responsibility for disease in their analysis of the response to HIV/AIDS Buse and Martin suggest: 'Shared responsibility represents a normative ideal to which both individual stakeholders and the global community must subscribe [if our collective vision of an AIDS-free world is to be realised].'[8] Davies et al. recognise this normative ideal through their work on 'Shared Responsibilities of Disease Surveillance'.[9] Furthermore, Gostin et al. highlight in their analysis of global health that there is a 'shared responsibility for collective defence against transnational health threats'.[10]

Moreover, global leaders have also used this rhetoric of shared responsibility for disease control. Margaret Chan, Director General of the WHO stated: 'When the world is collectively at risk, defence becomes a shared responsibility of all nations'.[11] David Heymann, former Assistant Director General at the WHO, suggested that there is a 'shared responsibility for improving international public health security'.[12] During the EVD outbreak President Obama asked the global community to speed up the response, claiming: 'The world has a responsibility to act, to step up and do more'.[13] This language echoes that of Hillary Clinton in relation to HIV/AIDS, who declared 'America's commitment to shared responsibility as we all work together towards...creating an AIDS-free generation',[14] and of Onyebuchi Chukwu, Nigeria's Health Minister, saying 'African countries were on the right track by sharing the responsibility in health'.[15]

However, this global shared responsibility is most clearly manifested through the revisions to the International Health Regulations (IHR) completed in 2005. These marked a conceptual shift in the responsibilities of states, non-state actors and the WHO.[16] The aim was to develop a regulatory framework for states and non-state actors to meet certain core public health competencies to limit the transnational spread of infectious disease, championing this new understanding of global shared responsibility. To paraphrase Bruen et al., frameworks such as the IHR rearrange responsibilities to mimic the transition from a world of governments to a world of governance.[17] Under the IHR all states have a responsibility to develop, strengthen and maintain the capacity to detect, assess, notify and report (an outbreak) to the WHO.[18] Furthermore, they also have a responsibility beyond their own borders, first in maintaining a degree of vigilance over the health of others,[19] but also in supporting other states in meeting their core capacities: 'State parties shall undertake to collaborate with each other in... the development, strengthening and maintenance of the public health capacities required under the regulations'.[20]

The involvement of a wider set of stakeholders beyond just states further reflects the normative shift to global disease governance and the framing of shared responsibility for disease control. For example, under the IHR the WHO has a responsibility to help states meet the core capacity requirements, collaborate in surveillance, verification and response (Articles 5, 8 and 10) and even to share information with other states if necessary for public health benefit (Article 10). Moreover, under Article 9, other actors (broadly defined) are able to notify the WHO of unusual health events, if member states fail to do so in a timely manner. This represented a normative change from previous iterations of the IHR, which only allowed for reporting between states and the WHO. Articles 14 and 44 suggest that states and the WHO should coordinate their activities in infectious disease control multilaterally with other states, through regional networks, international organisations and with other competent international bodies.[21]

On first viewing such articles of the IHR may seem to show quite clearly defined responsibilities for individual actors. However, framed holistically as part of the wider discourse of shared responsibility, a tension has arisen with their enforceability. An inherent problem with a collective governance arrangement is that it is incapable of bearing shared responsibility for any particular outcome when no individual member of that community is individually accountable for their part.[22] As highlighted by Gostin and Friedman, 'the IHR do not allocate responsibility'.[23] There may be defined activities for each actor to carry out, but there are no means to ensure actors uphold their responsibilities. What underlies the power of any governance mechanism is enforceability; even where broad norms are accepted in rhetoric (as with global shared responsibility) and even formalised in treaties (such as the IHR) their enforcement remains problematic.[24] This may be the result of multilateral horizontal governance arrangements creating chains of accountability that are less clear and direct than within more vertical systems such as domestic politics.[25] This paper suggests that the outbreak of EVD highlights the fact that the framing of global shared responsibility offers an unclear allocation of responsibility. Where this allocation is present (under IHR), global shared responsibility lacks a clear chain of enforceability and accountability. Major failures of governance normally call for a review of the status quo and a reconfiguration of the arrangements to ensure that such a crisis does not reoccur. This paper suggests that, to provide greater security from the threat of disease, global shared responsibility should be reframed in terms of multiple responsibilities of individual actors.

Multiple responsibilities

Accountability for one's responsibilities can be understood as the condition of being answerable to someone for one's activities or performance. It is often underpinned by principal–agent logic, in that there is a lead actor (principal) to set responsibilities for agents to carry out, and judge whether they have fulfilled them.[26] However, global health does not always lend itself to readily identifiable principals and agents, as this binary relationship does not reflect the multiple actors, relationships and power in a multi-actor governance framework such as global disease governance.[27] One suggestion might be that the rhetoric of global shared responsibility for disease infers that the agents are the multiple actors involved in the framework. However, designating the principal of such a collective arrangement proves more difficult. If taking a globalist view, this principal might be the global population, which seeks to benefit from the reduction in disease incidence and give multiple organisations the responsibility for delivering on that.[28] A statist approach might suggest that Western states are the principal, as they champion the global disease governance framework to ensure their own health security. However, while either of these principals would be able to judge whether the global health community had fulfilled its responsibilities, neither is able to truly hold the many actors to account for their failings. Ebrahim and Weisband identify this common analytical problem of accountability and responsibility as 'a rift between how it is imagined and how it actually operates… [for] definitions and framings of responsibility tend to be driven by normative agendas rather than by empirical realities'.[29] As such, the normative agenda may call for a global shared responsibility, but the empirical reality – as we shall see through an analysis of EVD – does not reflect this framing of responsibility; rather it suggests a myriad of differing principal–agent relationships which need to be recognised and incorporated into global disease governance to improve its efficacy.

Many actors recognise disease as a security threat. However, the way in which they conceive of this security may vary. For example, some may understand the referent object of threat to be the state (national security threat), others the population (human security threat), or economic interests (socioeconomic threat).[30] If there is no true common understanding of the ways in which disease constitutes a security threat, then it is probable that conceptions of global shared responsibility to combat the threat will not be alike either. Therefore it may be that there is never a clear alignment of what this shared responsibility may entail, and other accountability chains may be prioritised. Accordingly, what might be seen is that, fundamentally, collective responsibility cannot and does not take precedence over actors' individual interests.[31] In the case of EVD each actor made a rational calculation of their interests in and responsibility for disease control and of whom they felt accountable to for this responsibility, such as their electorate, their international donors or economic interest groups, rather than prioritising this notion of global shared responsibility.

Moving away from this notion of global shared responsibility, this paper seeks to show that in fact there were multiple responsibilities and accountability relationships present during the outbreak concurrently. The paper suggests that the actions of three key sets of actors can be shown to represent the failure of shared responsibility: E3 states (Sierra Leone, Liberia and Guinea), the WHO and Western states. This is not an exhaustive list and several other actors involved in the global disease governance network could equally be placed here. However, these three have been selected as three of the most prominent actors involved in the response, both financially and from a hands-on perspective. Furthermore, these three sets of actors appeared during the outbreak to reject the norm of global shared responsibility either by favouring their own domestic priorities (the E3 and Western states), or because of structural and financial limitations (the WHO). It is important to understand why they were unable to uphold the normative ideal of global shared responsibility, and to reflect on their competing priorities and understandings of domestic and international accountability chains in an effort to strengthen the global disease governance framework ahead of future outbreaks.

E3 states

Individual states (at least in democratic political systems) have a clear principal–agent accountability relationship between state functions and elected officials, and the electorate. As part of the social contract states have a responsibility to safeguard and protect the health of their populations, and to take the necessary steps to ensure the health security of their citizens.[32] This includes providing access to essential goods and services under the concept of the right to health.[33] Thus it should have fallen to the E3 states to have sufficient resources to detect and respond to the outbreak in the first instance. The structural weakness of their health systems has been highlighted as a key factor in their failure to do so.[34] Liberia, Guinea and Sierra Leone rank among the lowest in the world on the Human Development Index (176, 179 and 183, respectively, out of 187 countries).[35] As such, it is not surprising that they do not have a health system able to cope with the extra capacity required to handle a mass epidemic.[36] An outbreak of cholera in 2012 in Guinea and Sierra Leone demonstrated that the health systems in this region were incapable of handing any sort of health emergency, with the WHO reporting on its website soon after that several health care facilities did not even have running water or electricity. [37]

Several functions of a health system which would normally be required to limit the spread of a communicable disease were not present. There was a severe dearth of qualified health care workers (for example Liberia has 0.1 physicians, 1.7 nurses and midwives and eight hospital beds for every 10,000 people);[38] disease surveillance was rudimentary at best (it is estimated that it took three months for the Guinean Ministry of Health to become aware of the outbreak in the first instance); and there was little wherewithal for surge capacity resources to respond to such an outbreak. This lack of capacity was compounded by the governments of the affected countries initially being in denial over the occurrence of the disease and, consequentially, relinquishing responsibility for the care of infected patients to overworked NGOs, while simultaneously issuing incoherent directives, such as the closures of markets and borders.[39] This highlights the fact that the E3 states had already failed in their responsibilities to offer health security to their citizens well before this outbreak emerged, quickly becoming overwhelmed when cases presented at hospitals. This suggests a first failure of responsibility – that of the elected organs of state failing to meet their safeguarding responsibilities to their citizens.

The E3 states are also accountable to international donors who have provided funding for their post-conflict reconstruction efforts, although not always in ways that delivered positive results. Kentekelenis et. al have shown that IMF loans with attached conditionalities have undermined government funding for the health systems in E3 states, and that these have contributed to the weak health systems which have proven wholeheartedly insufficient to cope with the outbreak.[40] This shows an interesting accountability prioritisation at play, in that these states have appeared to prioritise their relationships with Western donors, and the responsibilities they feel to them to meet certain governance requirements, rather than the accountability they feel towards their citizens to limit the spread of disease.

Under the IHR states are required to strengthen their disease control capacities, including in the areas of policy, surveillance, response, preparedness, human resources and lab capacity. However, an analysis in 2013 showed that none of the E3 states had met their IHR requirements. Nor, in fact, had any African nation.[41] Herein lies a key problem with the IHR as they stand. The IHR assume that states shall utilise their existing national structures and resources to meet their core capacity requirements. However, such requirements implicitly assume that states already have a relatively well functioning public health infrastructure to which these additional requirements can be attached.[42] The IHR, while offering best-practice disease control policies, include no financial allowance to help states attain the required infrastructure. More notably there is little enforceability if states fail to meet the requirements. Based on normative understandings (such as shared responsibility), it was hoped that states would strive to meet these competencies, yet there are no sanctions for not attempting to do so. E3 states therefore did not have infrastructure in place to be able to detect, report or respond to the EVD outbreak.[43] However, this may not necessarily suggest that the E3 states have not internalised the normative understandings of global shared responsibility and global disease governance; rather they do not have the resources to implement any public health improvements.

Interestingly a considerable amount of academic literature in global health since the IHR revisions has focused on the normative requirement of states to report an outbreak in a timely manner, irrespective of this capacity. It has been suggested that, despite a lack of strict enforceability, states would do so for fear of being named and shamed by the international community.[44] In this outbreak the fact that Guinea did not report an outbreak to the WHO under the IHR instrument for almost four months has not been subject to the aforementioned 'naming and shaming' that was witnessed during SARS. This may be because other actors recognise the lack of capacity in this region to detect an outbreak either through state or non-state infrastructure, or it may represent the fact that the global disease governance agenda has recognised that there is little enforceability of such a norm in the real world. Nevertheless, E3 states have violated their responsibilities both to their citizens to offer freedom from the threat of disease and to global shared responsibility global shared responsibility under the IHR to meet certain competencies.[45]

WHO

With the framing of disease as a security threat in recent decades, the WHO has continued with its 'central and historic responsibility for the control of the international spread of disease',[46] and has sought to take on the leadership duties enshrined within it. However, as the following discussion will show, throughout the EVD outbreak the WHO fell short of its leadership responsibilities for disease control, something it recognised itself through an open apology and an interim assessment panel highlighting its failures.[47] This is an interesting turn for understanding responsibility in global disease control, as the WHO's accountability relationship should (in strict principal–agent logic) be to its member states, and yet it recognises that it has also failed in its responsibilities to individuals affected by the outbreak.[48]

First and foremost, the WHO has been was widely criticised for inactivity in the first months of the outbreak. Although it was effective in its epidemiological analysis of the outbreak,[49] its initial approach failed to take into account the attributes of the location (in a densely populated area) with numerous travel routes across borders, suggesting the outbreak could have considerable reach. The *New York Times* (April 1, 2014) reported that the WHO dismissed the outbreak as 'it's quite difficult to transmit…you have to touch someone. Fortunately for the greater population, the risks are quite small'. Similarly the institution was quoted by *Reuters* (April 1, 2014): 'this is relatively small still…we need to be very careful about how we characterise something which is up until now an outbreak with sporadic cases'. In the initial months after notification of the outbreak, the WHO did little to elicit a response, relying on its regional AFRO office and the E3 WHO country offices to keep abreast of developments.[50]

Following on, the WHO sought to deflect any responsibility onto the overwhelmed governments of the E3 for not being able to manage such an outbreak on their own. Although it cannot be held accountable for the delay in reporting the outbreak by the E3 ministries of health, the WHO can be held to account for not understanding the gravity of the situation, in that it took it until 8 August 2014 to declare the outbreak a Public Health Emergency of International Concern (PHEIC), despite having received the initial report of the outbreak in March 2014, as well as a number of warnings from officials and NGOs in E3 states (*New York Times*, January 6, 2015). By this stage a WHO online interim report was suggesting that the disease had already infected 1779 cases, with 961 deaths. It could be suggested that the delay in declaring a PHEIC was as a result of being preoccupied with MERS-CoV, H7N9, H5N1 and polio, but it may also have been a reaction to its over-cautious response to the H1N1 pandemic in 2009.[51] The WHO may have been cognisant of the criticism it faced for overreacting to that outbreak, not wanting to cause undue global alarm, not to mention the organisation's concerns about the economic impact on West Africa (*Guardian*, March 20, 2015). However, such inactivity may suggest that the WHO failed in its responsibility to its member states to lead an effective response to the outbreak. More explicitly it failed in its prescribed role in the IHR to assist with verification and response to an outbreak (Articles 8 and 10) and in its responsibilities to cooperate, coordinate and collaborate with states and non-state actors in the ensuing response (Articles 14 and 44).

However, it is not greatly surprising that the WHO has failed in its responsibility to its member states in the outbreak of EVD when roles and responsibilities are not clearly defined within the organisation. This may have led to different levels of the organisation (HQ, regional and country) passing the buck, as there was no clear division of labour, nor of accountability.

Interestingly a review process in 2014 showed that 'there were different understandings and interpretations by managers and even senior leaders on their respective roles and responsibilities'.[52] Furthermore, the WHO has suffered from substantial budget cuts in recent years. The budget for responding to outbreaks was reduced to $228 million in 2014–15, compared with $469 million in 2012–13.[53] Its budget is now a third of that of the US Centers for Disease Control (CDC), something which Gostin and Friedman have described as 'incommensurate with its [ie the WHO's] responsibilities'.[54] More alarmingly there are no core funds reserved for emergency outbreaks, which does not allow for an appropriate base from which to start a response.[55] Even if the WHO had declared a PHEIC sooner, it would still have been missing the much needed financial resources required for managing the outbreak. The WHO subsequently had to put out a series of calls for increased emergency funding.[56] Before this outbreak Fidler questioned whether the consequences of WHO budget cuts would fall disproportionately on countries least able to manage dangerous disease events,[57] which appears to have been exactly what has happened in the E3 states, as the organisation they were supposed to rely on to offer leadership in their global shared responsibility for global disease control failed to support them in their time of need. However, responsibility for this lack of finances available to handle an outbreak can also highlight the failings of the reverse – the accountability relationship between the WHO and states, as the latter have consistently failed to meet their committed donations each year, hampering their agent's ability to carry out the necessary activities.

Western states

Western states have also been criticised for their response to the EVD outbreak. The USA has committed over $350 million, the UK £437 million, France €20 million and China $120 million to the response. To contextualise this, the USA spent a total of $321 million between 2012 and 2014 on emergency response and pandemic preparedness.[58] The Western response has included deploying personnel from several government departments, building EVD treatment units, providing diagnostic kits and laboratory facilities, training healthcare workers and provision of medical equipment.[59] However, these interventions have been heavily criticised because of the self-interested nature of the responses from Western states. Their involvement coincided with the first infections manifesting themselves in the USA and Europe, many months after the start of the outbreak in West Africa. Nevertheless, if we take the same principal–agent logic of accountability that was applied to E3 states, namely that these governments understand their responsibility to their population in the same terms, in that they are responsible to their electorates for ensuring that the threat of EVD does not reach their shores, then this is not surprising. By extension, examining the response of Western states to the EVD outbreak, it could be that their involvement shows that their understanding of a global shared responsibility is more aligned to a global shared responsibility for (their own) national health security. There is no coincidence to this; perhaps the self-interested nature of their response further highlights the inadequacies of the shared responsibility discourse championed by the global disease governance regime.[60]

The Western community could further be held responsible for the onslaught of media hysteria surrounding the outbreak. In highlighting the threat of EVD, and framing it as a deadly plague, the media spawned public fear in several Western countries. These states were then required to take what could be seen as placebo measures to reassure their citizens that they were not at risk of EVD, and that the government had a functioning preparedness plan, should it reach their shores. This plan included the USA, UK, France and Canada implementing heightened airport screening for potential EVD cases – a biosecurity measure which has been widely criticised by the public health community for its limited efficacy, because of the long incubation period of the pathogen, meaning that travellers may not show any symptoms.[61] Ironically, had the financing provided for airport screening been used to resource the on-going response in the E3 or to meet these countries' WHO funding commitments, rather than within Western states, it could have had a considerably greater impact.

A number of national airline carriers also suspended flights to E3 states in an effort to stop the international spread of the disease (including British Airways, Emirates, Air France), despite UN resolution 2177 asking for states to not impose such travel changes. Although this was at the discretion of each airline, rather than Western states, such action by Western carriers severely restricted the economies of these E3 states further through barriers to international travel and trade. This is in spite of the fact that such measures would do little to limit the spread: projections suggest that only 2.8 people per month were likely to be infected with EVD and leave the E3 by air.[62] This highlights a further accountability relationship, the accountability that the Western community feels towards its business and economic interests.

The Committee on Social, Economic and Cultural Rights has declared that cooperation in health is not only an obligation of all states, but for all those in a position to assist others.[63] However, according to Gostin et al. in their review of national and global responsibilities in health, one of the least understood obligations is the responsibility of Western states to augment the capacity of low and middle-income states to ensure their populations' health.[64] In the case of the EVD outbreak Western governments could be seen to be shirking their responsibilities in this area by failing to support the strengthening of the E3 health systems.

The IHR, though not offering provision for financing to help states meet their core competencies, does strongly encourage states to provide each other with technical cooperation and logistical support to help develop the core competencies sought through the legislative framework. However, as aforementioned, the E3 states suffered from an exhausted and woefully under-resourced health infrastructure, which was barely able to handle endemic diseases in the region, let alone an outbreak of this scale. Although the ultimate responsibility for not developing a functioning disease control mechanism must fall on the E3 states themselves (and on the flawed IHR funding and enforceability mechanisms), Western states should also bear some responsibility for their shortfalls in contributing to helping these states meet these requirements, as per the IHR articles 14 and 44. This argument has suggested that, had Western states invested in greater health system strengthening in the E3 countries before the outbreak, rather than focusing on issues of Western biosecurity, the outbreak might not have become the humanitarian crisis that has been witnessed.

The end of shared responsibility

> The [global] community must show the collective responsibility absent at the start of this out-break to bring it to an end.[65]

As set out in the preceding discussion, the EVD epidemic has exposed a fragmented disease control governance framework in which the institutions do not function as a coherent whole.[66] Moreover, it has highlighted the fact that global health does not always offer readily identifiable principals and agents, as this does not reflect the multiple responsibility relationships that actors contend with.[67] It is a combination of multiple failures in individual responsibilities that led to the collective failure of the global health community to be able to limit the spread of the EVD outbreak in a reasonable timeframe. The framing of responsibility as a shared concept muddied the waters of responsibility and made it less clear what each actor's role (and the duties of such role) are at the global level and to whom each is accountable.

This paper does not wish to suggest that actors should go it alone, or that there should be an end to global cooperation in disease control and response. In the interconnected world in which we exist, such action would be unfeasible. With mass travel and transport it is inevitable that diseases will cross borders, and that the mutual vulnerability to the threat of disease is ever present. As such, multiple actors will need to continue to work together to manage the threat. Gostin and Friedman have called for a new global health framework, one in which there are 'clearer roles and responsibilities for all stakeholders…Including effective legal methods to establish clear accountability (and shared responsibility to build core capacities)'.[68] This paper actively supports such a position, but suggests that a core problem with the global health framework as it stands is the very concept of shared responsibility.

Interestingly other areas of global health governance have clearer definitions of delineated responsibility. For example, the Framework Convention on Tobacco Control has a code on responsibility and the Global Health Workforce Alliance has defined membership responsibilities. As such, there seems to be a precedent for the production of clearer divisions of labour, which should be embraced by the global disease governance community. Fundamentally the global health architecture must find a way be able hold individual stakeholders accountable in order for global efforts in disease control to be effective.[69] There should be delineated roles and responsibilities, where each actor in the framework has a designated position within the global disease control matrix and understands what their responsibilities are for and to whom. It has been suggested that significant impetus or political shock must be present to change the status quo of any international law.[70] The crisis of the EVD outbreak and the evident failure of global shared responsibility may hopefully provide such an impetus, in the same way that SARS acted as a catalyst for the updating of the IHR in 2005.

As an interconnected globe there is a need to work together to face the spread of infectious disease, yet individual actors need more tangible individual responsibilities for which they can be held to account. Developing a more coherent responsibility and governance framework will be a difficult challenge. Although this paper cannot provide all the answers, it seeks to offer three recommendations for consideration in any new approach.

Learning from other governance frameworks

One recommendation would be to reflect on other global governance arrangements. An assessment of global environmental governance has shown that the most successful engagement between actors happens at a more devolved level of activity.[71] Furthermore, reflecting on the Sustainable Development Goals and the Millennium Development Goals, it can be seen that a goal-setting approach with effective progress monitoring has raised public and policy support, as well as being a mechanism to channel funds to areas in urgent need.[72] As such, multiple devolved arrangements with clearer tangible goals between actors bilaterally or multilaterally could provide a more fruitful result than broader normative calls for global shared responsibility for improving global health security.

Offering greater financing mechanisms

A key factor in this EVD outbreak and around the IHR more generally has been a lack of financing to implement disease control measures.[73] Western states will fundamentally need to offer greater financing mechanisms to ensure health security. This could be done bilaterally between states or through increased contributions to the WHO, allowing for a strengthened role for the lead global organisation for health. In the case of EVD, it did not appear that the E3 states were fundamentally unwilling to internalise the normative understanding of responsibility for global health security or to improve their domestic disease control capacities – they simply lacked the resources to do so. Accordingly, one such devolved responsibility relationship could, based on Articles 14 and 44 of the IHR, be for Western states to help build disease control infrastructure in developing states. The EVD crisis has demonstrated that improving disease control is very much in the interest of Western states that seek to protect their own populations and economies from the threat of disease, and therefore such a relationship may suit both parties.

Obviously there are a number of issues with such a recommendation that would need to be addressed, notably that it would reinforce unequal power relationships between states. Furthermore, it would depend on the willingness of Western states to bear the costs accordingly. Moreover, if done bilaterally, it would not adequately account for the WHO's activities in global health, or necessarily offer it an empowered role, as championed by Gostin and Friedman.[74] Who should decide on how these new multiple accountability relationships are formed or financed is a greater question, and would open its own Pandora's box. However, individual relationships have developed through previous outbreaks, as well as through the former colonial links re-emerging in the EVD crisis (which raises its own concerns), suggesting that actors could arrange themselves organically. Simply put, this paper calls for greater financing mechanisms, whether from Western states or other Bretton Woods institutions,[75] to help developing states, such as the E3, build effective disease control infrastructure.

Addressing issues of enforcement

Enforcement is another issue, and one that deserves considerable thought to explore effective mechanisms for ensuring that each actor in the framework takes its responsibilities seriously and meets any designated goals, in whatever formation these may appear. Although this is a recurrent problem in international law, the IHR and normative goals of global disease governance have not proven strong enough to generate global action. One example might be to include independent monitoring of country compliance into the IHR, rather than the status quo of self-assessment.[76] An alternative approach could include withholding institutional privileges at the WHO, such as voting rights at the World Health Assembly, for those actors who fail to meet their individual requirements. Another option would be to move away from conceptualising enforcement, and to consider incentivising states to adhere to their global health responsibilities. This could include a new financing mechanism for disease outbreaks, an insurance scheme or other innovative approaches.[77]

Conclusion

The EVD outbreak proves an excellent case study for highlighting a concern with the global disease governance landscape, in that imagining a governance framework in which every actor shares in the same collective security and collective responsibility to combat the threat is naïve. Although states and non-state actors have, for the most part, been complicit in constructing a discourse of global shared responsibility for disease control through the IHR and rhetorical changes to policy, each actor conceives of this threat and responsibility differently and has a multiple of different accountability relationships. These, in part, may have contributed to the 'perfect storm' of the failed response to the EVD outbreak in West Africa. This paper has suggested that, instead of working within a framework where accountability is unable to fall onto any one actor, it is better to reframe the responsibility for disease control as a series of differentiated responsibilities. Furthermore, the global health landscape should define clearer roles and responsibilities for each actor in the global health mosaic and understand how they can be held to account for them, rather than to continue by championing a global shared responsibility.

The paper does not seek to provide a definitive solution to the weaknesses of global shared responsibility. It has simply endeavoured to show that the framing of responsibility at a global level has itself become a factor in the inadequate response to the EVD outbreak, as there have not been clear lines of accountability between actors, who have thus been able to pass the buck to others for their failures to respond appropriately. The paper has offered a potential new framing of responsibility – that of multiple responsibilities for global disease control – but as there are inherent flaws in these too, further development of notions of responsibility and governance for disease control must be sought in an effort to strengthen global health security.

Disclosure statement

No potential conflict of interest was reported by the author.

Acknowledgements

An earlier version of this paper was presented at the BISA Annual Conference, 16 June 2015. Particular thanks go to Simon Rushton and Laura Hakimi for their insightful comments on earlier drafts.

Notes

1. Camacho et al., "Potential for Outbreaks of Ebola," 71.
2. Dhillon et al., "Controlling Ebola," 1409.
3. Piot, "Ebola's Perfect Storm," 1221.
4. Ibid.
5. Louis, "Global Health Surveillance," 16.
6. UN, *Millennium Declaration*, 1.
7. UN, *A More Secure World*, 1–2.
8. Buse and Martin, "AIDS," 2.
9. Davies et al., "The Shared Responsibility," 667–669.
10. Gostin et al., "The Joint Action and Learning Initiative," 2.
11. Margaret Chan, Speech on World Health Day 2007, http://www.who.int/dg/speeches/2007/020407_whd2007/en/.
12. Heymann, "SARS and Emerging Infectious Diseases," 350.
13. Schechinger, "Global Health Issues."
14. Hillary Clinton, remarks at UNAIDS, 2012, http://www.cfr.org/world/clintons-remarks-unaids-shared-responsibility-event-september-2012/p29164.
15. Onyebuchi Chukwu, speech at the Global Fund Conference, 2013, http://globalfund.org/en/mediacenter/newsreleases/2013-12-03_Replenishment_Partners_Talk_Shared_Responsibility.
16. Davies and Youde, *The Politics of Surveillance*, 2.
17. Bruen et al., "A Concept in Flux," 6.
18. WHO, *International Health Regulations*.
19. Youde, *Biopolitical Surveillance*, 165.
20. Ibid.
21. WHO, *International Health Regulations*.
22. Miller and Makela, "The Collectivist Approach," 634.
23. Gostin and Friedman, "Ebola," 1342.
24. Ebrahim and Weisband, *Global Accountabilities*, 7.
25. Mason, "The Governance of Transnational Environmental Harm," 11.
26. Bruen et al., "A Concept in Flux," 2.
27. Bruen et al., "A Concept in Flux," 3.
28. See Davies, *Global Politics of Health*, 23.
29. Bruen et al., "A Concept in Flux."
30. McInnes and Lee, *Global Health and International Relations*, 130–157.
31. Peltonen, *International Responsibility*, 42.
32. Gostin, L. O. and E. A. Friedman, Towards a Framework Convention on Global Health: a transformative agenda for global health justice, Yale Jounral of Health Policy, Law and Ethics, (2013), 13: no 1, 1-75.
33. Gostin et al., "National and Global Responsibilities for Health," 719.
34. O'Hare, "Weak Health Systems and Ebola," 71; Kieny et al., "Health-system Resilience," 850; and Piot et al., "Ebola in West Africa," 1034–1035.
35. UNDP, *Human Development Report 2014*.
36. Gostin, "Ebola," 49.
37. WHO (2012).
38. Tomori, "Ebola in an Unprepared Africa," g5597.
39. Ibid.
40. Kentikelenis et al., "The International Monetary Fund," 69.
41. Kasolo et al., "Implementation of the International Health Regulations," 11–13.
42. Youde, *Global Health Governance*, 128.
43. Gostin, "Ebola: Towards a Fund," 49.
44. Davies and Youde, *The Politics of Surveillance*.
45. Brigit, "The Ebola Crisis."
46. WHO, *International Health Regulations*, 1.

47. WHO, "Report of the Ebola Interim Assessment Panel."
48. Ibid.
49. Team, "Ebola Virus Disease in West Africa," 1483.
50. WHO, Report of the Ebola Interim Assessment Panel, 15.
51. WHO (2011).
52. WHO, "Roles, Responsibilities and Matrix Management."
53. The Lancet, 'Ebola: Failure of collective action', 637.
54. Gostin and Friedman, "Ebola."
55. Ibid.
56. WHO, "Ebola Virus Disease Response Plan."
57. Fidler, "Ebola and Global Health Governance."
58. Kaiser Foundation, "US Government Funding."
59. White House, "Fact Sheet"; Embassy of France in the United Kingdom, "France outlines Efforts"; Sanchez, " What Countries have pledged to Fight Ebola"; and UK Government, "Ebola Virus."
60. Smith, "Global Health Security," 2249.
61. Heymann, quoted in Taylor, "Health Experts question Effectiveness."
62. Bogoch et al., "Assessment of the Potential for International Dissemination," 29.
63. UNHCHR, "The Nature of State Parties' Obligations," Art 2 para 1: 14/12/1990, CESCR General Comment 3.
64. Heymann, "SARS and Emerging Infectious Diseases."
65. Philips and Markham, "Ebola."
66. Gostin and Friedman, "A Retrospective and Prospective Analysis," 1903.
67. Bruen et al., "A Concept in Flux."
68. Ibid.
69. Gostin et al., "The Joint Action and Learning Initiative," 3.
70. Diehl et al., "The Dynamics of International Law," 57.
71. Sandberg et al., Lessons for Global Health, 6.
72. Kanie et al., "Green Pluralism," 27; Griggs et al., "Sustainable Development Goals," 305–306.
73. Gostin and Friedman, "Ebola," 1323; and "Ebola: What are the Lessons?," 1321 Gostin, L. O. (2014).
74. Gostin and Friedman, "Ebola," 1324; and Bruen et al., "A Concept in Flux," 1903.
75. WHO, "Report of the Ebola Interim Assessment Panel," 11.
76. Bruen et al., "A Concept in Flux," 1906.
77. WHO, "Report of the Ebola Interim Assessment Panel," 12.

Bibliography

Bogoch, I., Creatore, M., Cetron, M., Brownstein, J., Pesik, N., Miniota, J. and Tam, T. "Assessment of the Potential for International Dissemination of the Ebola Virus via Commercial Air Travel during the 2014 West African Outbreak." Lancet 385, no. 9962 (2014): 29–35.

Brigit, T. "The Ebola Crisis: Challenges for Global Health Law." Shares Blog. 2015. http://www.sharesproject.nl/the-ebola-crisis-challenges-for-global-health-law/.

Bruen, C., R. Burgha, A. Kageni, and F. Wafula. "A Concept in Flux: Questioning Accountability in the Context of Global Health Cooperation." Globalisation and Health 10 (2014): 1–15. doi: http://dx.doi.org/10.1186/s12992-014-0073-9.

Buchanan, A., and M. DeCamp. "Responsibility for Global Health." Theoretical Medicine and Bioethics 27, no. 1 (2006): 95–114.

Buse, K., and G. Martin. "AIDS: Ushering in a New Era of Shared Responsibility for Global Health." Globalization and Health 8, no. 1 (2012): 1–3.

Camacho, A., A. J. Kucharski, S. Funk, J. Breman, P. Piot, and W. J. Edmunds. "Potential for Large Outbreaks of Ebola Virus Disease." Epidemics 9 (2014): 70–78.

Davies, S. Global Politics of Health. Cambridge: Polity, 2009.

Davies, S., and J. Youde. The Politics of Surveillance and Response to Disease Outbreaks. Aldershot: Ashgate, 2015.

Davies, S. E., J. Youde, and R. Parker. "The Shared Responsibility of Disease Surveillance." *Global Public Health* 7, no. 7 (2012): 667–669.

Dhillon, R., D. Srikrishna, and J. Sachs. "Controlling Ebola: Next Steps." *Lancet* 384, no. 9952 (2014): 1409–1411.

Diehl, P., C. Ku, and D. Zamora. "The Dynamics of International Law: The Interaction of Normative and Operating Systems." *International Organization* 57, no. 1 (2003): 43–75.

"Ebola: What are the Lessons for the International Health Regulations?" *Lancet* 384, no. 9951 (2014): 1321.

Ebrahim, A., and E. Weisband. *Global Accountabilities, Participation, Pluralism & Public Ethics*. Cambridge: Cambridge University Press, 2007.

Embassy of France in the United Kingdom. "France outlines Efforts to combat Ebola." 2014. http://www. ambafrance-uk.org/Minister-outlines-France-s-efforts.

Fidler, D. "Ebola and Global Health Governance: Time for the Reckoning." Chatham House Expert Comment, September 22, 2014. https://www.chathamhouse.org/expert/comment/15811.

Gostin, L. O., and E. A. Friedman. "Ebola: A Crisis in Global Health Leadership." *Lancet* 384, no. 9951 (2014): 1323–1325.

Gostin, L. O., and E. A. Friedman. "A Retrospective and Prospective Analysis of the West African Ebola Virus Disease Epidemic: Robust National Health Systems at the Foundation and an Empowered WHO at the Apex." *Lancet* 385, no. 9980 (2015): 1902–1909.

Gostin, L., E. Friedman, G. Ooms, T. Gebauer, N. Gupta, D. Sridhar, L O. Gostin, G. Ooms, M. Heywood, J. Haffeld, S. Mogedal, J-A. Rottingen and E. Friedman. "The Joint Action and Learning Initiative: Towards a Global Agreement on National and Global Responsibilities for Health." World Health Organization, Background paper for the World Health Report. 2010. 53.

Gostin, L. O. (2014). Ebola: towards an international health systems fund. *The Lancet, September*.

Gostin, L. O., M. Heywood, G. Ooms, A. Grover, J. A. Røttingen, and W. Chenguang. "National and Global Responsibilities for Health." *Bulletin of the World Health Organization* 88, no. 10 (2010): 719–719a.

Griggs, D., M. Stafford-Smith, O. Gaffney, J. Rockstrom, M. Ohman, P. Shyamsundar, et al. "Sustainable Development Goals for People and Planet." *Nature* 495 (2013): 305–307.

Heymann, D. L. "SARS and Emerging Infectious Diseases: A Challenge to Place Global Solidarity above National Sovereignty." *Annals Academy of Medicine Singapore* 35, no. 3 (2006): 350–353.

Kaiser Foundation. "US Government Funding for Emerging Infectious Diseases." 2014. http://kff. org/global-health-policy/fact-sheet/the-u-s-government-global-emerging-infectious-disease-preparedness-and-response/.

Kanie, N., P. Haas, S. Andresen, G. Auld, B. Cashore, S. Chasek, et al. "Green Pluralism: Lessons for Improved Environmental Governance in the 21st Century." *Environment: Science and Policy for Sustainable Development* 55, no. 5 (2013): 14–30.

Kasolo, F., Roungou, J., Kweteming, F., Impouma, B., Yahaya, A., Bakyaita, N. and Aturuku, P. "Implementation of the International Health Regulations (2005) in the African Region." *African Health Monitor* 18 (2013): 11–13.

Kentikelenis, A., L. King, M. McKee, and D. Stuckler. "The International Monetary Fund and the Ebola Outbreak." *Lancet Global Health* 3, no. 2 (2015): e69–e70.

Kieny, M. P., D. B. Evans, G. Schmets, and S. Kadandale. "Health-system Resilience: Reflections on the Ebola Crisis in Western Africa." *Bulletin of the World Health Organization* 92, no. 12 (2014): 850–850.

Louis, M. S. "Global Health Surveillance." *Morbidity and Mortality Weekly Report (MMWR) Supplements* 61(Suppl.) (2012): 15–19.

Mason, M. "The Governance of Transnational Environmental Harm: Addressing New Modes of Accountability/Responsibility." *Global Environmental Politics* 8, no. 3 (2008): 8–24.

McInnes, C., and K. Lee. *Global Health and International Relations*. Cambridge: Polity, 2012.

Miller, S., and P. Makela. "The Collectivist Approach to Collective Moral Responsibility." *Metaphilosophy* 36, no. 5 (2005): 634–651.

O'Hare, B. "Weak Health Systems and Ebola." *Lancet Global Health* 3, no. 2 (2015): e71–e72.

Peltonen, H. *International Responsibility and Grave Humanitarian Crises: Collective Provision for Human Security*. Abingdon: Routledge, 2013.

Philips, M., and A. Markham. "Ebola: A Failure of International Collective Action." *Lancet* 384, no. 9949 (2014): 1181.

Piot, P. "Ebola's Perfect Storm." *Science*, September 12, (2014); 1221.

Piot, P., J. J. Muyembe, and W. J. Edmunds. "Ebola in West Africa: From Disease Outbreak to Humanitarian Crisis." *Lancet Infectious Diseases* 14, no. 11 (2014): 1034–1035.

Sanchez, R. 2014. "What Countries have pledged to Fight Ebola." *Telegraph*, October 22.

Sandberg, K., Hoffman, S., and Pearcey, M. *Lessons for Global Health from Global Environmental Governance*. Chatham House Research Paper. London: Royal Institute of International Affairs, January 2015.

Schechinger, J. "Global Health Issues and Shared State Responsibility: The Case of Ebola." Shares Blog. 2014. http://www.sharesproject.nl/global-health-issues-and-shared-state-responsibility-the-case-of-ebola/.

Smith, J. "Global Health Security: A Flawed SDG Framework." *Lancet* 385, no. 9984 (2015):2249

Taylor, M. "Health Experts question the Effectiveness of Airport EVD Screening." Al Jazeera America, October 14, 2014. http://america.aljazeera.com/articles/2014/10/14/health-experts-questioneffec tivenessofairportEVDscreening.html.

Team, W. E. R. "Ebola Virus Disease in West Africa – The First 9 Months of the Epidemic and Forward Projections." *New England Journal of Medicine* 371, no. 16 (2014): 1481–1495.

The Lancet, (2014) Ebola: A failure of international collective action, The Lancet Editorial, Vol 284, August 23rd 2014

Tomori, O. "Ebola in an Unprepared Africa." *British Medical Journal* 349 (2014): g5597.

UK Government. "Ebola Virus: UK Government Response." 2014. https://www.gov.uk/government/topical-events/ebola-virus-government-response/about.

United Nations. *A More Secure World: Our Shared Responsibility*. Report of the Secretary General's High Level Panel on Threats, Challenges and Change. New York, 2004.

United Nations. *United Nations Millennium Declaration*. Resolution of the General Assembly 55/2. New York, 2000.

United Nations Development Programme (UNDP). *Human Development Report 2014*. New York, 2014.

United Nations High Commissioner on Human Rights (UNHCHR). "The Nature of State Parties' Obligations." 1990. http://www.unhchr.ch/tbs/doc.nsf/(Symbol)/94bdbaf59b43a424c12563ed0052b664?Open document.

White House. "Fact Sheet: The US Response to the Ebola Epidemic in West Africa." 2014. https://www.whitehouse.gov/the-press-office/2014/10/06/fact-sheet-us-response-ebola-epidemic-west-africa.

World Health Organization (WHO). "Ebola Virus Disease Outbreak Response Plan." 2014. http://www.who.int/csr/disease/ebola/evd-outbreak-response-plan-west-africa-2014.pdf.

WHO. *International Health Regulations*. Geneva: WHO, 2005.

WHO. "Report of the Ebola Interim Assessment Panel." Presented at the 68th World Health Assembly 16.1 – A68/25, 2015.

WHO. "Roles, Responsibilities and Matrix Management." March 2014, as accessed 29th May 2015 http://www.who.int/about/who_reform/matrix-management/en/.

WHO (2012), Cholera in Sierra Leone: the case study of an outbreak as accessed: http://www.who.int/features/2012/cholera_sierra_leone/en/

WHO, (2011) Implementation of the International Health Regulations, Report of the review committee on the functioning of the International Health Regulations in relation to pandemic H1N1, A64.10, 5th May 2011 as accessed http://apps.who.int/gb/ebwha/pdf_files/WHA64/A64_10-en.pdf

Youde, J. *Biopolitical Surveillance and Public Health in International Politics*. Basingstoke: Palgrave Macmillan, 2010.

Youde, J. R. *Global Health Governance*. Cambridge: Polity, 2012.

Ebola at the borders: newspaper representations and the politics of border control

Sudeepa Abeysinghe

School of Social and Political Science, University of Edinburgh, UK

ABSTRACT

As well as a site of politics and public health action, the outbreak of Ebola in West Africa has been a focus of media representations. This paper examines print media narratives around border control in relation to Ebola in the UK, the USA and Australia from the start of the epidemic to May 2015. It shows that Ebola became mobilised as a frame through which domestic politics could be discussed. The disease was transformed from a problem for West Africa to a problem for the West. The context of West Africa and affected populations was homogenised and hidden. The focus of reporting centred upon domestic political actions and more local sources of threat.

Introduction

Infectious threats in one part of the world may rapidly spread to other regions. This is addressed at the policy level through international endeavours at infections disease control, such as global surveillance systems and the application of the revised International Health Regulations.[1] However, the global spread of disease also engenders public reactions, where fear of disease is often incarnated as fear of 'outsiders' and the closure of borders, both in the literal and socio-cultural sense of that term. The politics of borders therefore encompasses formal political concerns (around the integrity and maintenance of sovereign borders) and socio-cultural concerns (around defending the social group from contagion).

Border control and surveillance is a primary mechanism through which societies respond to threats of infectious disease. Collective understandings of infectious disease tend to produce narratives of intervention which reflect notions of threat, morality and blame.[2] Since contagion is transmitted through social interaction, social distancing, isolation and quarantine are often a major part of collective responses towards infectious disease.[3] The perception of contagion has led to policy and social actions around border control in both historical and contemporary cases,[4] and remains a persistent frame through which infectious disease is understood and managed.

Before the 2014–15 outbreak Ebola had remained a disease of isolated African communities; however, representations of Ebola have been persistent in the West. The brutal symptomology of the disease, accompanied by the exoticisation of affected communities, has resulted in Ebola being an important cultural reference around infectious disease, as evidenced by the range of popular culture sources. Earlier Ebola outbreaks have also produced wide media coverage in the West, reflecting and reinforcing this public imagery. Research on media representations of previous Ebola outbreaks shows that media narratives tend to accentuate the exotic and 'African' nature of the disease, and it reveals how the cultural practices of affected communities precipitate outbreaks.[5] This may serve as a distancing strategy, depicting the grim results of outbreaks but assuring that the West (through Western practices) remains safe from the disease.

However, the 2014–15 Ebola epidemic presents a break from previous events, not just in its scope and impact but also in relation to the experience of the disease in the West. While previous outbreaks were clearly separated from the West, the 2014–15 outbreak threatened to 'infect' the West. This triggered border control and surveillance practices. It also affected the nature of Western representations surrounding the disease. This paper examines the newspaper discourse surrounding the 2014–15 outbreak of Ebola Virus Fever in West Africa, focusing upon debates surrounding border control. The analysis demonstrates that the representation of this outbreak differs from earlier narratives of Ebola in a number of key ways. The contemporary discourse does highlight cultural practices of affected West African communities as an important factor in contributing to the outbreak. However, the paper argues that the Western media reports on Ebola displaced the disease as a problem of affected West African communities to instead focus on the impact in the West. In particular, Ebola becomes a frame through which domestic political concerns can be represented and fought out. The media thereby refocuses the issue to concentrate upon the domestic politics of Western countries, hiding global health debates and the effect on West Africa.

Methods

The paper uses a qualitative analysis of print media to investigate newspaper representation of Ebola in three case countries – the UK, the USA and Australia. The three most widely circulated print media sources of each of the three countries were selected. These were: the *New York Times*, *Wall Street Journal* and *USA Today* in the USA; the *Sun*, the *Daily Mail* and the *Daily Mirror* in the UK; and *The Australian*, the *Daily Telegraph* and the *Herald Sun* in Australia. Across the sample there was a range of broadsheet and tabloid sources. Further, while the sources were chosen in terms of the largest circulation for each case country, in each case the sources chosen included at least one publication which has traditionally endorsed the political left and one that has endorsed the right. Although style (tabloid/broadsheet) did not affect the nature of the discourse uncovered, it did influence the wording through which narratives were presented. Political orientation (left- or right-leaning) was generally negligible in terms of the overall portrayal of the key narratives discussed in this paper, with the important exception of discussions of the domestic politics of the USA.

The media search revolved around seeking out articles that focused upon Ebola and borders and/or security. The search was made excluding articles under 100 words of length (to remove summary reports of events), using the key search terms in either the headline or lead paragraphs. The search inclusions were all articles using the term 'Ebola' and (at least one use of) the terms 'screen', 'airport', 'security', 'border', or 'travel'. The search period was the period for two years up to 30 April 2015. Overall, after the initial exclusion of articles (eg excluding reporting on stock market effects, letters to the editor, and remaining summary articles), 323 articles remained. While the research captured the entire period of the Ebola outbreak until May 2015, the reporting centred strongly around August to November 2014 (with around three-quarters of the articles appearing during that period). This corresponded with both the heightened international interest around Ebola (eg the World Health Organization (WHO) declaring a Public Health Emergency of International Concern in August) and specific cases of Ebola patients in the USA and Europe. From this sample, the key themes and narratives were coded and analysed.

Representations

Across the range of the newspaper sources analysed a number of persistent themes appear. There were some key differences across the sample of the newspapers analysed. For example, as can be expected, tabloid newspapers far more often deployed more dramatic language, while some of the broadsheet reporting included more extended analysis and coverage. Further, as the examination below shows, the more domestic politics of each of the three countries from which the newspapers were drawn resulted in shifts in the framing of the issues, and allowed for competing frames between different newspaper outlets. That said, the dominant discourses around border control and fear were persistent across the sample under investigation. One key finding was that the newspaper narrative throughout the three countries focused on the language of border control rather than security. Although 'security' was a key search term, overwhelmingly the concept was present in the results in the context of descriptive reporting of Security Council events and reporting that the US president had designated Ebola as a key security threat. Further, although there was an acknowledgement that Ebola had made a deep impacted on the affected West African countries, these contexts were overwhelmingly absent from most of the reporting, except in generalised ways (as discussed below). This mirrors the fact that the Ebola outbreak reached prominence in the global heath arena only following the emergence of key cases in the West (the USA and Europe). The media discourse served to reconstruct Ebola as a problem for the West, ignoring and silencing the core context in West Africa, or representing 'Africa' in general terms.

Fear and contagion

Border maintenance became a key issue in all the three countries. The ability of infectious disease to cross borders and populations was highlighted throughout the newspaper accounts. The issue of border control was also strongly linked to the problem of fear, suggesting that what was under management was not simply the disease but also fundamentally the public reaction.

The importance of the border was clear throughout the accounts. Newspaper headlines pronounced that this 'Deadly disease crosses borders',[6] and that the crisis was a product of 'Hot Zones without Borders'.[7] The idea that 'Infectious diseases show no respect for international borders',[8] which has become something of a truism in public and policy accounts of contemporary infectious disease threats, was constantly brought to the fore.

Efforts to manage infectious disease in the West tend to place particular emphasis on the potential for contagion from the Third World. This is evident in many modern examples of infectious disease governance, including the 2009 H1N1/A Pandemic, SARS, HIV/AIDS and even past outbreaks of Ebola. Scholarship around these cases shows that discourses of contagion from the Third World dominate public accounts, and may also appear in policy accounts (for example, in the Australian government's policy surrounding H5N1 avian influenza).[9] Fear of the unknown other is closely linked with the fear of infectious disease and this can be amplified in the contemporary world. The dystopian effects of globalisation – in particular the porosity of borders and the high potential for the 'mixing' of populations and diseases – underpins much of the current Western focus on infectious disease security.[10]

This idea of globalised interconnection was evident within the newspaper narrative. It was suggested that 'Ebola is a bushfire that, in our interconnected world, threatens us all'.[11] The idea that Ebola would arrive in the West through travel was evident throughout:

> 'We're a global village,' said Howard Markel, a professor of the history of medicine at the University of Michigan. 'Germs have always travelled. The problem now is they can travel with the speed of a jet plane.'[12]

This was embedded in vivid imagery around the situation in West Africa potentially being transported into the West; for example, 'right now there are corpses in the streets of nations only a plane-flight away'.[13]

Physical distance had so far allowed Western publics to remain shielded from disease threats in the Third World. However, the protective effects of distance were undermined given that 'enforced isolation in not an easy option in a complex and deeply interconnected world'.[14] This idea of the reduced buffer of physical distance was narrated in accounts from all three countries, with suggestions from the UK media that 'The virus has shown that it is able to spread via air travel, contrary to past outbreaks',[15] and from Australian media that 'Australia's great distance from most other nations has previously given us something of a barrier to many diseases. Modern air travel, however, means that an ebola case may be only one flight away',[16] despite the fact that 'Australia has the benefit of being a 30-hour plane ride away from the outbreak's ground zero',[17] while the US media proclaimed that 'The reality is, in an era of globalization, the United States can't wall itself off from the world'.[18]

Ebola is a disease that is particularly underpinned by public fear. It has been the focus of various cultural representations, including in films and popular novels.[19] It is clear that, as one newspaper exclaimed, 'an Ebola epidemic is the nightmare scenario which inspires Hollywood disaster movie writers and keeps public health officials awake at night'.[20] The importance of the crisis was highlighted in official public health narratives – not just WHO accounts but also in the US president's linking of Ebola with a security threat and a US health official's suggestion that 'this has become the biggest health crisis since the emergence of Aids [sic] 30 years ago',[21] among others. Given this level of concern from public health and official sources, it is unsurprising that the media discourse picked up on the general public fear and uncertainty around the disease.

Representations of public fear were somewhat evident in the UK and US samples. However, the Australian newspaper representations revolve tightly around the party politics of the problem, and even the UK and US newspapers tended to highlight the issue as a problem of government rather than focusing upon accounts of the public. Where public fear was narrated, this was done in ways that generally highlighted public fears as an overreaction. The *Daily Mirror* recounted the 'Ebola terror at Gatwick as woman dies'[22] under the headline 'We're Petrified'.[23] However, most of the UK newspaper accounts of public fear highlighted the absurdity of reactions. It was suggested that 'the arrival of Ebola in the States has brought an almost hysterical reaction in many',[24] and that there was 'growing hysteria' around Ebola (here, in the context of a celebrity's travel cancellations).[25] Fearful reactions were made light of in the examples where 'Ebola survival kits are being flogged online to panicking Brits',[26] and 'Fear in the West over the risk of catching ebola has reached such a peak that an air pas-senger was pictured wearing a protective suit at an airport'.[27] The US newspaper narratives surrounding the public fear similarly tended towards critiques of the public reaction. It was suggested that:

> Sometimes disinformation can spread faster than a deadly virus, as proven in recent days by the hyperventilation about Ebola. Tuesday, while a man who had visited West Africa was screened for the disease…tabloids screamed about an 'Ebola scare'…[o]n Wednesday, officials said the man doesn't have the virus.[28]

The idea that 'Fear of Ebola is spreading faster than the disease itself, and [that this under-pinned] the growing paranoia in the United States' highlighted the management of public fear as an important site of Ebola politics.[29] It was understood that 'Ebola evokes irrational fears,'[30] and suggested that 'We live in a society almost perfectly suited for contagions of hysteria and overreaction'.[31] The relationship between the fear of Ebola and the wider politics of insecurity – and in particular the issue of globalisation – was highlighted:

> you've got a large group of people who are bone-deep suspicious of globalization, what it does to their jobs and their communities. Along comes Ebola, which is the perfect biological embodiment of what many fear about globalization.[32]

The fear around border control was explicitly linked to this:

> The Ebola crisis has aroused its own flavor of fear…It's a sour, existential fear. It's a fear you feel when the whole environment feels hostile, when the things that are supposed to keep you safe, like national borders and national authorities, seem porous and ineffective, when some menace is hard to understand.[33]

In this way the fear of Ebola became an important site of examination in and of itself within the US newspapers. As will be shown below, this can be linked to the particular politics that emerged around Ebola control in the USA.

The US domestic politics of border control also resulted in the finding that newspaper outlets of different broad party-political alignments presented the issue is divergent ways. Thus, while the *New York Times* accounted for the public reaction with suggestions that 'the line between vigilance and hysteria can be as blurry as the edges of a watercolor painting,'[34] outlets that tend towards conservative politics highlighted different aspects of the public fear. They stated that liberal media outlets (and the government) had downplayed the threat and misunderstood the public instinct:

> People are irrational in their assessment of risks, blah, blah. Yes, we can find here and there examples of American overreacting to Ebola. But more in evidence has been the media's own anti-hysteria hysteria.[35]

The issue of public fear, as with the wider narrative of border measures, became a key site of politics here.

Overall the narrative of fear and the public reflected the broader themes of the newspaper accounts of border control. It was clear that border management was a key point of interest in each of the three case countries. However, as will be shown below, the particular nature of these representations was highly dependent upon national political climates.

Ebola and the West

One of the most troubling aspects of the global health reaction surrounding the Ebola cri-sis has been the fact that concern and substantial mobilisation around the event failed to materialise until the disease entered the West. While crisis and aid organisations had been early responders to the outbreak, even the WHO only articulated its highest level of mobili-sation (designating the epidemic a Public Health Event of International Concern) following Western interest.

Overall the newspaper documents analysed demonstrate that the discourse around Ebola centred upon the West. The disease was transformed from a problem of the 'distant' area of West Africa to a domestic concern. Issues in the core impact zone were erased and under-emphasised, with only general discussions of 'Africa' (and Africans) appearing (see below), contrasted with specific and prolonged examination of cases in the West.

Overall the newspaper narrative made clear that this was a Western problem. This revolves around stories portraying the ability of the disease to be spread to the West, where:

> The epicentre of this perfect storm outbreak may be out-of-mind, out-of-sight West Africa, but as the cases in the US and Spain have confirmed, Western countries like Australia are not immune and all of us have a role to play in the global fight.[36]

The potential for spread to the West underpinned the discussion of the threat posed by the disease. However, the irony of this attention – where Ebola only became a global health issue after reaching the West – was also acknowledged. For example, it was noted that, following the case of an affected Spanish nurse, Ebola 'is now attracting coverage and seems to have finally sheeted home the horror of the disease for Western audiences';[37] and 'Months into the epidemic, Western governments suddenly started paying attention. This was no longer a problem of faraway villages.'[38]

Nevertheless, the potential effects of the disease in the West were a matter of constant media interest. This included numerous reports on policy and public health concern about this disease, such as the statements that 'It's deadly, it's on the loose, and Australian health authorities are concerned the frightening disease ebola could be headed our way' in the Australian newspapers,[39] or that 'Public Health England said that the outbreak was the most 'acute health emergency' facing Britain' and that 'Up to ten ebola cases could be seen in Britain by Christmas' in the UK.[40]

The media narrative around the disease therefore served to transform the issue as a problem for West Africa into a problem for the West. The almost exclusive focus on Western interest, and on the potential for contagion across Western borders, thereby underpinned the sustained discussion of the nature and function of the border control measures. The West is the centre of the media narrative and the centre of the representations of the disease.

The domestic politics of fear

Within the newspaper representations Ebola was transformed from a problem focusing around the outbreak in West Africa, to a problem of the movement of contagion into the West. Further, the disease became a site around which the politics of health was played out. While publics and public fear presented an important strand of the representation, the vast majority of the newspaper reports concerned politics and political actions. In particu-lar, both in Australia and the USA, party and electoral politics was the predominant frame through which Ebola management was cast. While this effect was less pronounced in the UK sample – which focused upon criticism of 'government' actions, rather than imputing different positions to different political parties – it was still clear that Ebola had become a frame through which domestic politics could be understood.

Much of the existing literature on media representations of border control around disease demonstrates the wider politics of borders, for example in terms of representing problems of globalisation and Western–Third World relationships. While these factors (as shown above, and in the discussions around the representations of West Africa below) are evident in the case of Ebola, this is not the primary form of politics presented. Instead, the data demonstrate the way in which domestic politics are used to explain reactions to Ebola. This is evident to differing extents – far less so in the UK reports, clear in the Australian newspapers and overwhelmingly dominant in the US sample. In all cases it was narrated that, while Ebola was (as above) a cause for reasonable concern, domestic political actors were harnessing public fear as a part of general political manoeuvring.

UK

The UK reporting presented the management of Ebola as an issue of government misman-agement. The reports emphasised confusion between different sources of official action and the generally unprepared state of the government in handling the epidemic. This represents an important point of difference from both the US and Australian samples, where party policy shines through as fundamental to the politics surrounding Ebola.

Early in the process of implementing screening measures, the newspapers emphasised the incompetence of the actions taken. For example, it was suggested that 'Britain's airport Ebola checks turned into a shambles yesterday,'[41] and that 'Britain's ebola screening plans remained in chaos yesterday as airports said they had been given no instructions'.[42] The inefficacy of British systems of control was highlighted in suggestions that 'Ebola screen-ing plans were in chaos yesterday, as it emerged travellers might be allowed to stroll into Britain without mandatory checks'.[43] Following the implementation of screening measures, the media claimed 'a day of confusion', in an article entitled 'Battling Ebola: Government U-Turn'.[44] Confusion around these early screening events, eg between different strands of the government, was emphasised ('Border chiefs yesterday said they could not force trav-ellers to be screened for Ebola – a claim later rebuffed by Downing Street'[45]) and in terms of general confusion and ineffectiveness ('Ministers were accused of a chaotic response to the ebola crisis last night after it emerged new screening measures amounted to little more than a questionnaire'[46]).

As became quite prominent in the UK sample, the newspapers suggested that the govern-ment was serving to manage the fear of Ebola rather than the fact of the disease. For example:

> Mr Vaz [Labour MP and chairman of the Home Affairs Select Committee] said: 'What we need to ensure is that the public feel there is confidence in our borders. This means we need to put in screening at our borders.'[47]

This reinforces the fundamental emphasis on managing public expectations. However, while the government and public processes generally were criticised in the UK case, the particular domestic politics of Ebola management did not come through as strongly as in the contexts of the US and Australian newspapers.

Australia

Australian newspaper accounts focused upon the competing positions of politicians from opposing parties in their stance towards Ebola management. Politically the Australian case is of particular interest. The (Liberal) Australian government refused to send medical personnel to the Ebola-affected region. This became a point of contention between the government and various international health organisations, and set the tone for the discourse surrounding Ebola management.

It was suggested that 'Tony Abbott [the Australian prime minister] remains concerned about putting Australian personnel in harm's way when there is no commitment they could be safely evacuated and treated'.[48] Various statements of this position were reiterated throughout the newspaper sample.

However, opposition positions were depicted as a site of political tension in respect to Ebola management. Ebola was described as having been used as a political tool in defining party positions:

> Tanya Plibersek is using fear of Ebola coming to Australia, compassion about thousands of deaths in west Africa and growing global alarm to differentiate [opposition leader] Bill Shorten's Labor from Tony Abbott on national security. Concern about Ebola, issues such as border checks or quarantine, whether to try to stop the virus in Africa and whether Australia is dealing with the disease are all grounds to make new arguments and mark out new political territory.[49]

The quote above demonstrates the way in which the newspaper narrative centres upon Ebola management as a site of domestic politics.

This division was highlighted by the newspapers. In an article entitled 'Political split gives nation the jitters' it was reported that:

> Bipartisanship on the national security threat posed by the Ebola virus has been ripped up. At a time of great anxiety caused by war and pestilence without borders, Australia's political leadership has split on strategy and threatened to deepen that national alarm and confusion.[50]

In this way the unease around Ebola is at least in part attributed to political divisions and tensions. The idea that national security ought to be a bipartisan issue (evident also in the US case) was used to suggest that using Ebola 'politically' is one of the fundamental problems of the country's management of the issue.

USA

While the Australian sample begins to highlight the linking of Ebola management to domestic politics, this issue was a central and defining theme of the US newspaper reporting. Here party politics, particularly surrounding the then-upcoming elections, dominated the coverage. The Ebola crisis was leveraged as an axel for domestic political action. As was noted in the media the situation 'was turning into a political as well as a public health crisis.'[51]

Border control issues were central to the politics here. It was reported that a 'chorus of Republicans calling for the heightened foreign travel restriction,'[52] which also directed the concern over Ebola to more local points of tension. An example of this occurred when 'Scott Brown, the Republican candidate for Senate in New Hampshire, recently said that the spread of the Ebola virus should prompt the US government to seal the border with Mexico'.[53] Because of the forthcoming midterm elections political tensions were evident around discussion of the disease. The situation was exacerbated by moves from New York and New Jersey to implement border measures (quarantine) which were not part of federal government policy.

What was evident throughout the newspaper sample under analysis here – and noticeably distinct from the UK and Australian accounts – was that the newspaper outlets themselves divided in partisan lines in reporting on the border control issue. This was evident in the nature of editorial and opinion pieces published by the various outlets. For example, articles from the *Wall Street Journal* and *USA Today* (tending towards conservative policy options) report that:

The lesson is that government bureaucracy should be treated, at every level, as inherently and inescapably incompetent. And that expert opinion should be viewed as mistaken until proven otherwise.[54]

New York and New Jersey shouldn't be making Ebola policy, but if Washington leaves a vacuum, it will be filled. And leaving vacuums is becoming an Obama administration specialty.[55]

Strict border measures were clearly advocated by these outlets, suggesting that the administration and expert knowledge was untrustworthy:

The popular New England Journal of Medicine claimed that 'hundreds of years of experience show that to stop an epidemic of this type requires controlling it at its source.' That's dead wrong. In the 19th century cholera, yellow fever and smallpox were stopped from spreading widely in the US and Europe by travel bans.[56]

And in comparing the Ebola crisis to historical examples of isolation policy:

Allied nations had no hesitancy in banning private travel to and from Europe in the early 1940s as they dispatched considerable resources to end the Nazi menace. In exactly the same spirit, a travel ban on the affected West African nationals may be in order even as outside governments make a big investment in liberating those countries from the threat of mass death by Ebola.[57]

In this, these newspaper outlets mirrored Republican calls to strengthen border control measures and implement quarantine and travel ban measures.

In contrast, the New York Times reporting (often also employing historical analogy) tended towards emphasising that Ebola would be best managed in terms of control at its source:

overreacting might just be the way to spread the disease instead of contain it. It is a lesson we learned long ago. During the 14th century Black Death, Venice and other cities introduced a quarantine…to no effect…The city of Milan, well ahead of its time, avoided a major outbreak by isolating sick people and sealing off their houses.[58]

This outlet also often explicitly recognised the conservative discourse, where 'Some prominent conservative commentators dismiss the assurances of scientists, Obama administration officials and the news media as unreliable, elitist blather, contrasting its own reporting as a voice of rational authority on the subject.[59]

The US sample clearly showed that the Ebola outbreak was spoken of through the terms of domestic politics and political tensions. Ebola management served as a proxy through which debates between conservative and liberal politicians could be played out. This was also clearly evident in the Australian newspaper discourse, although here the media reported political positions rather than overtly speaking for particular viewpoints. In the UK, issues of government efficacy, rather than party politics, were highlighted. In all cases Ebola became an issue of the domestic politics of these countries, rather than an issue of either global politics or the affected West African region.

The spread of Ebola

Infectious disease spread tends to result in the blame and stigmatisation of affected populations. One of the reasons why border control and quarantine makes sense as a social and cultural reaction is that the population being protected is able to 'other' affected communities and band together in keeping members of these affected communities out of the social space under protection. Past outbreaks have seen the 'othering', stigmatisation and harassment of individuals and communities with links to affected areas. This can be seen, for example, in the case of Asian communities in the West during the SARS outbreak, of stigmatisation of communities during the rise of HIV/AIDS, as well as of historical examples surrounding

Spanish Influenza and other diseases. Work on media representations of earlier Ebola out-breaks also demonstrates the way in which 'Africa' became an 'othered' region.

It was clear that generalised depictions of West Africa were present throughout the arti-cles analysed here. These tended to emphasise the cultural factors that (from the perspective of the media discourse) underpinned the spread of Ebola in the region. However, simulta-neously, and in parallel with the emphasis on the domestic politics of borders, depictions of the agents of Ebola transmission tended to mirror more domestic concerns. The narrative around the spread of Ebola to the West focused not on West Africa but rather on more tra-ditional domestic concerns. These included fears around terrorism and immigration, and, in the USA, issues surrounding race. Again, the Ebola crisis simply became a frame through which domestic politics was played out.

Importers into the West

Issues of immigration and security were at the forefront of the narratives about the spread of Ebola into these three countries. In the UK sample Ebola was linked with illegal and unwanted immigration. The fact that 'An MP has called for Ebola screening at Dover over fears illegal immigrants could have the disease',[60] highlighted the link between Ebola and population movements. There were fears that these immigrants would spread Ebola into Europe, given that 'Desperate migrants from Ebola-stricken countries in Africa are attacking police and breaking through a major border to try to get to Europe'.[61] In addition, it was suggested that Ebola sufferers might travel specifically to the UK since 'Deadly Ebola could be brought here by health tourists, experts warn. They say victims may fly to the UK for NHS care.'[62] In this way the more persistent issue of immigration was discursively linked to the spread of Ebola.

Another mechanism through which Ebola might be spread to the West, it was suggested, was through terrorist activity. This concept was present throughout the three samples. Fear of bioterrorism was connected to fear of Ebola transmission. This was evident in representations surrounding the politics of border screening in Australia, where 'The Palmer United Party senator [Jacqui Lambie] also proposed screening of all airline passengers as a precaution against terrorist "suicide agents" carrying Ebola'.[63] Ideas around the use of Ebola as a terrorist weapon were a clear part of the media message:

> Islamic terrorists have discussed using the Ebola virus to attack the West, according to reports. Internet intelligence monitored by US agencies uncovered the plans to transmit the disease through biological warfare. The attacks could involve jihadists infecting themselves with Ebola before carrying out suicide attacks.[64]

As with the discussions around immigration, the Ebola crisis was represented in a way that chimed with more persistent domestic concerns.

In the USA, where (as shown above) politics between Democrats and Republicans pre-dominated in the discussion of Ebola, issues of race were also evident. This was clear in the coverage of right-wing criticism of the administration's policy through the frame of race:

> Ablow [a psychiatrist and Fox News contributor] implied that Obama hasn't imposed a travel ban on flights from the Ebola-afflicted countries…because of his race. 'His affinity, his affiliations are with them. Not us,' Ablow said.[65]

Issues of race were described as central to the decision-making process surrounding border control. In responding to criticism of the ethics of border measures, expert testimony (here, Gerald Weissman, research professor of medicine) was used:

'The objections are very humane and very lovely,' he said. 'They consider quarantine medieval, and think there's a touch of racism in this. It may be, but I wouldn't care if Ebola came from Sweden.'[66]

In addition, issues of race were evident in newspaper's explanations of the (inefficacy of) government positions:

If Washington's reason for resisting a travel ban from the hotzone countries is fear of being accused of racial profiling, politicians will be relieved by the rainbow coalitions of the afflicted [Ebola cases] in the US – two black, one Asian, one white.[67]

Just as in examples of the use of narratives of immigration and terrorism, the US newspapers' emphasis on issues of race reflected the juxtaposition of domestic political issues with concerns around Ebola.[68]

Representations of the carriers of Ebola into the West, just like depictions of the broader issue of border control, show that the newspaper discourse tended to present the epidemic through the lens of domestic and local concerns rather than international politics. Through the newspaper sample analysed, the discussion focused strongly on the Western nations themselves, giving often only passing reference to Ebola as a particular issue for an affected West African population or to the wider implications in terms of international security and global health.

Depictions of Africa

While narratives around West Africa were clearly marginal to the media discourse surrounding border control, the depiction of these populations highlights the fact that the media narrative focused upon the West. Here, it is clear that the media discourse presented the affected region in generalised terms, and focused upon particular 'cultural' aspects of Ebola transmission. African border control efforts were cited in a few cases,[69] both in highlighting cases of successful management (eg Senegal and Nigeria) and in terms of inefficacy of airport security as an example of 'Total chaos. Complete corruption.'[70] Border control measures within African were also represented as unwarranted:

Fear of the virus is rattling would-be tourists to the continent and is underlining the risks some associate with travel to Africa. Anxious African governments have potentially amplified those worries with their own draconian measures to keep the virus from breaching borders.[71]

This created a key contradiction with the depiction of (necessary) border control in the West. However, much of the narrative centred on West Africa as a site of transmission.

Past research on the depiction of Ebola in the Western media shows the way in which tropes of African exoticism, and horrifying visions of the virulent African jungle dominate the discourse.[72] These types of depiction are also prevalent in the wider cultural representation (eg books and films) around Ebola. This type of representation was certainly present within the newspaper sample, as shown in the following quote:

Some [Australian medical experts], wouldn't even entertain the thought that a traveller, suffering from ebola, or even the grim symptoms of the deadly blood disease, would travel 20-odd hours from the steaming jungles of West Africa, make their way through airport security and put Australians at risk.

However, while the above quote – criticising Australia's apparent complacency over the virus – provides an example of the use of these discourses, they did not tend to dominate the sample studied here.

Nevertheless, depiction of 'the jungle' and of West African populations were reinforced through repeated mention of the spread of the virus through bush-meat consumption, which was also suggested as a route of transmission to the West: 'The chief cause is the popularity of "bush meat"…Since bush meat is now being smuggled into London and Paris, scientists warn this could be another source of infection in Europe.'[73] In contrast, though to the same effect, it was also indicated that the West would not be shielded from the disease, and that the 2014–15 outbreak was more threatening:

> Just as well, then, that no one ever gets Ebola beyond a handful of unlucky souls in the remote rural villages of equatorial West and Central Africa, where locals ignore warning signs and still eat the fruit bats and monkeys that are the chief carriers of this disease. At least, that's what public health experts have been saying for years. Suddenly, though, they are changing their tune.[74]

While depictions of the 'uncivilised' practices of affected populations may not have been as prominent as in previous Ebola outbreaks, they were still evident. More conspicuous were general proclamations around the 'cultural norms' aggravating transmission.[75]

Not without some cause but clearly highlighted in the newspaper representations were issues surrounding the cultural practices around burial and care of the sick, such that:

> sustained outbreaks would not occur in the US because cultural factors in the developing world that spread Ebola – such as intimate contact while family and friends are caring for the sick and during the preparation of bodies for burial – aren't common in the developed world.[76]

Transmission through the rites surrounding the deceased was emphasised in the media,[77] alongside other depictions of the exacerbating nature of 'African' culture.

For example, critiques of the role of traditional healers, rumour, distrust of authority and of modern medicine, and conspiracy theories, were all prominent parts of the newspaper narrative.[78] While these issues undoubtedly impeded control of the disease in some contexts, the newspapers over-emphasised the role of these factors. For example, the narrative concentrated upon traditional features of the affected communities and cultures. There was only a single article pointing out that aspects of modernisation – population movement and travel, the concentration of people in urban areas, etc – had played an important role in the particular form of the 2014–15 outbreak.[79] Instead, the newspaper narrative dwelt upon 'traditional' cultural features, referred to the population as inhabiting a homogeneous monolithic 'culture' and provided descriptions of the African 'jungle' rather than the contemporary urban space.

These generalised depictions of Africa, and African culture, served to reinforce rather than negate the general tendency of the media reporting. While the disease originated in West Africa, it is clear that the primary focus of the newspaper representation revolved particularly around domestic issues. The representations of the spread and management of Ebola through the frames of immigration, bioterrorism and (in the USA) racial politics simply highlight the fact that Ebola had become transformed from a generalised 'African' health issue to a platform through which domestic politics could play out.

Conclusion

This study has centred upon newspaper deployment of the language of security and border control. For this reason other important narratives (eg the deployment of aid, the politics of affected countries or international organisations, accounts of events within the affected West African region) were not uncovered by this analysis. Nonetheless, it is clear that the problem of borders and security was a key frame through which the newspaper media related the events surrounding the Ebola outbreak.

The transgression and control of borders is often central to the media representation of infectious disease. Borders are both historically and contemporarily key to the management of contagion, acting as both geopolitical and symbolic boundaries between the ill and the healthy. Much of the previous research around the newspaper representation of infectious disease shows the othering and exoticising narratives about the (practices and threat produced by) affected populations in the Third World; developing countries are shown as a key site of contagion. While these ideas were present in the reporting around Ebola, this study has shown that the representations in the UK, USA and Australia instead focused on the disease as a frame through which domestic politics was acted out. Rather than the macro-politics of international borders, the border control measures in these countries were narrated in the particular context of domestic party politics and government.

Cultural reactions to border maintenance can be mobilised as a means to engage in domestic politics. Here, concerns around the intrusion of outsiders were evident in the reporting around Ebola. However the outsiders in question were more 'local' in nature. Domestic factors took precedence in the discourse over the more distant problems of West Africa. Thus, to the extent that othering occurred, it involved issues of immigration, terrorism and (national discussions of) race and ethnicity. West Africa itself was largely absent from discussions, and only presented in a general and passing manner.

What is clear from this newspaper analysis is that the Ebola outbreak was used within newspaper representations as a frame through which domestic politics could play out. In all three countries the media centred its focus on the government and party politics, rather than on the disease locus of West Africa. Further, even publics in the West did not appear as central aspects of the discourse, except as the source of the fear that political actors were harnessing; both the public and the wider global context disappear here. Within this sample, Ebola ceased to be an issue of global health – or even necessarily a problem of the health of domestic populations – but became a lens through which political action played out and government competence could be measured. In contrast to many previous studies of border control and the media, portrayals of Ebola did not appear to depict it primarily as an issue of transgression of national and social borders; rather, it was an issue around which public fears could be harnessed and mobilised as an avenue for domestic politics.

Disclosure statement

No potential conflict of interest was reported by the author.

Notes

1. Baker and Fidler, "Global Public Health Surveillance," 1058–1065; and Fidler, and Gostin, "The New International Health Regulations," 85–94.
2. Bashford, "At the Border," 345–348; King, "Security, Disease, Commerce," 763–789; and Nelkin and Gilman, "Placing Blame for Devastating Disease."
3. Abeysinghe and White, "The Avian Influenza Pandemic," 311–326; Foege, "Plagues"; Gensini, "The Concept of Quarantine in History," 257–261; and Herzlich and Pierret, *Illness and Self in Society*.
4. Auge and Herzlich, *The Meaning of Illness*; Bashford and Strange, "Isolation and Exclusion in the Modern World"; Eichelberger, "SARS and New York's Chinatown," 1284–1295; Foege, "Plagues"; Hooker and Ali, "SARS and Security," 101–126; and Wald, *Contagious*.
5. Haynes, "Still the Heart of Darkness," 133–145; Joffe and Haarhoff, "Representations of Far-flung Illnesses," 955–969; and Ungar, "Hot Crises and Media Reassurance," 36–56.
6. *Daily Telegraph*, October 10, 2014.
7. *Wall Street Journal*, September 20, 2014.
8. *The Australian*, September 19, 2014.
9. Abeysinghe and White, "The Avian Influenza Pandemic," 311–326.
10. Washer, *Emerging Infectious Diseases and Society*.
11. *Daily Telegraph*, October 26, 2014.
12. *New York Times*, October 9, 2014.
13. *Daily Telegraph*, October 19, 2014.
14. *The Australian*, October 18, 2014.
15. *Daily Mirror*, August 2, 2014.
16. *Daily Telegraph*, October 11, 2014.
17. *Daily Telegraph*, October 14, 2014.
18. *USA Today*, October 23, 2014.
19. For example, Peterson, *Outbreak*; and Preston, *The Hot Zone*.
20. *Daily Mail*, July 29, 2014.
21. *Daily Mail*, October 10, 2014.
22. *Daily Mirror*, August 4, 2014. See also *Sun*, August 4, 2014.
23. *Daily Mirror*, August 4, 2014.
24. *Daily Mirror*, October 11, 2014.
25. *Sun*, October 21, 2014.
26. *Sun*, October 14, 2014.
27. *Daily Mail*, October 17, 2014.
28. *USA Today*, August 7, 2014.
29. *New York Times*, October 18, 2014.
30. Ibid.
31. *New York Times*, October 21, 2014.
32. Ibid.
33. Ibid.
34. *New York Times*, October 20, 2014.
35. *Wall Street Journal*, October 26, 2014.
36. *Daily Telegraph*, October 10, 2014.
37. Ibid.
38. *The Australian*, October 4, 2014.
39. *Daily Telegraph*, July 31, 2014.
40. *Daily Mail*, July 31, 2014; and *Daily Mail*, October 14, 2014.
41. *Sun*, October 15, 2014.
42. *Daily Mail*, October 11, 2014.
43. *Daily Mail*, October 15, 2014.
44. *Daily Mail*, October 10, 2014.
45. *Sun*, October 15, 2014.
46. *Daily Mail*, October 10, 2014.

47. *Sun*, October 9, 2014.
48. *The Australian*, October 17, 2014.
49. *The Australian*, October 17, 2014.
50. *The Australian*, October 18, 2014.
51. *New York Times*, October 17, 2014.
52. *Wall Street Journal*, October 17, 2014.
53. *USA Today*, October 16, 2014.
54. *Wall Street Journal*, October 21, 2014.
55. *Wall Street Journal*, October 29, 2014.
56. *USA Today*, October 31, 2014.
57. *Wall Street Journal*, October 25, 2014.
58. *USA Today*, October 10, 2014.
59. *New York Times*, November 1, 2014.
60. *Sun*, October 16, 2014.
61. *Sun*, November 23, 2014.
62. *Sun*, October 11, 2014.
63. *The Australian*, October 23, 2014.
64. *Sun*, October 10, 2014.
65. *USA Today*, October 21, 2014.
66. *New York Times*, October 18, 2014.
67. *Wall Street Journal*, October 26, 2014.
68. Mirroring previous accounts, see, for example, Murdocca, "When Ebola came to Canada," 24–31.
69. *New York Times*, August 13, 2014; and *Wall Street Journal*, October 24, 2014.
70. *Sun*, October 19, 2014.
71. *Wall Street Journal*, August 20, 2014.
72. Jones, "Ebola, Emerging," 1–6; and Haynes, "Still the Heart of Darkness," 133–145.
73. *Daily Mail*, July 29, 2014.
74. Ibid.
75. *Wall Street Journal*, September 20, 2014.
76. *Wall Street Journal*, August 4, 2014.
77. See also the *Sun*, August 7, 2014.
78. *The Australian*, October 4, 2014; *New York Times*, August 7, 2014; *New York Times*, October 19, 2014; and *Daily Mail*, June 4, 2014.
79. *New York Times*, August 10, 2014.

Bibliography

Abeysinghe, S., and K. White. "The Avian Influenza Pandemic: Discourses of Risk, Contagion and Preparation in Australia." *Health, Risk & Society* 13, no. 4 (2011): 311–326.

Auge, M., and C. Herzlich. *The Meaning of Illness: Anthropology, History and Sociology*. Paris: Harwood Academic Press, 1995.

Baker, M. G., and D. P. Fidler. "Global Public Health Surveillance under New International Health Regulations." *Emerging Infectious Diseases* 12, no. 7 (2006): 1058–1065.

Bashford, A. "At the Border: Contagion, Immigration, Nation." *Australian Historical Studies* 120 (2002): 345–348.

Bashford, A., and C. Strange. "Isolation and Exclusion in the Modern World." In *Isolation: Places and Practices of Exclusion*, edited by C Strange and A Bashford, 1–19. London: Routledge, 2003.

Eichelberger, L. "SARS and New York's Chinatown: The Politics of Risk and Blame during an Epidemic of Fear." *Social Science & Medicine* 65 (2007): 1284–1295.

Fidler, D. P., and L. O. Gostin. "The New International Health Regulations: An Historic Development for International Law and Public Health." *Journal of Law, Medicine & Ethics* 34, no. 1 (2006): 85–94.

Foege, W. H. "Plagues: Perception of Risk and Social Responses." In *In the Time of Plague: The History and Social Consequences of Lethal Epidemic Disease*, edited by A Mack, 9–21. New York: New York University Press, 1991.

Gensini, G., M. Yacoub, and A. Conti. "The Concept of Quarantine in History: From Plague to SARS." *Journal of Infection* 49 (2004): 257–261.

Haynes, D. M. "Still the Heart of Darkness: The Ebola Virus and the Meta-narrative of Disease in the Hot Zone." *Journal of Medical Humanities* 23, no. 2 (2002): 133–145.

Herzlich, C., and J. Pierret. *Illness and Self in Society*. London: Johns Hopkins University Press, 1987.

Hooker, C., and S. H. Ali. "SARS and Security: Health in the 'New Normal.'" *Studies in Political Economy* 84 (2009): 101–126.

Jones, J. "Ebola, Emerging: The Limitations of Culturalist Discourses in Epidemiology." *Journal of Global Health* 1 (2011): 1–6.

Joffe, H., and G. Haarhoff. "Representations of Far-flung Illnesses: The Case of Ebola in Britain." *Social Science & Medicine* 54, no. 6 (2002): 955–969.

King, N. B. "Security, Disease, Commerce: Ideologies of Postcolonial Global Health." *Social Studies of Science* 32, nos. 5-6 (2002): 763–789.

Murdocca, C. "When Ebola came to Canada: Race and the Making of the Respectable Body." *Atlantis* 27, no. 2 (2003): 24–31.

Nelkin, D., and S. Gilman. "Placing Blame for Devastating Disease." In *In Time of Plague: The History and Social Consequences of Lethal Epidemic Disease*, edited by A Mack, 39–56. New York: New York University Press, 1991.

Peterson, W., dir. *Outbreak*. Burbank, CA: Warner Bros., 1995.

Preston, Richard. *The Hot Zone*. New York: Anchor, 1999.

Ungar, S. "Hot Crises and Media Reassurance: A Comparison of Emerging Diseases and Ebola Zaire." *British Journal of Sociology* 49, no. 1 (1998): 36–56.

Wald, P. *Contagious: Cultures, Carriers, and the Outbreak Narrative*. Durham, NC: Duke University Press, 2008.

Washer, P. *Emerging Infectious Diseases and Society*. London: Palgrave Macmillan, 2010.

Infectious injustice: the political foundations of the Ebola crisis in Sierra Leone

Emma-Louise Anderson and Alexander Beresford

Politics and International Studies (POLIS), University of Leeds, UK

ABSTRACT

This article identifies the long-term political factors that contributed to the Ebola crisis in Sierra Leone, factors which are largely overlooked by the emerging international focus on building resilient health systems. We argue that the country exhibits critical symptoms of the recurrent crises of a gatekeeper state, including acute external dependency, patron–client politics, endemic corruption and weak state capacity. A coterie of actors, both internal and external to Sierra Leone, has severely compromised the health system. This left certain sections of the population acutely at risk from Ebola and highlights the need for political solutions to build stronger, inclusive health systems.

Introduction

According to the World Health Organisation (WHO), one of the core reasons the Ebola Virus Disease (EVD) spread so extensively in Sierra Leone, Liberia and Guinea was that their health systems 'lacked resilience' and that, as a result, 'when the crisis struck, the countries had no reserve capacity to mount an effective and timely response'. The WHO argued that these countries' health systems suffered from particular structural weaknesses, including an insufficient number of health workers, who were poorly distributed across the country, and inadequate surveillance and information systems for oversight. The report identified further weaknesses such as 'absent or weak rapid response systems, few laboratories mainly located in cities, unreliable supply and procurement systems for PPEs [personal protective equipment] and other supplies, lack of electricity and running water in some health facilities and few ambulances'.[1]

This article focuses on Sierra Leone, where the number of infections eclipsed those of other countries (reaching 13,683) and where new cases continue to be reported in September 2015.[2] Indeed, the weakness of Sierra Leone's health infrastructure was exposed by the EVD epidemic. Hospitals were already understaffed and under-resourced to cope with everyday health challenges, including maternal health and endemic malaria. In 2008 there were only 95 physicians and 991 nurses and midwives, equating to two physicians and 18 nurses and midwives per 100,000 people.[3] As a result, some of Sierra Leone's health indicators, including life expectancy (45 years) and death rate (17 per 1000 people), remain persistently among the worst in the world.[4]

The international community's response to the EVD epidemic was to promote a containment strategy. The president of Sierra Leone, Ernest Bai Koroma, ordered the quarantine of EVD 'epicentres' and military personnel were deployed to establish roadblocks; clinics were built to try and isolate infected people. The UK was among the countries leading the international response, which was directed largely by its armed forces with the support of health organisations such as Médecins Sans Frontières (MSF). The virus was eventually contained and by August 2015 a successful trial of the VSV-EBOV vaccine was hailed as a 'game-changer' by one Assistant Director-General of the WHO.[5]

However, the eventual success of the containment strategy should not provoke celebration but instead a prolonged period of detailed introspection among the actors involved. Indeed, the scale of the crisis is argued to present an opportunity to galvanise renewed commitment to long-term health systems strengthening (HSS). In this vein the WHO Executive Board on the Ebola Emergency argued that 'Media interest, technical support, and financial resources have surged into these countries. This creates a *window of opportunity* for reinforced action on health systems strengthening that lays the groundwork in the affected countries for universal access to safe, high quality health services.'[6] This sentiment is echoed by those on the ground who led the emergency response, including the head of the MSF mission in Sierra Leone, who contended that:

> It is clear that the work to improve healthcare in Sierra Leone will not end with the epidemic. Even before Ebola, Sierra Leone suffered from an acute shortage of skilled staff, limiting access for the population to key life-saving services. After the loss of more than 220 health workers to Ebola, there is a real need, not for just funding and promises, but for skilled clinicians on the ground across the country.[7]

Building more resilient health systems has thus become almost an article of faith for international donors and NGOs.[8]

Our concern here is with the need to broaden the scope of these reflections to include a focus on the political foundations of the EVD epidemic.[9] In short, the task before us is not simply to enhance short-term resilience to health crises, but to tackle the very roots of endemically weak health systems in the first place. The IR scholarship and much of the Global Health scholarship more specifically are traditionally ill-equipped to respond to this challenge: as Harman and Brown argue, this is not simply a question of Africa's omission;[10] there is often a disconnection between the 'discipline's theoretical constructs and African realities'.[11]

We will elucidate below how the weakness of the health system reflects an extreme manifestation of the recurring political crises afflicting many of Africa's 'gatekeeper states', including acute external dependency, patron–client politics, endemic corruption and a weak state unable to provide basic services and protections to its population.[12] Since the country's devastating civil war (1991–2002), Sierra Leone has become what Harris describes as a 'laboratory' for liberal experiments in state building and governance.[13] We argue that, as powerful external actors endeavour to protect their investments and decentralise power, the creation of multiple parallel health systems complicates health provision and entrenches dysfunction. Within this context the potential for rent-seeking among politicians and local health professionals is particularly acute in a sector that attracts such high volumes of external resources. The lack of capacity for oversight has reproduced an environment in which local actors invert external interventions – including, in this case, those designed to contain the

EVD epidemic – for private gain. Therefore, while the vast majority of Sierra Leoneans working to combat the spread of EVD have done so with great courage and at considerable personal risk, the rent-seeking behaviour of some government officials and health care professionals has nonetheless diverted substantial resources away from this effort. Furthermore, the manner in which the epidemic spread in Sierra Leone highlights the structural violence that permeates society: where social structures (including economic, political, legal, religious and cultural structures) engender inequality, they prevent individuals or groups from achieving their full potential and expose them to risk.[14]

The core challenge ahead remains to augment stronger, inclusive health systems. While the latest emphasis on health system 'resilience' may help contain future outbreaks, such a focus ultimately reflects a desire to manage the public health risks generated from the fallout of late capitalism and the global inequities that it produces. Broad-based HSS, on the other hand, is a much more ambitious project of social transformation, tackling, as best it can, the roots of structural violence. This requires long-term commitment to finding political solutions to health problems, solutions that address the reasons why populations are at risk in the first place.

The recurrent crises of the gatekeeper state

Like their colonial predecessors, Africa's postcolonial elites often struggled to extend their power and control over the entirety of their states. First, these states were weak from their very inception as a result of seemingly arbitrary demarcation of their borders, which reflected the European colonial rivalries of the late 19th century, rather than the political and social realities of African societies. Second, Africa's postcolonial leaders inherited economies that had been orientated towards servicing external demands for African resources and rarely generated sufficient economic growth to sustain industrial diversification or an expansionary fiscal programme that was not entirely dependent on external aid, loans and other forms of development assistance. As Cooper notes, a 'gatekeeper state' complex therefore prevails in many African states. Political elites in office attempt to reproduce their power as best they can by controlling the internationally recognised state (the 'gate') and regulating access to the resources channelled into it from outside. This includes controlling the allocation of development assistance, jobs, status, authority and access to markets.[15] Public resources are thus distributed in a private, discretionary fashion as a form of political patronage in exchange for political support. Beresford argues that the kind of 'gatekeeper politics' that emerges 'is therefore not synonymous with corruption, though corruption is a pervasive symptom of it. Instead, it reflects something much broader: political and social structures through which authority and power are cultivated, disseminated, and contested.'[16] It is important to recognise that this kind of patronage-based political system is not a uniquely 'African' form of political aberration and breakdown, however.[17] Furthermore, scholars have noted the need to be careful to identify the varying degrees to which such politics prevails across different African countries and the different forms it can take, which can in large part depend on the strength of the central state and the dynamics of capitalist development in each particular state.[18]

We will argue here that Sierra Leone exhibits one of the more extreme manifestations of the 'recurrent crises' described by Cooper that afflict some of Africa's gatekeeper states, which we characterise as having several interconnected symptoms:

- a weak economy premised primarily upon primary resource extraction;
- external dependency on international resources;
- volatile gatekeeper politics based on political patronage, producing a weak state vulnerable to political upheavals;
- an inability to provide basic services or perform basic social functions for the population.

Such an analysis stands in contrast to an emerging narrative among Western donors and investors celebrating 'Africa's rising', pointing to a continent of 'hopeful economies' exhibiting relatively high levels of GDP growth rates, emerging middle classes and an increasingly large market of African consumers.[19] This narrative has also been embraced, with considerably less credibility, to celebrate Sierra Leone's recent economic record since the war, including GDP growth of over 20% before the EVD epidemic.[20] The country's most recent Poverty Reduction Strategy Paper (PRSP), the 'Agenda for Prosperity (2013–2018)', aims to build on what it calls the 'tremendous progress' achieved as a result of the previous 'Agenda for Change (2008–2012)' and to contribute towards Sierra Leone's 'epic journey to become a middle income country'.[21] While mindful of the challenges that still confront the country, the World Bank has consistently noted the 'remarkable strides and reforms' it has witnessed since the end of the civil war in 2002, and that as a result of its recent programmes of reform, 'progress has been made, albeit at different levels, on most indicators of growth, poverty, MDGs, fragility, investment climate, and governance'.[22]

The 'Africa rising' narrative contains severe deficiencies, however. As Taylor notes, 'the dynamics which are accompanying a notional "rise" of Africa' are 'actually contributing to the continent being pushed further and further into maldevelopment and dependency'.[23] Sierra Leone has historically been endowed with natural resources, including iron ore, titanium ore, bauxite, cocoa, rutile and diamonds, as well as relatively fertile land with plenty of rainfall. However, as Zack-Williams observed back in the 1980s, little had been achieved since independence in terms of diversifying the economy and decreasing the dependence on primary resource exports.[24] Indeed, Sierra Leone's recent growth is underpinned by a continued dependence on exporting iron ore in particular,[25] highlighting the country's narrow export base and its vulnerability to changes in the terms of trade.[26] Little has therefore been achieved in terms of the long-term structural transformation of the economy and, as the IMF has recently argued, the recent 'twin shocks' of the EVD epidemic and a sharp drop in iron ore prices have 'dealt a severe blow' to this dependent economy.[27] What growth has been achieved has done little to generate a sustainable tax base that could underpin an expansionary state agenda and Sierra Leone remains acutely dependent on external resources, which account for 80% of gross national income and reflect more than double the amount of annual government expenditures.[28]

Furthermore, Mkandawire argues that it is not simply the presence of growth alone that confirms Africa's 'rise', and that we should remain critical of the kinds of economic growth that are taking in place, particularly when these exacerbates vast inequalities and social stress.[29] Despite rapid economic growth in Sierra Leone, any notion that this has 'trickled down' to the poorest in society is highly questionable. Sierra Leone continues to have some of the worst development statistics in the world and glaring social inequalities. 53% of the population were living below the poverty line in 2011 and this was particularly acute in rural areas, at 66%. It ranks close to the bottom of the Human Development Index (HDI), which assesses long-term progress in living a long and healthy life, access to knowledge and a decent standard of living. 77% of the population are living in multidimensional poverty, in that they experience multiple deprivations in education, health and standard of living.[30] Furthermore, rural populations, the poor, youth and women bore the brunt of the negative implications of externally supported neoliberal Structural Adjustment Programmes (SAPs).[31]

While relations of global dependency have undoubtedly contributed to Sierra Leone's enduring political and social crisis, we should nonetheless be careful not to overlook or downplay the manner in which African elites have participated in the processes which have inserted African societies as dependent partners in the global economy, as well as the manner in which the prominence of patron–client relations have exacerbated inequalities within these societies themselves.[32] Harris argues that, from the outset, the under-resourced colonial state was forced to forge linkages with traditional institutions such as the chieftaincy and to distribute the resources of the new state as a form of patronage in exchange for their loyalty.[33] Indeed, authors have long observed the distribution of public goods in Sierra Leone within private networks of political patronage and how this has remained an enduring feature of elite survival strategies since independence.[34] Reno argues that these patrimonial networks have remained essential to the exercise of power by the postcolonial elites through what he describes as the 'shadow state': a dense collection of 'informal commercially orientated networks' between global and local actors which operate alongside official government bureaucracies and formal state structures.[35] Indeed, a ubiquitous feature of Sierra Leonean politics – like that of so many African states – has been entrenched structural violence in which livelihoods are premised upon the quality of access to these private, informal channels of resource and opportunity distribution, controlled by a coterie of gatekeepers strategically placed within the parallel realms of the authority of the state bureaucracy and traditional institutions like the chieftaincy.[36]

By the early 1990s this form of gatekeeper politics had become increasingly volatile. Economic decline and endemic corruption generated a crisis for the state as the resources available for patronage networks began to dry up.[37] The state elites responded by assuming an increasingly predatory and violent posture in relation to the wider population, while the state's retreat from offering even basic social services to the population magnified existing social exclusion, generating resistance and, eventually, rebellion.[38]

By the time the war ended in 2002, the country's already weak infrastructure and governmental capacity had been decimated. International attention was focused on Sierra Leone's post-conflict reconstruction, making it a 'test laboratory' for liberal peace building.[39] However, the economy is still heavily dependent on the outside world and on the relatively small incomes it receives from the enclave extraction of minerals and, as discussed above, little has been achieved to address this. Despite intensified liberal interventions promoting greater accountability and anti-corruption campaigns, political elites have proved remarkably adept at balancing donor demands for good governance and neoliberal reforms with the political prerogative of managing access to donor resources to further their political survival.[40] According to Transparency International, Sierra Leone was ranked 119 out of 175 territories and countries and scored 31 out of 100 in the Corruption Perceptions Index (2014), based on data from expert and business surveys.[41] Meanwhile, donors have supported the state's attempts to re-establish the powers of the traditional authorities (particularly the paramount chiefs) as part of efforts to promote the decentralisation of authority and encourage local accountability. While these traditional authorities enjoy a degree of legitimacy among Sierra Leoneans, there are widespread concerns that they will continue to play the role of local gatekeepers whose discretionary control over access to resources and opportunities can reproduce social exclusion for those not included within their networks of patronage.[42]

This brief account of Sierra Leone's political and economic fortunes therefore offers little to support the celebratory tone of the 'Africa rising' commentary. Instead, it offers an insight into a particularly acute manifestation of the recurrent crises of the gatekeeper state. The concern for the rest of this paper is how this contributed not only to the weakness of the state, and the consequent weakness of the country's health system, but also to the structural violence experienced by its population, which enabled the virus to spread so rapidly.

A dependent health system in crisis

In 2012 the WHO offered an optimistic outlook for Sierra Leone's health system, arguing that 'macroeconomic stability and economic growth will help reduce poverty, increase equity and enable the Government of Sierra Leone to allocate additional resources to the health sector'.[43] However, once again, the limitations of this *a priori* assumption that economic growth would necessarily contribute to improving health provision are revealed when one analyses the enduring symptoms of the gatekeeper state crisis in Sierra Leone and the impacts this has on the health sector.

First, the health sector is acutely dependent on external aid. In 2007 78% of resources were derived from external sources, with US$12.9 million (42%) coming from the UK's Department for International Development (DfID). The other key donors include the Global Fund, World Bank, Asian Development Bank and United Nations Population Fund (UNFPA). Despite the 15% pledged by the Abuja Declaration, the Ministry of Health and Sanitation (MoHS) receives only 8% of the government's budget. Core health initiatives, such as the government's Free Healthcare Initiative (FHCI) to address maternal and infant health, are heavily dependent on external funding in the absence of sufficient government resources. The FHCI attracted considerable external resources: 87% of the estimated $$35 million cost was funded by the development partners.[44]

As a result of this dependency, the government's control over the health sector is severely compromised, as is its ability to set and coordinate a coherent health agenda at the national level. The government is influenced by the 'swinging pendulum' of the constantly shifting priorities of the international donors,[45] and has to remain malleable to embracing externally defined health agendas, including the Alma Ata Declaration, the Ouagadougou Declaration, the Millennium Development Goals and the IMF/World Bank PRSPs. Donors have promoted decentralisation and anti-corruption campaigns as a way of combating the misuse of funds in the health sector and increasing accountability.[46] Meanwhile, NGOs often attempt to circumvent the state because of fears over corruption by funding and delivering individual projects according to their own priorities. This has led to the fermentation of multiple parallel health systems, some funded and managed through the government and others run by traditional healers, faith-based organisations, international and local NGOs and also civil society organisations, which are often entirely reliant on either external funds or on collecting private service fees. For example, Gavi, the global Vaccine Alliance for creating equal access to new and underused vaccines, represents another major funder in the health sector since 2001, with $23.2 million of direct funding for vaccines and $4.1 million of cash-based support including for Immunisation Services Support (ISS) since 2001 and Health Systems Strengthening (HSS) from 2008.[47] Despite the suspension of Gavi funding channelled through the state in 2012 as a result of fears about corruption, considered further below, Gavi itself continued to provide vaccines through alternative supply mechanisms and, in other instances, DfID directly funded health workers' salaries rather than channelling assistance through the government.[48] These parallel structures of health care management and delivery have generated complexity and in some cases dysfunction, draining time and resources and reducing the capacity for oversight. For example, the Ministry of Health's 'National Health Sector Strategic Plan' identified 'weak sector coordination structures and arrangements at all levels' between health service providers, 'weak public private partnership (PPP) in the provision of comprehensive integrated health services' and 'weak mechanisms for public accountability.'[49] The government reports that a lack of harmonisation leads to 'fragmented individual projects', unpredictability, duplication and a general lack of accountability.[50] Amnesty International has also reported on the problems these parallel health systems present, arguing that 'the lack of monitoring and oversight within the system has created a context where corruption can flourish.'[51]

Second, as Brown notes, while the power imbalance between donors and African elites in office can severely curtail the state's autonomous control over policy, it is important to understand that this does not mean the entire 'politico-legal independence' of the state is being challenged.[52] Instead, we have to examine the manner in which state actors compensate for their limited power by navigating and even exploiting their external dependency, what Bayart refers to as the 'strategies of extraversion' – putting on a show of compliance with external agendas in order to preserve the flow of resources into the country.[53] African state and non-state actors can play up their situations of dependence, problems and poverty as leverage for attracting resources.[54]

In this respect, even though the capacity for autonomous policy action and initiatives in the health sector is restricted by external agendas, rent-seeking opportunities are abundant. This is because considerable amounts of resources are directed into the health sector. For example, international concerns with 'HIV exceptionalism' generated much donor attention and funding for HIV/AIDS prevention and care (despite the low, stable prevalence) at the expense of tackling more pressing health challenges. In response, the Sierra Leonean government (and some citizens) exaggerated this presentation of the country as one suffering from HIV in order to preserve this lucrative flow of resources for their own benefit.[55] At the same time the complexity of health care provision undermines accountability by limiting processes for monitoring and evaluation. It is also, of course, a sector which is too significant to fail, and a complete cessation of funding would be politically unfeasible for donors. This has generated some high-profile corruption scandals. For example, in March 2010 the former minister of health, Sheiku Tejan Koroma, was convicted of abuse of office, abuse of position and failure to comply with procurement procedures.[56] Even this seeming crackdown presented an opportunity in itself. With respect to the indictment of the minister in 2009, a cable from Freetown to the Economic Community of West African States (ECOWAS) suggests it was a strategy of extraversion:

> Sources told the Political Section that Koroma's indictment appears deliberately timed to make a good impression on the donors before the Consultative Group meeting. According to several contacts, the ACC presented the indictment to the Attorney General (AG), who buried it for two months before it was moved forward in the court.[57]

Corruption and rent-seeking are not the preserve of state elites with global connections alone, however. It is important to understand corruption as a multi-scaled phenomenon and that the gateways to resources extend well beyond the confines of the internationally recognised capital city. Reflecting the findings of studies elsewhere in Africa,[58] ordinary health professionals will navigate the aid industry in order to secure the most lucrative returns available to them, often at the expense of the strength of the health system. It is reported, for example, that the issue of low salaries encourages health workers to seek informal increments to their wages, such as by charging patients illicit fees. This may undermine new initiatives. As part of the new FHCI project to offer basic health services without charges, President Ernest Bai Koroma announced plans to tackle this issue directly, declaring that: 'Our doctors and nurses have been underpaid and overworked. As a consequence, it became a common practice for health workers to charge vulnerable patients inappropriately to make up for their inadequate salaries.'[59] Nonetheless, the FHCI was severely undermined by the persistence of rent-seeking by health practitioners, who continued to supplement their meagre salaries through the illegal sale of medicines and health services that were now supposed to be free.[60]

Indeed, bureaucratic positions within the health sector offer health administrators a gate-keeping role through their control over access to resources and opportunities. This can provoke a range of corrupt, rent-seeking behaviour, including the creation of long lists of 'phantom workers' connected to the gatekeeper, who claim salaries but who do not actually work in the health sector. In other cases we can see the manipulation of resource flows, such as the hiring of sub-contractors personally connected to health administrators for work in the health sector who subsequently over-charge for their work or fail to complete it.[61] While donors often threaten to withdraw funding in the face of this rent-seeking, it is extremely difficult to hold those responsible to account. For example, in 2012, the Gavi cash-based support was suspended after an external audit of the HSS programme. The MoHS was required to reimburse half a million dollars of misused funds, including for undocumented expenditure on training and workshops, overcharging for procurements (with three ambulances purchased for 80% higher than justifiable) and the misappropriation of at least 14 motorcycles intended for peripheral health units.[62] Funding from Gavi and DfID was subsequently suspended and was only resumed once the 'Billiongate' trial of the 29 public officials implicated in the misuse of the health systems funds commenced in March 2013. Ultimately, however, the trial illustrated the toothless nature of anti-corruption reforms and the capacity of political elites to resist pressures for greater accountability. Of the 29 accused, only two physicians were convicted in the High Court. Crucially the key public officials were acquitted, including the Chief Medical Officer, the Director of Primary Health Care, the Programme Manager Productive Health, the Director of Human Resources and Nurses Services, and the Permanent Secretary of the MoHS.[63] This was in spite of indirect evidence of large houses and expensive cars that were not consistent with official salaries, as well as kickbacks from suppliers.[64]

In summary, the acute dependence on external funding in the health sector undermines the state's control over its health policy and the multiplicity of donor agendas has generated a complex array of parallel health systems. Meanwhile, the volume of resources, combined with lack of accountability in the health sector provides rent-seeking opportunities for gate-keepers in positions of authority, which has exacerbated the weakness of the health system. These two trends have important consequences for containing the EVD epidemic.

Ebola and strategies of extraversion

When international attention focused on EVD – particularly with the fear of the threat it posed to the West – an influx of resources into the health sector followed, providing lucrative opportunities for rent-seeking and corruption. The government of Sierra Leone spent over Le84 billion ($20.7 million) in response to the outbreak and appealed to donors for support. The European Union duly pledged over €1 billion from March until November 2014, the European Commission provided over €350 million for humanitarian development and research funds,[65] the UK £205 million,[66] and the Gates Foundation provided $50 million. The government established the National Ebola Response Centre (NERC) and a Health Emergency Account for all donations and appropriations to finance the response.[67]

The regular 'Ebola Outbreak Updates' on the MoHS website and Facebook page (established in April 2014) were designed to offer greater transparency to a distrustful population but also to make direct appeals to external donors. Over time this included the 'important note' at the end of the update with the Emergency Account Details and an appeal for direct cash transfers from those willing to help. Similarly appeals were made from other sections of society for increased resources from outside. The *Sierra Leone Telegraph*, for example, directly appealed to global philanthropy in a piece entitled 'Ebola strikes first female doctor in Sierra Leone – appeal to Bill Gates for help':

> Please Mr Bill Gates and Mrs Miranda Gates [sic], help our doctor, sister, mother, colleague and friend, help Sierra Leone. We need 300,000 Euros to fly Dr Buck out of Sierra Leone and to pay for her treatment in Hamburg![68]

It has been widely reported that large proportions of the funding to combat EVD were siphoned off and misappropriated by a range of actors.[69] The government's auditors concede that 'Monies that have been set aside for the purpose of combating the Ebola outbreak may have been used for unintended purposes, thereby slowing the government's response to eradicate the virus'.[70] Throughout the epidemic the government has encountered problems with 'ghost workers' on its Ebola staff payrolls, with some people forging identities or claiming for payments twice. A government spokesperson complains that 'the issue of ghost workers has been disingenuous on the part of some Sierra Leoneans who think this is time to make money when we are in a crisis'.[71] The *Guardian* also reported that:

> Residents, journalists and an official told *The Guardian* that trucks carrying food aid were sometimes parked outside quarantine cordons, which intended recipients couldn't cross. The food was then looted by those meant to be distributing it. Burial teams have repeatedly gone on strike over unpaid hazard allowances.[72]

Indeed, Transparency International highlighted the fact that the 'Systemic corruption in the health sector in West Africa hurt the response to the Ebola epidemic'.[73] An in-depth 'Report on the audit of the management of the Ebola funds' by Sierra Leone's Auditor General for May to October 2014 catalogues a series of issues with the way government money was spent, including large payments and withdrawals of over Le14 billion ($3.5 million) made from the Emergency Health Response and Miscellaneous Accounts 'without *any* supporting documents to substantiate the utilisation of such funds' (emphasis in the original); a 'complete disregard for the law' during the public procurement of contractors and service providers to help contain EVD, meaning that the price paid was often overly inflated and poorly accounted for; the duplication of payments to politicians for their work communicating to their constituents about EVD; illegitimate claims by police and armed forces for hazard payments from hospitals; Le26 billion ($6.4 million) paid out for healthcare workers' 'incentives' not accounted for; poorly documented loans granted where 'concern' was expressed that these were being received by individuals and not the charities combating EVD; and the withholding of Le525 million ($130,000) tax payments by suppliers and contractors. Following the audit the ACC commenced its investigations and identified 39 individuals, who included high-profile public officials required to report to them in relation to the management of funds and associated issues.[74]

The opportunities generated by the surge in external resources being channelled into Sierra Leone's health sector during the EVD epidemic thus reflected what might be characterised as a windfall moment within the context of an extended, recurrent crisis of the gatekeeper state. Access to the gateway of resources was suddenly and dramatically widened and extended to a range of individuals who, as best they could, sought to 'do well' out of the crisis. This windfall event was particularly conducive to rent-seeking behaviour because the rubric of crisis necessitated an urgency which over-stretched an already weak state capacity to enforce accountability. However, we should not crudely dismiss this as some sort of uniquely 'African' moral aberration. First, the vast majority of Sierra Leoneans who engaged in efforts to contain EVD did so with great courage and at considerable personal risk, with little or no prospect of material reward. Second, to understand rent-seeking behaviour we need to focus on the political economy of 'everyday corruption' in Africa.[75] In a situation where poverty and inequalities are vast and opportunities scarce, rent-seeking can be an integral feature of livelihoods strategies and, as Harris notes, in Sierra Leone 'nepotism, diversion of resources and low levels of productivity can be explained by workers with moral communal obligations…to those they support and loyalties…to those who orchestrated their post in the first place'.[76]

Structural violence in a predatory state

The recurrent political crises exacerbate structural violence by reproducing a 'semi-permanent state of exclusion'[77] in Sierra Leone. Those able to successfully navigate patronage networks for their own benefit may profit from them (albeit to varying degrees), while those excluded from access to resources have severely diminished opportunities (particularly the youth, rural population and women). The EVD laid bare the violence and exclusionary nature of the country's gatekeeper politics: where it disproportionately affected certain segments of society, it highlighted the existing social, economic and cultural patterns of exclusion.[78]

One aspect of this exclusion relates to gender. Women are a resource within neoliberal development: their unpaid labour mitigates the impact of Structural Adjustment and they become 'shock absorbers' in times of crisis.[79] In Sierra Leone women's unpaid labour in the care economy fills the gaps in the health system and women have taken on much of the burden of care in the EVD outbreak. This has direct implications for their risk of contracting EVD and yet, as Harman argues, women are 'conspicuously invisible' in much of the commentary on EVD, which obscures their multiple roles.[80]

Another aspect is the entrenched rural–urban divide, which is crucial to understanding the state's failure to respond effectively to contain the initial outbreak. The rural–urban cleavages are rooted in the legacies of the government's 'urban bias' policies, which were intended to stimulate development but 'became a mechanism for the transfer of resources from rural peasants to the country's elite'.[81] These structural inequalities were exacerbated by external interventions: the rural poor were disproportionately disadvantaged by the introduction of user fees for health services because they pay disproportionately more for health care as compared to wealthier households in terms of the percentage of their incomes.[82] Even with the FHCI there were challenges in terms of accessing health care facilities in rural areas and, as we have already discussed, illicit costs for services that should be free. This has implications for containing EVD in rural areas. Farmer's observations during the outbreak reveal the dearth of health centres in rural areas.

> In Zwedru, we visited the Grand Gedeh's only hospital. Although there have been stories of doctors and nurses fleeing their posts, the fact is that many remain. But without personal protective equipment or other supplies, there isn't a lot they can do…In Ziah Town, a small village a couple of hours away, we met some community health workers…They were the front line in the struggle against Ebola, the ones who could bring information and services to the rural poor. But they were isolated and badly equipped.[83]

The real momentum to respond to the outbreak came with the shift in the infections from the East to the West of the country and the spread to urban areas. As Batty highlights, this laid bare deep mistrust between rural Sierra Leoneans and the government, including the widely held assumptions that the response to the crisis was politically driven:

> Many wonder if the virus would have been approached differently if it had emerged in the northwest, where most of the senior [ruling party] APC officials, including the president, call 'home'. Indeed, only as the disease crossed from the southeast into other parts of the country did the crisis response intensify and the government finally enlist the help of the international community to help fight Ebola.[84]

Exclusion and isolation has engendered what the UN Development Programme (UNDP) describes as a 'pervasive distrust of politics',[85] which had important consequences for the EVD epidemic.[86] Government messages telling people how to recognise and avoid the disease, to go to hospital for treatment and about safe burial practices were largely ignored by the local populations. There were also reportedly fears among the local populations that the government and aid agencies were intentionally spreading the virus and that the government wanted to sell patients' blood or use limbs for rituals, which prompted a lack of cooperation with medical teams.[87] In addition, there were public perceptions of corruption surrounding EVD and conspiracy theories circulating that the virus was a government ruse to bring in donations,[88] or that so-called 'eastbola' was a strategy to depopulate the East of the country, which is the power-base of the opposition.[89] Lind and Ndebe note that the EVD epidemic has thus 'unmasked persisting deep public suspicion and mistrust of the state, laying bare the limits of post-conflict reconstruction to transform state–society relations'. They argue that the response has exacerbated social exclusion because 'quarantines, aggressive policing, closed borders and other restrictions on people's movements, hark back to military controls deployed during the region's long wars, thereby further eroding trust and confidence in public authorities'.[90]

Despite the civil war ending, Sierra Leone is not at peace in the broadest sense. Structural violence shifts our gaze to the 'everyday violence' of the enduring, lived reality of 'small wars and invisible genocides' that are a normalised feature of post-war West Africa.[91] Ultimately the EVD epidemic was not simply a medical crisis but an infection that spread along the fault lines of the injustice generated by recurring political crises and deeply rooted structural violence.

Conclusion: a way forward?

Now that the immediate task of containing the virus has almost been achieved, the EVD epidemic is argued to constitute an 'opportunity' for a serious rethink of how global health risks can be dealt with more effectively in future. On the one hand, UK Prime Minister David Cameron worked with US President Barrack Obama to table a resolution to the WHO, which called for the formation of a 'global health emergency workforce' that could respond to future epidemics and which would be 'composed of comprehensive emergency medical response teams that can be deployed effectively and quickly with adequate resources'. The WHO Secretariat subsequently proposed this initiative as part of a wider reconfiguration of the international community's capacity to intervene in health emergencies.[92] On the other hand, it is recognised that building resilient health systems requires much more than material resources. The WHO recognises in its rethinking of the 'key principles' of building health system resilience in the aftermath of the EVD outbreak that this includes the coordination of development partners' work; building each country's core capacities to 'detect, report and respond to public health emergencies'; enhancing 'community trust, engagement and ownership'; and reducing the financial costs of accessing health services. Its report also called for more 'predictable' financial support for health systems that should not affect the country's debt burdens.[93]

However, at its core, the prevailing emphasis on building health system 'resilience' as a means of facilitating the effective containment of future epidemics reflects a fundamental shortcoming in both the *political understanding* and *political ambition* needed to build stronger, inclusive health systems. It is not simply the case that the main actors are unaware of these political dynamics, and it is likely that there are political reasons that they have to focus on the technical 'resilience-building' approach. Since the end of the civil war we have witnessed a hybrid form of liberal peace building in Sierra Leone, informed to a large extent by an emerging mentality of 'make do and mend' among donors. The emphasis is placed on the need to reign in liberal expectations and settle for 'good enough governance' or 'second best solutions'.[94] This involves the continued promotion of liberal institutions but also the belief that the success of the project is premised upon securing popular legitimacy for these institutions, not least the 'buy-in' of local power brokers. In Sierra Leone this includes the resurrection of illiberal institutions such as the chieftaincy which, paradoxically, has been a focal point of societal tension throughout its history but also commands a degree of popular legitimacy that liberal state institutions might not.[95] It has also meant an awkward embrace of the idea of working 'with the grain' of the logics of patron–client networks by identifying individuals in state authority who can be worked with to drive through change, and directing authority and resources towards them, even if this does not preclude, and could even exacerbate, ongoing patronage politics. This hybrid liberal project offers little to challenge the structural inequity of the global system that entrenches the external dependency and enclave economic activity contributing to the weakness of the state in the first place. Moreover, Harris notes that the tensions generated by this donor-driven hybrid approach are 'abundantly clear' and that elites have displayed remarkable dexterity in their capacity to adjust to the 'ever-evolving calculation' of how to balance external demands for reform with their political prerogative of maintaining power through dispensing patronage.[96] Labonte argues that this reproduces social exclusion by leaving non-elites with little option other than to navigate 'between liberal and illiberal governance institutions to accrue the kinds of public goods, justice and/or other necessities they need to survive'.[97]

This structural violence generated by the patched-up post-war political status quo in Sierra Leone has a debilitating impact on the health system and is acutely highlighted by the EVD epidemic. A less ambitious project of building health systems 'resilience' around the status quo therefore does little to address the more fundamental structural transformation required to build more inclusive and socially just health systems in future. Such a project would require a much broader conversation about HSS and an ambition to address a range of interconnected issues, including Sierra Leone's dependent position in the world economy and its reliance on mineral exports; the need for a sustained redistribution of global wealth to underpin an expansionary state programme for the sectors fundamental to the health system, in particular higher education and health infrastructure; measures to decrease the 'brain drain' of skilled medical staff by ending externally promoted austerity measures that limit medical staff salaries; and ending user fees for medical services and medicines. This is by no means an exhaustive list. It nonetheless seeks to illuminate the kinds of wider conversations that would be needed to shift away from the emerging agenda of building coping mechanisms and health systems 'resilience' towards a long-term, more ambitious agenda of HSS through tackling some of the great challenges posed by the recurrent crises of the gatekeeper state and the injustice it reproduces.

Disclosure statement

No potential conflict of interest was reported by the authors.

Acknowledgements

The authors would like to thank the anonymous reviewers for their comments. We also appreciate the feedback we received on earlier versions from the participants at the events on the Ebola outbreak at the Universities of Leeds, York and Sussex, as well as from the Global Health scholars at the BISA Conference, 2015.

Notes

1. WHO, *Building Resilient Health Systems*, 1.
2. WHO, *Ebola Situation Reports*.
3. See WHO, *World Health Statistics*; WHO, "Sierra Leone"; and WHO Regional Office for Africa, "African Health Workforce Observatory."
4. World Bank, http://data.worldbank.org/country/sierra-leone.

5. James Gallagher, "Ebola Vaccine is 'Potential Game-changer.'" BBC, July 31, 2015. http://www.bbc.co.uk/news/health-33733711.
6. WHO, *Building Resilient Health Systems*, 1 (our italics).
7. MSF, "Ebola."
8. Kieny, *Ebola and Health Systems*; Kim, "What Ebola Taught the World"; and Cairns, *Ebola is Still Here*, 2.
9. See Wilkinson and Leach, "Briefing"; and Lind and Ndebe, "Return of the Rebel."
10. See, for example, Lavelle, "Moving in from the Periphery."
11. Harman and Brown, "In from the Margins?," 71. See also Death, "Introduction," 1; Brown, "A Question of Agency"; and Chabal, and Daloz, *Africa Works*, 142.
12. Cooper, *Africa since 1940*, 157.
13. Harris, *Sierra Leone*.
14. Galtung, "Violence, Peace, and Peace Research."
15. Cooper, *Africa since 1940*, 157.
16. Beresford, "Power, Patronage and Gatekeeper Politics," 229.
17. Ibid., 226.
18. Ibid; and Erdmann and Engel, "Neopatrimonialism Reconsidered."
19. Severino and Ray, *Africa's Moment*.
20. World Bank, *Global Economic Prospects*, 14.
21. GoSL, *Agenda for Prosperity*, xi; and GoSL, *Agenda for Change*, xx.
22. World Bank, *International Development Association…Country Assistance Strategy*, 1.
23. Taylor, "Why Africa is not Rising."
24. Zack-Williams, "Sierra Leone," 22.
    IMF, "IMF Executive Board."
25. IMF, *Sierra Leone*, 4.
26. IMF, "Sierra Leone gets $102 Million."
27. Ibid.
28. Kaldor with Vincent, *Evaluation*, 4.
29. Mkandawire, "Can Africa turn from Recovery?," 171.
30. UNDP, *Human Development Report*, 2–3.
31. Zack-Williams, "Sierra Leone."
32. Bayart, "Africa in the World," 220.
33. Bøås, "Liberia and Sierra Leone."
34. Luke, "The Politics of Economic Decline."
35. Reno, *Corruption and State Politics*, 4.
36. Fanthorpe, "On the Limits of Liberal Peace."
37. Richards, *Fighting for the Rainforest*.
38. Ibid.
39. Harris, *Sierra Leone*.
40. Bøås, "Liberia and Sierra Leone."
41. Transparency International, *Corruption Perceptions Index*.
42. For discussion, see Fanthorpe, "On the Limits of Liberal Peace."
43. Africa Health Observatory, http://www.aho.afro.who.int/profiles_information/index.php/Sierra_Leone:Health_financing_system.
44. Ibid.
45. Lee, "The Pit and the Pendulum."
46. Labonte, "From Patronage to Peacebuilding?," 91.
47. Gavi Alliance, *Sierra Leone*, 4.
48. "British Aid Money to Sierra Leone Investigated after Claims of Misuse." *Huffington Post*, April 15, 2013. http://www.huffingtonpost.co.uk/2013/04/15/sierra-leone-aid-money_n_3083057.html.
49. GoSL, *National Health Sector Strategic Plan*, 14.
50. GoSL, *Health Compact*, 4.
51. Amnesty International, *At a Crossroads*, 17.
52. Brown, "Sovereignty Matters," 262.

53. Bayart, "Africa in the World."
54. Ellis, *Season of Rains*.
55. Benton, *HIV Exceptionalism*.
56. ACC, "Monitoring Court Report."
57. Wikileaks, "Minister of Health Indicted."
58. Kingsley, "NGOs, Doctors, and the Patrimonial State."
59. Cited in Yates, *Insight*.
60. Adam Nossiter, "Sierra Leone's Health Care System becomes a Cautionary Tale for Donors." *New York Times*, April 13, 2013. http://www.nytimes.com/2013/04/14/world/africa/sierra-leone-graft-charges-imperil-care-and-aid.html?pagewanted=all&_r=0.
61. Donnelly, "How did Sierra Leone?," 1396.
62. Gavi Alliance, *Sierra Leone*, 5–6, 22.
63. ACC, "News – ACC Indicts"; and ACC, "News – High Court Acquits."
64. Nossiter, "Sierra Leone's Health Care System."
65. European Commission, "Ebola Response."
66. Monica Mark, "Sierra Leone: Journalist Arrested after Questioning Official Ebola Response." *Guardian*, November 5, 2014. http://www.theguardian.com/world/2014/nov/05/ebola-journalist-arrested-over-criticism-sierra-leone-government-response.
67. Audit Service Sierra Leone, *Report on the Audit*.
68. "Ebola strikes first Female Doctor in Sierra Leone." *Sierra Leone Telegraph*, September 11, 2014. http://www.thesierraleonetelegraph.com/?p=7352.
69. Hitchen, "Mismanagement." In the press, see for example, Lisa O'Carroll, "Sierra Leone investigates alleged Misuse of Emergency Ebola Funds." *The Guardian*, February 17, 2015. http://www.theguardian.com/world/2015/feb/17/sierra-leone-investigates-alleged-misuse-of-emergency-ebola-funds; O'Carroll, "A Third of Sierra Leone's Ebola Budget unaccounted for says Report." *Guardian*, February 16, 2015. http://www.theguardian.com/world/2015/feb/16/ebola-sierra-leone-budget-report; and BBC, "Sierra Leone Audit claims Ebola Funds unaccounted For." BBC, February 13, 2015. http://www.bbc.co.uk/news/world-africa-31461564.
70. Audit Service Sierra Leone, *Report on the Audit*, 6.
71. Emma Farge, "Sierra Leone to prosecute Fraudulent Ebola 'Ghostworkers.'" Reuters, February 10, 2015. http://www.reuters.com/article/2015/02/10/us-health-ebola-fraud-idUSKBN0LE2M920150210.
72. Mark, "Sierra Leone."
73. Transparency International, *Ebola*.
74. ACC, "Public Notice," i.
75. Blundo and De Sardan, *Everyday Corruption*.
76. Harris, *Sierra Leone*, 156.
77. Bøås, "Liberia and Sierra Leone," 697–698; and Beresford, "Power, Patronage and Gatekeeper Politics," 226.
78. Baylies, "Cultural Hazards," 71; and Anderson, *Gender, Risk and HIV*. On Ebola, see Diggins and Mills, "The Pathology."
79. Moser, "Gender Planning."
80. Harman, "Ebola, Gender and Conspicuously Invisible Women."
81. Riddell, "Sierra Leone," 118.
82. Fabricant et al., "Why the Poor."
83. Farmer, "Diary."
84. Batty, "Reinventing 'Others.'"
85. Kaldor with Vincent, *Evaluation*, 4.
86. Oxfam International, "Mistrust and Confusion."
87. "Ebola in West Africa: Death and Disbelievers." *The Economist*, August 2, 2014. http://www.economist.com/news/middle-east-and-africa/21610250-many-sierra-leoneans-refuse-take-advice-medical-experts-ebola-death.
88. Wilkinson and Leach, "Briefing," 9.
89. "Ebola in West Africa"; and Batty, "Reinventing 'Others.'"

90. Lind and Ndebe, "Return of the Rebel," 3.
91. Scheper-Hughes, *Death without Weeping*.
92. WHO, *Ensuring WHO's Capacity*.
93. WHO, *Building Resilient Health Systems*, 2.
94. Harris, *Sierra Leone*, 157.
95. Fanthorpe, "On the Limits of Liberal Peace."
96. See Harris, *Sierra Leone*, 156.
97. Labonte, "From Patronage to Peacebuilding?," 114–115.

Bibliography

Amnesty International. *At a Crossroads: Sierra Leone's Free Health Care Policy*. London: Amnesty International, 2011. https://www.amnestyusa.org/sites/default/files/pdfs/sierral_maternaltrpt_0.pdf.

Anderson, Emma-Louise. *Gender, Risk and HIV: Navigating Structural Violence*. Basingstoke: Palgrave Macmillan, 2015.

Anti-Corruption Commission (ACC). "Public Notice in Respect of Ebola Funds." Freetown, February 17, 2015. http://www.anticorruption.gov.sl/show_news.php?id=462#sthash.zlr788lW.dpuf.

ACC. "Monitoring Court Report 31st March–1st April, 2015." Freetown, April 2015. http://www.anticorruption.gov.sl/index.php?p=102&pn=Concluded%20Criminal%20Cases.

ACC. "News – High Court acquits Dr Kizito Daoh and Four Others of Corruption Offences." Freetown, October 28, 2013. http://www.anticorruption.gov.sl/show_news.php?id=271.

ACC. "News – ACC indicts 7 Medical Practitioners and 22 Others for Various Offences relating to the Misuse of Gavi Funds and the 2011 Audit Service Report Findings." Freetown, March 7, 2013. http://www.anticorruption.gov.sl/show_news.php?id=188.

Audit Service Sierra Leone. *Report on the Audit of the Management of the Ebola Funds – May to October 2014*. Freetown, October 31, 2014. https://afrosai-e.org.za/sites/afrosai-e.org.za/files/report-files/assl-report-on-ebola-funds-management-may-oct-2014.pdf.

Batty, Fodei. "Reinventing 'Others' in a Time of Ebola." *Cultural Anthropology Online*, October 7, 2014. http://www.culanth.org/fieldsights/589-reinventing-others-in-a-time-of-ebola.

Bayart, Jean-François. "Africa in the World." *African Affairs* 99, no. 395 (2000): 217–267. doi:10.1093/afraf/99.395.183.

Baylies, Carolyn. "Cultural Hazards facing Young People in the Era of HIV/AIDS." In *The Political Economy of AIDS in Africa*, edited by Alan Whiteside and Nana Poku, 71–84. Aldershot: Ashgate, 2004.

Benton, Adia. *HIV Exceptionalism: Development through Disease in Sierra Leone*. Minneapolis: University of Minnesota Press, 2015.

Beresford, Alexander. "Power, Patronage and Gatekeeper Politics in South Africa." *African Affairs* 114, no. 455 (2015): 226–248. doi: 10.1093/afraf/adu083.

Blundo, Giorgio, and Olvier De Sardan. *Everyday Corruption and the State in Africa*. London: Zed Books, 2006.

Bøås, Morten. "Liberia and Sierra Leone – Dead Ringers?" *Third World Quarterly* 22, no. 5 (2001): 697–723. doi:10.1080/01436590120084566.

Brown, William. "A Question of Agency." *Third World Quarterly* 33, no. 10 (2012): 1889–1908. doi:10.1080/01436597.2012.728322.

Brown, William. "Sovereignty Matters: Africa, Donors and the Aid Relationship." *African Affairs* 112, no. 447 (2013): 262–282. doi:10.1093/afraf/adt001.

Cairns, Edmund. *Ebola is Still Here*. Oxford: Oxfam International, February 2015. http://policy-practice.oxfam.org.uk/publications/ebola-is-still-here-voices-from-liberia-and-sierra-leone-on-response-and-recove-345644?cid=em_LKET_0215.

Chabal, Patrick, and Jean-Pascal Daloz. *Africa Works*. Bloomington: Indiana University Press, 1999.

Cooper, Frederick. *Africa since 1940: The Past of the Present*. Cambridge: Cambridge University Press, 2002.

Diggins, Jennifer, and Elizabeth Mills. "The Pathology of Inequality: Gender and Ebola in West Africa." *IDS Practice Paper in Brief* 23 (2015). http://opendocs.ids.ac.uk/opendocs/handle/123456789/5856#.VjjJ1KpOdBl.

Death, Carl. "Introduction: Africa's International Relations." *African Affairs* adv041 (2015): 1–6. doi: 10.1093/afraf/adv041.

Donnelly, John. "How did Sierra Leone provide Free Health Care?" *Lancet* 377, no. 9775 (2011): 1393–1396. doi:10.1016/S0140-6736(11)60559-X.

Ellis, Stephen. *Season of Rains: Africa in the World.* Chicago, IL: University of Chicago Press, 2011.

Erdmann, Gero, and Ulf Engel. "Neopatrimonialism Reconsidered." *Commonwealth and Comparative Politics* 45, no. 1 (2007): 95–119. doi:10.1080/14662040601135813.

European Commission. "Ebola Response: EU scales up Aid with Planes, Material Aid and Research Support." Press release, November 6, 2014. http://europa.eu/rapid/press-release_IP-14-1462_en.htm.

Fabricant, Stephen J., Clifford W. Kamara, and Anne Mills. "Why the Poor pay More: Household Curative Expenditures in Rural Sierra Leone." *International Journal of Health Planning and Management* 14 (1999): 179–199. doi:10.1002/(SICI)1099-1751(199907/09).

Fanthorpe, Richard. "On the Limits of Liberal Peace." *African Affairs* 105, no. 418 (2006): 27–49. doi:10.1093/afraf/adi091.

Farmer, Paul. "Diary." *London Review of Books,* October 23, 2014, 38–39. http://www.lrb.co.uk/v36/n20/paul-farmer/diary.

Galtung, Johan. "Violence, Peace, and Peace Research." *Journal of Peace Research* 6, no. 3 (1969): 167–191. doi:10.1177/002234336900600301.

Gavi Alliance. *Sierra Leone: Audit of Health Systems Strengthening (HSS) Support Disbursed in the Period 2008–2010.* Geneva, April 2013. http://www.google.co.uk/url?sa=t&rct=j&q=&esrc=s&source=web&cd=1&ved=0CCEQFjAA&url=http%3A%2F%2Fwww.gavi.org%2Flibrary%2Fgavi-documents%2Flegal%2Faudit-report–sierra-leone—april-2013%2F&ei=vg1iVPDuNpXasASp1IDgBQ&usg=AFQjCNGfG8s62qlHldQ2vjU0jkJtQ8VQvw&sig2=r3YQ7Inq-Jj02KnSTzgflA&bvm=bv.79189006,d.cWc.

Government of Sierra Leone (GoSL). *Agenda for Change (2008-2012).* Freetown: GoSL, 2008. http://unipsil.unmissions.org/portals/unipsil/media/publications/agenda_for_change.pdf.

GoSL. *Agenda for Prosperity: The Road to Middle Income Status (2013–2018).* Freetown: GoSL, 2013. http://www.sierra-leone.org/Agenda%204%20Prosperity.pdf.

GoSL. *Health Compact.* Freetown: GoSL, December 2011. http://www.internationalhealthpartnership.net/fileadmin/uploads/ihp/Documents/Country_Pages/Sierra_Leone/Government%20of%20S.%20Leone%20Health%20Compact.pdf.

GoSL. *National Health Sector Strategic Plan (NHSSP) – 2010–2015.* Freetown: GoSL, November 2009. http://www.internationalhealthpartnership.net/fileadmin/uploads/ihp/Documents/Country_Pages/Sierra_Leone/NationalHealthSectorStrategicPlan_2010-15.pdf.

Harman, Sophie, "Ebola, Gender, and Conspicuously Invisible Women in Global Health Governance." *Third World Quarterly* (2016). doi:10.0.4.56/01436597.2015.1108827.

Harman, Sophie, and William Brown. "In from the Margins?" *International Affairs* 89, no. 1 (2013): 69–87. doi:10.1111/1468-2346.12005.

Harris, David. *Sierra Leone.* Oxford: Oxford University Press, 2014.

Hitchen, Jamie. "Mismanagement of Sierra Leone's Ebola Spending." Africa Research Institute blog, February 20, 2015. http://www.africaresearchinstitute.org/blog/mismanagement-ebola-spending/.

International Monetary Fund (IMF). "Sierra Leone gets $102 Million in Extra IMF Financing, Debt Relief." *IMF Survey Magazine: Countries & Regions,* March 24, 2015. http://www.imf.org/external/pubs/ft/survey/so/2015/car030315a.htm.

IMF. *Sierra Leone: Staff Report for the 2013 Article IV Consultation and Request for a Three-year Arrangement under the Extended Credit Facility – Debt Sustainability Analysis.* October 18, 2013. https://www.imf.org/external/pubs/ft/dsa/pdf/2013/dsacr13330.pdf.

IMF. *IMF Executive Board Concludes the 2013 Article IV Consultation with Sierra Leone.* November 24, 2013. http://www.imf.org/external/np/sec/pr/2013/pr13450.htm.

Kaldor, Mary, with James Vincent. *Evaluation of UNDP Assistance to Conflict-affected Countries: Case Study Sierra Leone.* New York: UNDP, 2006. http://web.undp.org/evaluation/documents/thematic/conflict/SierraLeone.pdf.

Kieny, Marie-Paule. *Ebola and Health Systems.* Geneva: WHO, December 2014. http://www.who.int/mediacentre/commentaries/health-systems-ebola/en/.

Kim, Jim Yong. "What Ebola taught the World one year Later." *Time*, March 24, 2015. http://time. com/3755178/ebola-lessons/?xid=emailshare#3755178/ebola-lessons/.

Kingsley, Pete. "NGOs, Doctors, and the Patrimonial State: Tactics for Political Engagement in Nigeria." *Critical African Studies* 6, no. 1 (2014): 6–21. doi:10.1080/21681392.2013.852029.

Labonte, Melissa T. "From Patronage to Peacebuilding?" *African Affairs* 111, no. 442 (2012): 90–115. doi:10.1093/afraf/adr073.

Lavelle, Kathryn. "Moving in from the Periphery: Africa and the Study of International Political Economy." *Review of International Political Economy* 12, no. 2 (2005): 364–379. doi:10.1080/09692290500105946.

Lee, Kelley. "The Pit and the Pendulum." *Development* 47, no. 2 (2004): 11–17. doi:10.1057/palgrave. development.1100025.

Lind, Jeremy, and Johnny Ndebe. "Return of the Rebel." Practice Paper in Brief 19 (2015). http://opendocs. ids.ac.uk/opendocs/bitstream/123456789/5852/1/ID560%20Online.pdf.

Luke, David Fasthole. "The Politics of Economic Decline in Sierra Leone." *Journal of Modern African Studies* 27, no. 1 (1989): 133–114. doi: 10.1017/S0022278X00015676.

Médicins Sans Frontières (MSF) "Ebola: We must Finish the Job." London, July 7, 2015. http://www.msf. org.uk/article/ebola-we-must-finish-the-job.

Mkandawire, Thandika. "Can Africa turn from Recovery to Development?" *Current History*, May (2014): 171–177. http://www.currenthistory.com/Article.php?ID=1153.

Moser, Caroline O. "Gender Planning in the Third World." *World Development* 17, no. 11 (1989): 1799–1825. doi:10.1016/0305-750X(89)90201-5.

Oxfam International. "Mistrust and Confusion are allowing Ebola to Thrive." Press release, October 27, 2014. https://www.oxfam.org/en/pressroom/pressreleases/2014-10-27/mistrust-and-confusion-are-allowing-ebola-thrive-west-africa.

Reno, William. *Corruption and State Politics in Sierra Leone*. Cambridge: Cambridge University Press, 1995.

Richards, Paul. *Fighting for the Rainforest: War, Youth and Resources in Sierra Leone*. Oxford: James Currey, 1996.

Riddell, Barry. "Sierra Leone: Urban-elite Bias, Atrocity & Debt." *Review of African Political Economy* 32, no. 103 (2005): 115–133. doi:10.1080/03056240500121032.

Scheper-Hughes, Nancy. *Death without Weeping*. Oakland: University of California Press, 1993.

Severino, Jean-Michel, and Olivier Ray. *Africa's Moment*. Cambridge: Polity Press, 2011.

Taylor, Ian. "Why Africa is not Rising." *Review of African Political Economy*. Forthcoming.

Transparency International. *Ebola: Corruption and Aid*. Berlin: Transparency International, February 2015. http://www.transparency.org/news/feature/ebola_corruption_and_aid.

Transparency International. *Corruption Perceptions Index*. Berlin: Transparency International, 2014. https://www.transparency.org/country#SLE.

UNDP. *Human Development Report: The Rise of the South*. Geneva: UNDP, 2013. http://www.gm.undp. org/content/dam/undp/library/corporate/HDR/2013GlobalHDR/English/HDR2013%20Report%20 English.pdf.

WHO. *Building Resilient Health Systems in Ebola-affected Countries*. Geneva: WHO, January 2015. http:// apps.who.int/gb/ebwha/pdf_files/EBSS3/EBSS3_INF2-en.pdf.

WHO. *Ensuring WHO's Capacity to Prepare for and Respond to Future Large-scale and Sustained Outbreaks and Emergencies*. Geneva: WHO, January 2015. http://apps.who.int/gb/ebwha/pdf_files/EBSS3/ EBSS3_3-en.pdf.

WHO. "Sierra Leone: WHO Statistical Profile." http://www.who.int/gho/countries/sle.pdf?ua=1.

WHO. *Ebola Situation Reports – Archive*. September 9, 2015. http://apps.who.int/ebola/ebola-situation-reports-archive.

WHO. *World Health Statistics*, Geneva: WHO, 2013. http://www.who.int/gho/publications/world_health_ statistics/EN_WHS2013_Full.pdf.

WHO Regional Office for Africa. "African Health Workforce Observatory HRH Fact Sheet Sierra Leone." Brazzaville, 2006. http://www.hrh-observatory.afro.who.int/en/country-monitoring/87-sierra-leone. html.

Wikileaks. "Minister of Health indicted on Corruption Charges." November 4, 2009. https://www. wikileaks.org/plusd/cables/09FREETOWN435_a.htm.

Wilkinson, Annie, and Melissa Leach. "Briefing: Ebola – Myths, Realities, and Structural Violence." *African Affairs* 114, no. 454 (2014):136–148. doi:10.1093/afraf/adu080.

World Bank. *Global Economic Prospects: Sub-Saharan Africa.* June 2015. http://www.worldbank.org/content/dam/Worldbank/GEP/GEP2015b/Global-Economic-Prospects-June-2015-Sub-Saharan-Africa-analysis.pdf.

World Bank. *International Development Association International Finance Corporation and Multilateral Investment Guarantee Agency Country Assistance Strategy Progress Report for the Republic of Sierra Leone.* Washington, DC: World Bank, July 2012. http://www-wds.worldbank.org/external/default/WDSContentServer/WDSP/IB/2012/07/23/000333037_20120723002431/Rendered/INDEX/699130CASP0P130Official0Use0only090.txt.

Yates Rob. *Insight on Free Health Care Launch in Sierra Leone.* London: DFID Human Development Resource Centre, April 2010. http://hdrc.dfid.gov.uk/wp-content/uploads/2012/09/272216_LR-Scoping-Mission-_CPHF__Report-Sierra-Leone.pdf.

Zack-Williams, Alfred B. "Sierra Leone: The Political Economy of Civil War 1991–98." *Third World Quarterly* 20, no. 1 (1999): 143–162. doi:10.1080/01436599913965.

The race for Ebola drugs: pharmaceuticals, security and global health governance

Anne Roemer-Mahler and Stefan Elbe

Centre for Global Health Policy, University of Sussex, Brighton, UK

ABSTRACT
The international Ebola response mirrors two broader trends in global health governance: (1) the framing of infectious disease outbreaks as a security threat; and (2) a tendency to respond by providing medicines and vaccines. This article identifies three mechanisms that interlink these trends. First, securitisation encourages technological policy responses. Second, it creates an exceptional political space in which pharmaceutical development can be freed from constraints. Third, it creates an institutional architecture that facilitates pharmaceutical policy responses. The ways in which the securitisation of health reinforces pharmaceutical policy strategies must, the article concludes, be included in ongoing efforts to evaluate them normatively and politically.

Introduction

Reflecting on the past two decades of global health governance, scholars highlight two major trends – especially in relation to lethal infectious disease outbreaks. First, there is a growing political tendency to frame such outbreaks as security threats. Driven by concerns about emerging and re-emerging infectious diseases, drug-resistant strains of known diseases and the proliferation of biological weapons, health threats are argued to have an impact on national and international security. The stated reasons for this include the fact that high levels of morbidity and mortality can affect the operations of the state, disturb the global economy by interrupting travel and trade, and threaten military operations. Beginning in the 1980s in the USA, the discourse on 'health security' was soon picked up by other governments, notably in Australia, Canada and Western Europe, as well as by international organisations, including the World Health Organization (WHO). In response to these events the framing of health as a security issue has become an important field of study, with scholars analysing the processes through which health issues are 'securitised', the extent to which this trend is normatively and politically desirable and – more recently – the complex interplay between dynamics of securitisation and de-securitisation in global health policy.

That notable trend towards securitisation in global health governance has also been accompanied by a second one – a growing recourse by policy makers to pharmaceutical responses and solutions in managing such global health issues. This second trend largely centres on the provision of medicines and vaccines as a key instrument of global health governance. Thus increasing the availability of – and international access to – pharmaceuticals is now a core mandate of many of the global health institutions that have emerged in the past 25 years. These include the US president's Emergency Plan for AIDS Relief (PEPFAR), the Global Fund to Fight AIDS, Tuberculosis and Malaria, GAVI, more than two dozen product development partnerships, the WHO Prequalification Programme, and the WHO Global Pandemic Influenza Action Plan.

At the national level, furthermore, the USA has taken the lead by creating the so-called Public Health Emergency Medical Countermeasures Enterprise (PHEMCE), which promotes the development and national procurement of medicines and vaccines against health-based threats.[1] Other governments, notably from Australia, Canada, various European counties and Japan, have followed suit and created their own policy frameworks on health security, which include measures to facilitate the use of medicines and vaccines to counter global health security threats. This growing emphasis on pharmaceutical response strategies means that global health policy is today not just a site of securitisation alone, but simultaneously a site of 'pharmaceuticalisation' as well.

The twin trends towards securitisation and pharmaceuticalisation in global health governance are now becoming increasingly well understood in their own terms, with separate groups of scholars exploring each trend respectively. What has so far escaped scholarly attention, however, is how these two pivotal dynamics are also profoundly interlinked in practice, and indeed tend to reinforce one another. This lacuna is the result, in part, of the fact that the scholarship on securitisation and pharmaceuticalisation has different disciplinary origins and roots, with scholars in both fields tending to work independently of one another. At the risk of oversimplifying, scholars of securitisation have simply not paid much attention to the growing role pharmaceuticals now play in global health policy, while scholars of pharmaceuticalisation in turn have not focused on recent developments in security policy and the rise of health security. Against that backdrop, this article undertakes the first analysis of how the dual processes of securitisation and pharmaceuticalisation are linked in contemporary global health governance. In particular, the article examines whether the securitisation of health issues promotes or facilitates pharmaceutical responses to infectious disease outbreaks, and – if so – how.

The international response to the recent Ebola outbreak in West Africa emerges as a critical site for carrying out such an analysis. As the article will show at the outset, the dynamics of both securitisation and pharmaceuticalisation have been pervasive in the international response to the recent Ebola outbreak. Efforts to respond to the outbreak mobilised a number of securitisation strategies, while at the same time also being an important site for the development of new pharmaceutical strategies for responding to the Ebola outbreak. Based on a detailed analysis of the international response, the article then goes on to identify three ways in which securitisation processes tend to facilitate pharmaceutical responses to infectious disease outbreaks. First, we argue, securitisation encourages technological policy responses, which in the field of global health policy tend to give pharmaceutical strategies greater salience. Second, securitisation also creates an exceptional political space in which the development, approval and administration of new pharmaceutical interventions can be freed from many constraints. Third, the framing of health as a security issue over the past two decades has created a set of policies and legal institutions that facilitate the use of pharmaceuticals as a key instrument of global health policy. These ways in which the securitisation of infectious diseases reinforces pharmaceutical policy responses in global health governance must, the article concludes, be included in the ongoing process of their normative and political evaluation.

Déjà Vu: Ebola as the latest securitisation of infectious disease

On 8 August 2014 WHO declared the Ebola outbreak a Public Health Emergency of International Concern. The Emergency Committee convened by WHO under the International Health Regulations (2005) advised that heads of states with Ebola transmission 'should declare a national emergency,[2] something several countries in West Africa did in the following weeks, including the worst affected countries – Sierra Leone, Liberia and Guinea – but also Nigeria, where only 19 people would become infected overall. Liberia and Sierra Leone also used military units to enforce quarantines and suppress riots.

The language of security was also employed by political leaders outside the immediately affected region. On 7 September US President Obama called the outbreak a 'national security priority';[3] shortly afterwards he announced plans to send 3000 military personnel into the region. In the following weeks China, France and the UK similarly announced the deployment of military personnel and equipment to West Africa. Even NGOs such as Médecins Sans Frontières and Oxfam, usually critical of military intervention, could see no other way forward than calling for the deployment of military medical capability. Importantly the United Nations Security Council declared on 18 September 2014 that the Ebola outbreak constituted 'a threat to international peace and security'.[4]

The securitisation of the international Ebola response is consistent with a much longer trend in global health governance. In fact, the rapid expansion of security agendas to incorporate health-based threats has received extensive scholarly attention.[5] The framing of global health as an issue of security has mostly been analysed through the lens of securitisation theory,[6] which uses the insights of speech act theory to analyse security issues.[7] Specifically securitisation theory analyses what effects it has when an issue is framed as a security threat. The theory emphasises that 'language can [...] do much more than just convey information' and 'constitute a form of action or social activity'.[8] Securitising an issue, in other words, means more than saying something, it *does* something.

Existing scholarly literature on securitisation in the field of global health has highlighted some of the political effects of securitisation processes on policy priorities, policy procedures and even the institutional structure of global health governance.[9] Furthermore, that scholarship has explored the extent to which the securitisation of infectious diseases is politically desirable, ie whether the trend towards securitisation should be encouraged.[10] More recently it has also begun to analyse the interplay between dynamics of securitisation and de-securitisation in the area of global health policy.[11] Viewed against the background of this growing body of scholarship, the international response to Ebola emerges as the most recent manifestation of the securitisation of global health, and as one consistent with a longer history of securitising infectious diseases already seen in the cases of HIV/AIDS, SARS and pandemic flu. In the case of Ebola, however, that is only part of the story.

Where are the drugs and vaccines? The pharmaceutical response to Ebola

The international response to Ebola is also consistent with a second major trend in global health governance – the growing recourse to pharmaceutical logics and responses in global health policy. Thus, and in parallel to framing the Ebola outbreak as a security issue, an international pharmaceutical response also began to unfold rapidly. On 11 August, only three days after WHO had declared a Public Health Emergency of International Concern, the Organisation convened a meeting to decide whether it would be ethical to treat Ebola patients with experimental drug compounds that had never been tested in humans. Given the disease's high mortality rate, the meeting concluded that it was.[12] Now the race was on among governments, companies and nongovernmental organisations to find a pharmaceutical solution to the Ebola outbreak.

A further WHO meeting held in early September then agreed on a list of experimental drugs and vaccines whose development should be prioritised.[13] Funding for taking things forward was provided by a range of organisations – including national governments, research councils, philanthropic organisations and partnerships for financing health development.[14] To plan and coordinate clinical trials in Africa, Europe and the USA, new public–private partnerships, spanning organisations from several countries, were created.[15] Yet further efforts went into creating the regulatory pathways necessary for the accelerated development of new drugs and vaccines. Rules and standards were discussed for how to run clinical trials in emergency situations and how to harmonise regulation for the approval of clinical trials and end products internationally to enable simultaneous development and distribution of new drugs and vaccines.

In some respects this intense focus on a pharmaceutical response is puzzling, because it seemed highly unlikely that any of these drugs and vaccines could actually be used in the outbreak.[16] All of them were in the very early stages of development, and even the most optimistic forecasts did not envisage that they would become available for widespread use during the outbreak. Moreover, many public health experts pointed out that contact tracing and isolation had been the key methods of success in the containment of previous outbreaks – leading to the question of why – largely unavailable – drugs and vaccines attracted so much attention in the latest Ebola outbreak.

This intense focus on pharmaceutical strategies means that the international response to Ebola has not just been a site of securitisation, but also one of pharmaceuticalisation. The international Ebola response, in other words, shows evidence not just of a proliferation of security logics, but also points towards an intensification – and indeed international expansion – of pharmaceutical logics, rationalities and interventions in global health policy. The pharmaceuticalisation in global health governance has not received nearly as much attention in the scholarly literature as the securitisation phenomenon. However, an emerging literature is now beginning to capture and analyse this phenomenon. For example, Elbe et al show that the securitisation of health has 'intensified government interest in acquiring pharmaceutical defenses for their populations'.[17] The key role pharmaceuticals have come to play as a policy instrument in global health security[18] – and in global health governance more widely[19] – has been explored mainly through the conceptual lens of 'pharmaceuticalisation'.

This concept was first developed by scholars from sociology and anthropology, who observed an increase in recourse to pharmaceutical products in various areas of social life and who analyse these dynamics and their drivers and implications.[20] The literature has postulated a number of potential drivers of pharmaceuticalisation. For example, scientific and technological advances in biomedicine are identified as an important factor, because they enable novel pharmaceutical products to be developed.[21] The sheer possibility that exists today of addressing health problems through pharmaceutical products that were not available previously has helped propel drugs and vaccines to the top of the health policy agenda. Second, Peter Conrad also argues that a broader 'medicalization of existence' is a relevant driver of pharmaceuticalisation because it encourages a tendency to address complex issues through recourse to pharmaceutical therapies.[22] Finally, several studies have emphasised that marketing and direct-to-consumer advertising by pharmaceutical companies can increase the societal penetration of pharmaceutical products.[23]

Some of this scholarship on pharmaceuticalisation even looks directly at how various *political* factors can contribute to pharmaceuticalisation processes. Williams et al and Abraham highlight the role of expedited approaches to the approval of pharmaceuticals pursued by some government regulatory agencies, and how this is making more pharmaceuticals available.[24] Elbe et al also show how national governments, international organisations, philanthropic organisations and cross-sectoral partnerships have facilitated the use of pharmaceuticals in global health policy by providing financial and regulatory incentives to encourage pharmaceutical companies to invest in the development of pharmaceuticals for which limited commercial opportunities exist.[25] In a different article Elbe and his colleagues looked beyond specific policy and regulatory incentives to analyse the underlying rationalities of political rule within which pharmaceuticals have emerged as such attractive policy instruments. Drawing on Michel Foucault's notion of a 'crisis of circulation', they argue that pharmaceuticals are such an attractive policy option because they allow for the rapid interception of 'bad' and, in this case, pathogenic systems of circulation without disrupting the 'good' circulatory systems that are deemed critical for maintaining population welfare, such as mobility, commerce and trade.[26]

Notwithstanding this interest in the political drivers of pharmaceuticalisation, however, neither scholars of securitisation nor those of pharmaceuticalisation have so far been able to capture and analyse how these two parallel dynamics are interlinked in practice. Do securitisation processes tend to favour pharmaceutical responses to infectious diseases outbreaks? If so, what are the principal mechanisms or trajectories along which they do this? Focusing specifically on the analysis of the International Ebola response, we identify three such underlying mechanisms linking the framing of health as a security problem with a policy response focused on pharmaceuticals: (1) provoking a greater impetus for technological policy solutions; (2) creating an exceptional political space where the processes of pharmaceutical development, approval and administration can be freed from many constraints; and (3) creating a lasting institutional architecture that facilitates the recourse to pharmaceuticals as a key instrument of global health policy.

Searching for a quick fix: the race for technological solutions

In the first instance securitisation processes tend to encourage 'quick-fix' and therefore often technologically driven responses. As has been widely noted by securitisation theorists, processes of securitisation invoke a sense of imminent danger. Buzan and Waever point out more generally that 'a security issue is posited (by a securitising actor) as a threat to the survival of some referent object (national, state, the liberal economic order, the rain forests), which is claimed to have a right to survive...a question of survival necessarily involves a point of no return at which it will be too late to act'.[27] In other words, the process of securitisation promotes the perception of an immediate, potentially irreversible danger that creates a perceived need for rapid response. In a situation perceived as an emergency alternative policy options, such as a long-term engagement with complex socioeconomic issues and political negotiations, for instance, appear less suitable. Demand increases for a quick fix to avert the imminent danger.

That securitisation processes privilege certain policy pathways over others has already been noted in the literature. Nunes argues that 'framing issues as threats to security entails the establishment of a political modality for dealing with them'.[28] Craig Calhoun highlights the rise of emergency as a mode of justification for urgent global intervention.[29] Such emergency interventions, he argues, are short-term and focus on mitigating a temporally circumscribed event. Although the field of health was not one of the initial sectors studied by early securitisation theorists, there is evidence that this effect takes place in global health policy as well. There, too, securitisation processes have promoted such an emergency mode of governance or, as Weir and Mykhalovskiy put it, a 'World on Alert'.[30] Indeed, Stephen Collier and Andrew Lakoff argue that the securitisation of health has fostered an 'emergency modality of intervention'.[31] In addition to creating a sense of urgency and emergency, they also show that the securitisation of global health has promoted interventionist policy responses. More specifically it has promoted interventions that can be launched rapidly and are applicable in different contexts by using standardised protocols and technologies. In that sense, the field of global health remains consistent with the broader findings of securitisation theory.

The need, then, to rapidly intervene and urgently stop the threat is one way in which securitisation processes tend to emphasise technological responses in the area of global health – rather than encouraging longer-term strategies of dealing with underlying socioeconomic and political drivers. It is, however, not the only the reason. For, in the field of global health policy, such interventionist policies are particularly difficult to implement because the source of the threat is often located in other countries. As McInnes points out, the link between health and security has been 'generally cast in terms of a response to exogenous developments, that new risks have emerged and have acquired added salience in the context of accelerated globalization'.[32] Increasing economic interconnectedness, the accelerated mobility of people and goods, and international military operations have played a crucial role in the construction of health as a security issue.[33] Indeed, even the first international conferences linking health and security were driven by states' concerns about cross-border disease spread that was caused by and would create problems for the growing international traffic of goods and persons.[34] Given that the problem of health security is perceived as 'global', an effective response has to be global too.

Yet the problem with implementing interventionist policies on a global scale is that they create particular political sensitivities with regard to national sovereignty. In the field of global health security this has been observed in particular with regard to developing countries. Several studies have pointed out that the security interests behind the securitisation of global health are mainly those of governments in North America and Western Europe, while the origin of the problem is considered to reside largely in the developing world.[35] When an infectious disease becomes securitised, there is thus a tension between the perceived need for rapid intervention across countries, on the one hand, and a legal–political world order that is still largely based on the principle of national sovereignty, on the other.

Technological solutions become particularly attractive in this context not only because they are hoped to work rapidly, but because they may appear politically more neutral, minimising the risk of difficult political confrontations. In this political context there is a turn towards technological measures, such as 'medical response, standardized protocols for managing global health crises, surveillance and reporting systems, or simple technological fixes like mosquito nets or drugs'.[36] Even a cursory glance at the global health governance architecture that has emerged in the past 20 years reveals a plethora of institutions providing technological health interventions. In the field of global health this impetus for technological solutions is certainly not confined to pharmaceuticals. Surveillance systems, for example, are another prominent technological response. Such disease surveillance systems have been established and expanded at both at the national level and international levels.[37]

However, if pharmaceuticals are clearly not the only technological response, they remain a highly significant one. Indeed, policies and institutions to promote the international provision of pharmaceuticals have proliferated in the past 15 years. Prominent examples include the Global Fund to Fight AIDS, Tuberculosis and Malaria, GAVI, the WHO Prequalification Programme (to serve as an international reference point for good-quality medicines and vaccines), the WHO Global Pandemic Influenza Action Plan (to increase the supply of vaccines), the Directly Observed Treatment, Short-Course (DOTS) programme at the heart of WHO's Stop TB Strategy, and a range of cross-sectoral partnerships for the development of new pharmaceuticals, such as Aeras, DNDi, the Medicines for Malaria Venture, PATH and the TB Alliance, to name but a few.

Technological interventions are an attractive policy instrument not only because they promise a quick-fix and a politically more neutral solution but also because such interventions can immensely reduce 'the scale of intervention, from global political economy to laboratory investigation and information management'.[38] For governments in North America and Western Europe, in particular, it is much easier to mobilise resources and domestic political support for interventions that seemingly focus on a precise target in a circumscribed event with direct security relevance for domestic populations, rather than for long-term engagement with complex socioeconomic problems whose domestic relevance is uncertain.

Such a process was also evident in the international response to the Ebola outbreak in West Africa. The portrayal of the epidemic as a security threat invoked the sense of imminent danger and perceived need for rapid action that Buzan and Weaver have pointed out. Specifically the securitisation of the outbreak created a focus on containment and control strategies, which privileged a policy pathway based on rapid, largely technological interventions to enhance surveillance, diagnosis and treatment.[39] Technologies provided by the international community included laboratories and treatment centres, infection and prevention control capacity, personal protective equipment, and diagnostics. Furthermore, governments – especially those in the USA and Europe – WHO and several NGOs emphasised the development of new medicines and vaccines as an important element of outbreak containment and control. It was suggested that 'the window of opportunity for containing the epidemic, using "classical" control tools was closing',[40] and that new medicines and vaccines would both 'dramatically strengthen the ability to counter the disease' and 'act as an insurance policy against future outbreaks'.[41] As described elsewhere in this article, measures to accelerate the development of new pharmaceuticals were among the first steps taken after the Ebola outbreak had been declared a Public Health Emergency of International Concern, and several hundred million US dollars were mobilised in the following months.

The Ebola outbreak in West Africa illustrates once more how the securitisation of a health issue can contribute to a pathway of policies that focus on technological – and often pharmaceutical – fixes, rather than encouraging a more long-term approach that deals with the socioeconomic and political determinants of the problem. The Ebola crisis emerged in the context of stark inequalities – both local and global – and has been interpreted as a manifestation of 'structural violence'.[42] The international community has accepted that structural factors such as weak national health systems have contributed to the crisis, and committed to strengthening health systems in developing countries. Yet this commitment has so far focused on technical capacity building, while neglecting the political and socioeconomic context that has brought about those weaknesses. Almost two years after the beginning of the outbreak, long-term approaches to 'fixing' some of the structural conditions in which the crisis emerged are yet to take a prominent place in the international Ebola response.

Exceptions: extraordinary measures for pharmaceutical innovation

Securitisation processes create space 'to use extraordinary means or break normal rules for reasons of security'.[43] The use of extraordinary measures in the context of health security has already received much attention in the literature. Some scholars have noted that the securitisation of health has contributed to the extraordinary mobilisation of money, resources and political commitment.[44] Nevertheless, the space created for extraordinary measures can also be used to weaken civil liberties, human rights and democratic procedures.[45] In the Ebola outbreak three such exceptional measures have been critical for the pharmaceutical response: extraordinary amounts of funding were mobilised to promote the development of Ebola drugs and vaccines, experimental medicines that had never been tested in humans were given to Ebola patients, and candidate drugs and vaccines were rushed into clinical trials.

First, in recognition of the threat that some infectious diseases also pose to security, governments have mobilised enormous financial resources for the development of medicines and vaccines. In the first six months of the international Ebola response, the USA alone authorised more than $500 million to support accelerated development and manufacture, 'in keeping with the President's charge that we tackle Ebola as a national security priority'.[46] The largest UK medical science funding organisation, the Wellcome Trust, provided £3.2 million to fund a clinical trial consortium to tackle 'one of the most virulent infectious agents known to man, [which] has been declared a threat to international peace and security'.[47] The EU Innovative Medicines Initiative provided €215 million to fund eight vaccine development projects for the Ebola 'emergency',[48] and GAVI pledged to provide $300 million to purchase up to an estimated 12 million doses of a vaccine once it was ready and recommended by WHO.[49]

Moreover, most of the drugs and vaccines that were rushed into clinical development had already benefitted from health security funding released in the aftermath of the terrorist attacks in the USA in 2001. The pharmaceutical response to the Ebola outbreak, therefore, came against the background of governments mobilising much larger sums of funding over the past 15 years to encourage the development of new medicines and vaccines against a range of health security threats. For example, the US government had provided $5.6 billion for the purchase and stockpiling of medicines and vaccines against diseases considered a health security threat through the Project Bioshield Act in 2004.[50] Before that the US Congress had already increased the bio-defence budget of the US National Institutes of Health (NIH) from $53 million in 2001 to $1.7 billion in 2005, although NIH funding essentially flat between

2004 and 2014.[51] PEPFAR has been provided with some $60 billion since 2003,[52] while $7.5 billion was pledged to GAVI in 2015.[53] In the name of security, therefore, governments have increasingly intervened in the play of normal market forces – which control the development of routine medicines and vaccines - and have channelled public funds into programmes for the development and procurement of pharmaceuticals against perceived health security threats.

Second, the sense of urgency created by framing the Ebola outbreak as a security threat created exceptional policy space to facilitate the use of drugs that had never been tested in humans. At a very early stage in the international Ebola response, at the 11 August WHO meeting, a consensus was 'reached…that it is ethical to offer unproven interventions with as yet unknown efficacy and adverse effects, as potential treatment or prevention'.[54] Moreover, WHO, the US government, researchers and funding bodies urged national regulators to consider new regulation on how to approve experimental drugs and vaccines.[55] Regulation on the use of experimental drugs beyond the area of research exists only in a few countries, such as in Europe and the USA, which allow for the use of unapproved pharmaceuticals in emergency situations. Under normal circumstances the rules governing the use of new drugs and vaccines require their extensive testing in humans in lengthy clinical trials. There are several reasons for this. Only about 10% of drugs and vaccines that show promising results in the laboratory and animal studies are found to be safe and effective in humans.[56] Giving experimental drugs and vaccines to patients may therefore cause severe health damage. Furthermore, doing so can be a waste of resources if it deflects attention from other, potentially more effective interventions. Finally, giving experimental drugs to patients outside clinical trials can compromise the systematic collection of data about their effects. Yet, in the weeks following the WHO meeting, several patients received experimental treatments in Europe, Liberia and the USA. Most patients received one or more experimental drug – including brincidofovir, convalescent blood and plasma, favipiravir, TKM-Ebola and ZMapp.[57] That use of experimental treatments in Ebola patients led to both extensive public attention being paid to the new 'miracle drugs' and to considerable controversy about the use of experimental drugs for Ebola.[58]

Third, the emergency environment around Ebola created exceptional possibilities for exploring how the development and distribution of medicines and vaccines could be accelerated – even before their efficacy and safety was fully understood. A series of meetings and teleconferences was held at WHO on how to speed up clinical development, including unblocking some of the ethical, financial and regulatory issues involved.[59] According to WHO, the discussions were characterised by 'a high sense of urgency'.[60] Indeed, almost all available meeting documents make reference to the emergency nature of the situation, to the fact that it was 'unprecedented in scale and geographical distribution',[61] to the 'escalating scale and mortality of the outbreak',[62] and to the need for 'immediate action'.[63]

The key question was how to accelerate to only a few months a process that would usually take several years. One idea was that, rather than running the different stages of drug development – such as designing clinical studies, applying for ethical and regulatory review, conducting the studies, licensure and distribution – sequentially, they had to be done largely in parallel.[64] This required the rapid mobilisation of resources, mentioned above, and an unprecedented level of coordination between industry, regulators, scientists and funders, which was achieved though the rapid formation of large consortia of organisations from different sectors and countries.

Accelerating clinical development and approval also required greater international har-monisation of regulation. In November the African Vaccine Regulators Forum agreed to conduct joint ethical and regulatory reviews of clinical trials in Africa.[65] This was put into practice one month later by the national ethics and regulatory authorities in Cameroon, Ghana, Mali, Nigeria and Senegal, which held a joint review for the approval of an advanced vaccine trial. Meanwhile, WHO began work on an emergency regulatory pathway for Ebola vaccines,[66] but specific requirements had not been announced by the time of writing.

Finally, accelerating the development and approval of medicines and vaccines also required an acceptance by all parties that decisions had to be made in situations of con-siderable uncertainty with regard to the reliability of the data that could be collected from clinical trials and, ultimately, the safety of the products. The need 'to balance the imperative for immediate action to control the outbreaks with ensuring that measures employed were appropriate, safe, and effective'[67] was recognised in several discussions. All groups empha-sised that patient safety, good science and reliable data were paramount.[68] Yet, at the end of the day, it was also recognised that compromises would have to be made with regard to trial design and regulatory approval, for instance to be able to speed up development and, moreover, to do this in a situation of an acute outbreak with extremely high mortality rates.[69]

The extraordinary measures implemented to both facilitate the use of experimental drugs and accelerate the clinical development of drugs and vaccines thus employed risk calcula-tions that differed from the respective procedures used under non-emergency conditions. The assessment of the risks weighed against the potential benefits of these measures had changed. In a situation of a perceived 'emergency' and 'threat to security', it seems easier to justify risks as acceptable. This observation has also been made by others studying the implementation of new technologies in the context of health security interventions. In a study on the Smallpox Vaccination Programme in the USA, Dale Rose found that, under the new security rationale, there was a willingness to accept a much higher risk of side-effects of the vaccine than had been acceptable from a public health rationale.[70] A similar logic seems to have been at play when decisions were made to expand the use of pharmaceutical interventions in the international Ebola response.

Not only do securitisation processes encourage technological solutions, then, but the political urgency associated with them facilitates the implantation of extraordinary meas-ures, notably the mobilisation of public funds for pharmaceutical development, the use of drugs that have never been tested in humans and the acceleration of pharmaceutical development. That is a second way in which securitisation processes have encouraged and facilitated pharmaceutical response strategies.

Institutionalising pharmaceutical responses to health security threats

The extraordinary measures taken to facilitate the pharmaceutical response to Ebola did not have to start from 'scratch'. Rather, they could draw on an existing set of policies and legal institutions that had been created in the past two decades to facilitate the use of pharma-ceuticals as a key instrument against health security threats. In other words, the securitisa-tion of health has not only created space for extraordinary measures but it has also – over time – created a set of lasting institutions. Some of these have facilitated – indeed made possible – a pharmaceutical response to the Ebola outbreak.

The fact that, when the outbreak occurred, experimental drugs and vaccines against Ebola existed that could be moved into clinical testing, was largely a result of the expansion of bio-defence policies in the USA since the early 2000s. As mentioned above, most of the drugs and vaccines rushed into accelerated clinical trials had initially been developed through NIH bio-defence funding streams. For commercially operating pharmaceutical companies investment in Ebola medicines and vaccines is of little interest because of a lack of commercial opportunities.[71] And, while there were complaints that NIH budget cuts since the mid-2000s had hampered the development of Ebola pharmaceuticals,[72] without public funding for health security hardly any drug or vaccine would have been ready for clinical testing when the outbreak occurred.

In addition to bio-defence funding for pharmaceutical development, three other rules created in the USA to facilitate pharmaceutical responses to health emergencies played a role in the Ebola response: the Emergency Use Authorization (EUA), the Animal Efficacy Rule, and legal liability protection for pharmaceutical companies. The EUA was established as part of the Project Bioshield Act and the Pandemic and All-Hazards Preparedness Reauthorization Act (2013). It can provide authorisation for the use of pharmaceuticals and medical devices that have not yet been fully tested for safety and efficacy.[73] During the Ebola outbreak, several diagnostic tests were authorised under this rule.[74] Before Ebola the EUA was invoked for a drug against anthrax, and for several products during the influenza A (H1N1) pandemic of 2009.[75] Other governments are also looking into introducing similar regulation. In Europe an agreement on strengthening health security reached in 2013 'provides for the possibility that the Commission recognises a situation of public health emergency for the purposes of conditional marketing authorisations for medicinal products'.[76] This would allow accelerated marketing of medicinal products or vaccines in an emergency situation.

Another legal institution that has been referred to in the international Ebola response is the so-called Animal Efficacy Rule introduced in the USA in 2002. The Animal Efficacy Rule responds to the problem that many diseases that are considered health security threats occur only rarely – or not at all – in nature. Medicines and vaccines against such threats can often not be approved on the basis of human clinical trials. The reason for this is that disease outbreaks may be too short or involve too few people for large-scale clinical testing to be organised, and deliberately exposing humans to pathogens merely for the purpose of pharmaceutical development is considered unethical.

Under the Animal Efficacy Rule the US Food and Drug Administration (FDA) can approve pharmaceuticals based on efficacy studies conducted with animal models rather than on human clinical trials. The product's safety, however, has to be demonstrated in human studies. So far the Animal Efficacy Rule has been used for only a small number of products, including one to treat pneumonic plague and another one against anthrax.[77] In Europe the European Medicines Agency (EMA) has initiated procedures for accelerating the availability of vaccines during an influenza pandemic, including a 'mock-up procedure' whereby a vaccine can be authorised on the basis of the virus strain that might cause a pandemic – before the pandemic has actually occurred; of an 'emergency procedure' that reduces the period of approval; and of a 'modification' procedure whereby a vaccine that was approved only for seasonal influenza can be modified and approved for pandemic influenza.[78]

At the time of writing neither the Animal Efficacy Rule nor the EMA initiatives has been used to approve drugs or vaccines against Ebola. Yet the Animal Efficacy Rule is actively being considered to approve some of the drugs and vaccines currently undergoing clinical trials.[79] Originally it was hoped that at least some of the trials could be completed during the outbreak. Approval could then have been obtained on the basis of the data gathered during these trials. However, infection rates have been decreasing rapidly since the end of 2014, which means that many trials have run out of patients, and those still ongoing may do so in the next few months – before sufficient data are generated. A report by the Center for Infectious Disease Research and Policy (CIDRAP) at the University of Minnesota and the Wellcome Trust therefore suggests that the Global Health Security Agenda, an international health security institution launched in February 2014, 'could provide an effective mechanism to accelerate regulatory review and deployment of Ebola vaccines in the future'.[80] Specifically the report calls on national regulators to harmonise regulation for pharmaceutical approval internationally, including by adopting measures like the Animal Efficacy Rule and the EUA.

Furthermore, it has been suggested that the WHO Prequalification Programme could be amended to also cover unapproved drugs and vaccines.[81] The WHO Prequalification Programme is a key global health institution in facilitating access to pharmaceuticals because it forms a single point of reference for drug quality. Global health organisations can therefore also purchase easily from low-cost manufacturers in developing countries where regulatory standards are weak. Yet, in its current form, the WHO Prequalification Programme cannot be used for experimental drugs and vaccines.

A third legal institution that has become of critical importance in the pharmaceutical response to the Ebola outbreak is the legal liability of manufacturers. This issue concerns the question of who pays for legal claims against pharmaceutical companies when side-effects or other injuries occur among people participating in accelerated clinical trials or receiving a medicine or vaccine that has been approved on the basis of only limited or no testing in humans. In 2005 the USA introduced protections against liability claims that may be brought against pharmaceutical companies that develop medicines and vaccines required in health emergencies. In the following years the mechanism was invoked in relation to anthrax botulism, to pandemic influenza and to smallpox.[82]

During the international Ebola response pharmaceutical companies, scientists, WHO, and the UK and US governments called for indemnity for the manufacturers involved in the development of Ebola medicines and vaccines.[83] The US government issued a declaration that extended liability protection for two years for three experimental Ebola vaccines and also shielded the manufacturer of an experimental drug from legal liability[84]. However, the US government can provide protection only for claims brought in a US court, not internationally. The US Secretary for Health and Human Services, Sylvia Burwell, therefore called on other governments to enact similar regulation. As Burwell explained, 'as a global community, we must ensure that legitimate concerns about liability do not hold back the possibility of developing an Ebola vaccine, an essential strategy in our global response to the Ebola epidemic in west Africa'.[85] To address this problem, WHO suggested that a group of donors, in collaboration with the World Bank, could be formed to establish an international liability fund.[86]

The international Ebola response shows, therefore, how policies and legal institutions established in the name of health security can facilitate the recourse to pharmaceutical policy strategies. The international Ebola response has built on existing institutions to pursue a pharmaceutical approach, such as national bio-defence funding and legislation to approve experimental drugs and protect manufacturers from legal liability. Moreover, the move towards greater international harmonisation of clinical trial and approval procedures, as well as liability protection, has further advanced the process of building institutions that facilitate the use of pharmaceuticals as a key instrument of global health governance.

Conclusion

This article has highlighted two pivotal dynamics that characterise the international Ebola response and indeed global health governance more broadly: (1) the framing of health as a security issue; and (2) the provision of pharmaceuticals as a key instrument of global health governance. In exploring the ways in which these two processes are linked in practice the article has identified three mechanisms or pathways through which the securitisation of infectious disease subtly, but powerfully, encourages pharmaceutical policy responses.

First, the framing of health as an issue of national and international security invokes a sense of imminent danger that creates a perceived need for immediate intervention and a quick fix. Alternative policy pathways, such as long-term socioeconomic changes, appear much less appropriate in a situation of perceived emergency. Moreover, as international intervention is difficult in a world order still dominated by national sovereignty, it creates a bias for interventions that are perceived as politically neutral. In that context technologies, including pharmaceutical technologies, become politically attractive. Although pharmaceuticals are certainly not the only technological 'solution' that comes into play in this context, they are one of the most important.

Second, the framing of health as a security issue has created an exceptional political space in which extraordinary funding could be mobilised for developing medicines and vaccines, not only against Ebola but against a range of health threats. Moreover, the securitisation of health has also created exceptional political space to break key norms and rules governing the development and approval of drugs and vaccines. Medicines that had never been tested in humans were given to Ebola patients, and procedures put in place to speed up clinical tests in ways that would not normally be possible.

Finally, the securitisation of health has created a lasting institutional architecture for pharmaceutical response strategies that the international Ebola response was able to draw upon, and which it has advanced further. Of particular importance here were national institutions in the USA such as the EUA, Animal Efficacy Rule and liability protection for manufacturers. During the Ebola outbreak this institution-building process has been pushed further ahead by efforts to increase the international harmonisation of regulation of clinical trials and approval procedures, as well as liability protection.

There is, of course, no doubt that improved access to pharmaceuticals enabled by various global health governance institutions in the past two decades has done much to improve people's health and saved countless lives, including through access to anti-retrovirals for HIV and to childhood vaccines. However, by focusing policy attention largely on providing access to drugs, vaccines and other medical technologies, there is also a danger of obscuring the complex socioeconomic and political determinants of health. Indeed, there is a risk of obscuring the fact that pharmaceutical and other technologies work in specific socioeconomic contexts that shape their efficacy.[87] The reason that infectious diseases, such as Ebola, tend to spiral out of control mostly in low-income countries is the result of weak health systems, poverty, legacies of war, and deeply unequal global power relations, to name but a few of the complex issues underlying this catastrophe. Indeed, these issues have been recognised in public and policy debates from the beginning of the outbreak. Moreover, there have always been significant doubts that the drugs and vaccines rushed into accelerated development would be ready to help the people affected by the Ebola outbreak.

Yet, despite the public acknowledgement of the socioeconomic dimensions of this epidemic, millions have been spent on a pharmaceutical response to the Ebola outbreak – and billions more in the past two decades on a pharmaceutical approach to strengthening global health security. Many scholars have pointed out that the global health security agenda is driven by the national interests of governments in North America and Western Europe, and that the policy focus therefore is on containment rather than the prevention of epidemics. Nevertheless, many public health experts have continued to express doubts that a pharmaceutical response was appropriate to achieve containment. Hence this explanation does not seem entirely satisfactory. To understand the focus on pharmaceuticals as a key instrument of global health policy, we need also to look at how the framing of health as a security threat has established political rationales, practices and institutions of governance. Moreover, the subtle but powerful ways in which the securitisation of infectious diseases reinforces pharmaceutical strategies in global health governance must be included in the ongoing process of their normative and political evaluation.

Disclosure statement

No potential conflict of interest was reported by the authors.

Funding

The research leading to these results has received funding from the EU's Seventh Framework Programme (FP/2007-2013) [ERC Grant Agreement no 312567].

Notes

1. Hoyt, *Long Shot*.
2. WHO, "Statement on the 1st Meeting."
3. Klein, "Ebola is a 'National Security Priority.'"
4. United Nations, S/RES/2177, 1.
5. Cooper, *Life as Surplus*; Elbe, *Virus Alert*; Elbe, "Haggling over Viruses"; Enemark, "Is Pandemic Flu?"; Lakoff and Collier, *Biosecurity Interventions*; McInnes and Lee, "Health, Security and Foreign Policy"; and Rushton and Youde, *Routledge Handbook*.
6. Buzan et al., *Security*.
7. Austin, *How to do Things*; and Searle, *Speech Acts*.
8. Elbe, *Security and Global Health*, 11.
9. Aldis, "Health Security"; McInnes, "HIV/AIDS and Security"; Rushton, "Global Health Security"; Weir, "Inventing Global Health Security"; Buzan et al., *Security*; Elbe, *Security and Global Health*; and Hanrieder and Kreuder-Sonnen, "WHO Decides on the Exception?"
10. Elbe, "Should HIV/AIDS be Securitized?"
11. McInnes and Rushton, "HIV/AIDS and Securitization Theory"; and Enemark, "Ebola in West Africa."
12. WHO, *Ethical Considerations*.
13. WHO, "Consultation on Potential Ebola Therapeutics."
14. White House, "Progress in our Ebola Response"; Wellcome Trust, *Ebola Treatment Trials*; Innovative Medicines Initiative, "First Innovative Medicines Initiative"; and WHO, *Second WHO High-level Meeting*.
15. NIH, "Liberia–US Clinical Research Partnership"; Wellcome Trust, "New Trial of TKM-Ebola Treatment"; WHO, "Trial of Vaccine"; Moran, "Chimerix"; NIH, "PREVAIL"; and Wellcome Trust, "Ebola Treatment Trials."
16. When the first candidate treatments and vaccines entered into clinical trials in late 2014, the height of the epidemic had indeed passed and several trials faced difficulty even recruiting sufficient patient numbers. Yet small outbreaks continued to occur in West Africa and in the summer of 2015 one trial indicated that a vaccine (rVSV-ZEBOV) might have been found that was highly efficacious in preventing Ebola. Henao-Restrepo, "Efficacy and Effectiveness of an rVSV-vectored Vaccine."
17. Elbe et al., "Medical Countermeasures," 265.
18. Elbe et al., "Medical Countermeasures"; and Elbe et al., "Securing Circulation."
19. Roemer-Mahler, "The Rise of Companies from Emerging Markets."
20. Abraham, "Pharmaceuticalization of Society"; Clarke et al., *Biomedicalization*; Gabe, *Pharmaceuticalization*; Lakoff, *Pharmaceutical Reason*; Petryna et al., *Global Pharmaceuticals*; and Williams et al., "The Pharmaceuticalisation of Society?"
21. Clarke et al., *Biomedicalization*.
22. Conrad, *The Medicalization of Society*.
23. Healy, *Let Them Eat Prozac*; Dumit, *Drugs for Life*; and Goldacre, *Bad Pharma*.
24. Abraham, "Pharmaceuticalization of Society"; and Williams et al., "Pharmaceuticalisation of Society?"
25. Elbe et al., "Medical Countermeasures"; and Roemer-Mahler, "The Rise of Companies from Emerging Markets."
26. Elbe et al., "Securing Circulation."
27. Buzan and Wæver, *Regions and Powers*, 71.
28. Nunes, "The Politics of Health Security," 64.
29. Calhoun, "The Imperative to Reduce Suffering."
30. Weir and Mykhalovskiy, *Global Public Health Vigilance*.
31. Collier and Lakoff, "The Problem of Securing Health."
32. McInnes, "The Many Meanings," 14.
33. Institute of Medicine, *Emerging Infections*; Brower and Chalk, *The Global Threat*; and WHO, *World Health Report 2007*.
34. Fidler, "The Globalization of Public Health"; and Kamradt-Scott, "Health, Security and Diplomacy."

35. Weir, "Inventing Global Health Security"; Rushton, "Global Health Security"; Aldis, "Health Security as a Public Health Concept"; Elbe, "Should HIV/AIDS be Securitized?"
36. Collier and Lakoff, "The Problem of Securing Health," 17.
37. Fearnley, "Redesigning Syndromic Surveillance"; Weir, "Inventing Global Health Security"; and Davies, "Securitising Infectious Diseases."
38. King, "The Scale Politics," 67.
39. See, for instance, United Nations, S/RES/2177, 1; WHO, "Statement on the 1st Meeting"; and WHO, "Ebola Response Roadmap."
40. WHO, *Second WHO High-level Meeting*, 6.
41. WHO, *Ethical Considerations*, 6; and WHO, *Second WHO High-Level Meeting*, 3.
42. Leach, "The Ebola Crisis"; and Wilkinson and Leach, "Briefing."
43. Buzan and Wæver, *Regions and Powers*, 6.
44. Singer, "AIDS and International Security"; and McInnes and Rushton, "HIV/AIDS and Securitization Theory."
45. Buzan et al., *Security*; and Elbe, "Should HIV/AIDS be Securitized?"
46. White House, "Progress in our Ebola Response."
47. Wellcome Trust, "Ebola Treatment Trials."
48. Innovative Medicines Initiative, "First Innovative Medicines Initiative"; and Innovative Medicines Initiative, "Innovative Medicines Initiative launches Ebola+."
49. WHO, *Second High-level Meeting*.
50. White House, "President Bush Signs Project Bioshield Act."
51. US Department of Health and Human Services, "Testimony of Anthony S. Fauci."
52. PEPFAR, "PEPFAR Funding."
53. GAVI, "Gavi's Resource Mobilisation Process."
54. WHO, *Ethical Considerations*.
55. Wellcome Trust and CIDRAP, *Recommendations*; and WHO, "Consultation on Potential Ebola Therapeutics."
56. Paul et al., "How to Improve R&D Productivity."
57. WHO, "Compassionate Use of Experimental Treatments."
58. Rid and Emanuel, "Ethical Considerations."
59. WHO, "Ebola Treatment and Interventions."
60. WHO, "High-level Meeting on Ebola Vaccines."
61. WHO, "Consultation on Potential Ebola Therapies."
62. WHO, "Agenda of the Meeting."
63. WHO, "Consultation on Potential Ebola Therapies."
64. Kieny, "Overview of Vaccine Development."
65. WHO. "Fast-tracking the Development"; and WHO, "African Regulators' Meeting."
66. WHO, *Second High-level Meeting*.
67. WHO, "Consultation on Potential Ebola Therapies."
68. WHO, *High-level Meeting*.
69. Ibid.
70. Rose, "How did the Smallpox Vaccination Program?," 103.
71. The number of people contracting Ebola in the past has been very small compared with other diseases. Moreover, Ebola outbreaks occur mostly in poor countries where people are often unable to pay for medicines. Conventional mechanisms for commercial investment in drug development, notably market size and intellectual property protection, are therefore not effective in the case of Ebola.
72. Stein, "Ebola Vaccine."
73. Stroud et al., *Medical Countermeasure Dispensing*, 5.
74. US Food and Drug Administration, "Ebola Virus EUA Information."
75. Stroud et al., *Medical Countermeasure Dispensing*, 25.
76. EU, "Presidency Confirms Agreement."
77. Elbe et al., "Medical Countermeasures."
78. European Medicines Agency, "Authorization Procedures."

79. US Food and Drug Administration, *Vaccines*; Hirschler, "Liberia Ebola Vaccine Trial"; and Burton, "NIH to Start Vaccine Study."
80. Wellcome Trust and CIDRAP, "Accelerating Development," 31.
81. Ibid; and Marinissen et al., "Strengthening Global Health Security."
82. Stroud et al., *Medical Countermeasure Dispensing*, 24.
83. Hirschler and Nebehay, "Drugmakers may need Indemnity"; and Wintour, "David Cameron Presses for Indemnities."
84. US Department of Health and Human Services, "Ebola Virus Disease Vaccines"; and US Department of Health and Human Services, "Ebola Virus Disease Therapeutics."
85. Quoted in McCarthy, "US provides Immunity."
86. WHO, "WHO High-level Meeting."
87. Koch, "Disease as a Security Threat."

Bibliography

Abraham, John. "Pharmaceuticalization of Society in Context: Theoretical, Empirical and Health Dimensions." *Sociology* 44, no. 4 (2010): 603–622.

Aldis, William L. "Health Security as a Public Health Concept: A Critical Analysis." *Health Policy and Planning* 23, no. 6 (2008): 369–375.

Austin, John. *How to do Things with Words*. Cambridge, MA: Harvard University Press, 1962.

Brower, Jennifer, and Peter Chalk. *The Global Threat of New and Reemerging Infectious Diseases: Reconciling US National Security and Public Health Policy*. Santa Monica, CA: Rand Corporation, 2003.

Burton, Thomas M. 2015. "NIH to start Ebola Vaccine Study with Glaxo, Merck." *Wall Street Journal*, January 23.

Buzan, Barry, and Ole Wæver. *Regions and Powers: The Structure of International Security*. Cambridge: Cambridge University Press, 2003.

Buzan, Barry, Ole Wæver, and Jaap de Wilde. *Security: A New Framework for Analysis*. Boulder, CO: Lynne Rienner, 1998.

Calhoun, Craig. "The Imperative to Reduce Suffering: Charity, Progress, and Emergencies in the Field of Humanitarian Action." In *Humanitarianism in Question: Politics, Power, Ethics*, edited by Michael Barnett and Thomas G. Weiss, 73–97. Ithaca, NY: Cornell University Press.

Clarke, Adele, L. Mamo, J. Fosket, J. Fishman, and J. Shim, eds. *Biomedicalization: Technoscience, Health and Illness in the US*. Durham, NC: Duke University Press, 2010.

Collier, Stephen J., and Andrew Lakoff. "The Problem of Securing Health." In *Biosecurity Interventions: Global Health and Security in Question*, edited by Andrew Lakoff and Stephen Collier, 33–60. New York: Columbia University Press, 2008.

Conrad, Peter. *The Medicalization of Society: On the Transformation of Human Conditions into Treatable Disorders*. Baltimore, MD: Johns Hopkins University Press, 2007.

Cooper, Melinda. *Life as Surplus: Biotechnology and Capitalism in the Neoliberal Era*. Seattle, WA: Washington University Press, 2008.

Davies, Sara E. "Securitising Infectious Diseases." *International Affairs* 82, no. 2 (2008): 295–313.

Dumit, Joseph. *Drugs for Life: How Pharmaceutical Companies define our Health*. Durham, NC: Duke University Press, 2012.

Elbe, Stefan. *Security and Global Health*. Cambridge: Polity, 2010.

Elbe, Stefan. "Haggling over Viruses: The Downside Risks of Securitizing Infectious Disease." *Health Policy and Planning* 25, no. 6 (2010): 476e–485.

Elbe, Stefan. *Virus Alert: Security, Governmentality and the AIDS Pandemic*. New York: Columbia University Press, 2009.

Elbe, Stefan. "Should HIV/AIDS be Securitized? The Ethical Dilemmas of Linking HIV/AIDS and Security." *International Studies Quarterly* 50, no. 1 (2006): 119–144.

Elbe, Stefan, Anne Roemer-Mahler, and Christopher Long. "Securing Circulation Pharmaceutically: Antiviral Stockpiling and Pandemic Preparedness in the European Union." *Security Dialogue* 45, no. 5 (2014): 440–457.

Elbe, Stefan, Anne Roemer-Mahler, and Christopher Long. "Medical Countermeasures for National Security: A New Government Role in the Pharmaceuticalization of Society." *Social Science & Medicine* 131 (2014): 263–271.

Enemark, Christian. "Ebola in West Africa as 'a Threat to International Peace and Security': A Tale of Desecuritisation." *Third World Quarterly* (under review).

Enemark, Christian. "Is Pandemic Flu a Security Threat?" *Survival* 51, no. 1 (2009): 191e–214.

EU. "Presidency confirms Agreement on Strengthening Responses to Serious Cross-border Health Threats." Press release. Brussels, May 15, 2013.

European Medicines Agency. "Authorization Procedures." http://www.ema.europa.eu/ema/index.jsp?curl=pages/special_topics/q_and_a/q_and_a_detail_000080.jsp (accessed December 16, 2015).

Fearnley, Lyle. "Redesigning Syndromic Surveillance for Biosecurity." In *Biosecurity Interventions: Global Health and Security in Question*, edited by Andrew Lakoff and Stephen Collier, 61–88. New York: Columbia University Press, 2008.

Fidler, David. "The Globalization of Public Health: The First 100 Years of International Health Diplomacy." *Bulletin of the World Health Organization* 79, no. 9 (2001): 842–849.

Gabe, Jonathan. *Pharmaceuticalization: The Wiley Blackwell Encyclopedia of Health, Illness, Behavior, and Society*, edited by William C. Cockerham, Robert Dingwall and Stella R. Quah, 1804–1810. Chichester: Wiley, 2014.

GAVI. "Gavi's Resource Mobilisation Process." 2015. http://www.gavi.org/funding/resource-mobilisation/process/.

Goldacre, Ben. *Bad Pharma: How Drug Companies mislead Doctors and Harm Patients*. London: Fourth Estate, 2012.

Hanrieder, Tine, and Christian Kreuder-Sonnen. "WHO decides on the Exception? Securitization and Emergency Governance in Global Health." *Security Dialogue* 45, no. 4 (2015): 331–348.

Healy, David. *Let Them Eat Prozac: The Unhealthy Relationship between the Pharmaceutical Industry and Depression*. New York: New York University Press, 2004.

Henao-Restrepo, Ana Maria, Ira M. Longini, Matthias Egger, Natalie E Dean, W. John Edmunds, Anton Camacho et al. "Efficacy and Effectiveness of an rVSV-vectored Vaccine Expressing Ebola Surface Glycoprotein: Interim Results from the Guinea Ring Vaccination Cluster-randomised Trial." *Lancet*. Published online July 31, 2015. http://dx.doi.org/10.1016/S0140-6736(15)61117-5.

Hirschler, Ben. "Liberia Ebola Vaccine Trial 'Challenging' as Cases Tumble." *Reuters*, January 24, 2015.

Hirschler, Ben, and Stephanie Nebehay. "UPDATE 2 – Drugmakers may need Indemnity for Fast-tracked Ebola Vaccines." *Reuters*, October 23, 2014.

Hoyt, Kendall, and Long Shot. *Vaccines for National Defense*. Cambridge, MA: Harvard University Press, 2012.

Innovative Medicines Initiative. "First Innovative Medicines Initiative Ebola Projects get Underway." Press release. January 16, 2015.

Innovative Medicines Initiative. "Innovative Medicines Initiative launches Ebola+ Programme." Press release. November 6, 2014.

Institute of Medicine. *Emerging Infections: Microbial Threats to Health in the United States*. Washington, DC: National Academies Press, 1992.

Kamradt-Scott, Adam. "Health, Security and Diplomacy in Historical Perspective." In *Routledge Handbook of Global Health Security*, edited by Simon Rushton and Jeremy Youde, 189–201. Abingdon: Routledge, 2015.

Kieny, Marie-Paule. "Overview of Vaccine Development Pathway." Presentation at the WHO consultation on Ebola vaccines, Geneva, September 29–30, 2014.

King, Nicholas B. "The Scale Politics of Emerging Diseases." *Osiris* 19 (2004): 62–76.

Klein, Betsy. "Ebola is a 'National Security Priority,' Obama Says." CNN, September 8, 2014.

Koch, Erin. "Disease as a Security Threat: Critical Reflections on the Global TB Emergency." In *Biosecurity Interventions: Global Health and Security in Question*, edited by Andrew Lakoff and Stephen J Collier, 121–146. New York: Columbia University Press, 2008.

Lakoff, Andrew. *Pharmaceutical Reason: Knowledge and Value in Global Psychiatry*. Cambridge: Cambridge University Press, 2005.

Lakoff, Andrew, and Stephen Collier (eds.). *Biosecurity Interventions: Global Health and Security in Question*. New York: Columbia University Press, 2008.

Leach, Melissa. "The Ebola Crisis and Post-2015 Development." *Journal of International Development* 27, no. 6 (2015): 816–834.

Marinissen, Maria Julia, Lauren Barna, Margaret Meyers, and Susan E. Sherman. "Strengthening Global Health Security by developing Capacities to deploy Medical Countermeasures Internationally." *Biosecurity and Bioterrorism: Biodefense Strategy, Practice, and Science* 12, no. 5 (2014): 284–291.

McCarthy, Michael. "US Provides Immunity from Legal Claims related to three Ebola Vaccines." *British Medical Journal*, no. 349 (2014): g7608. http://www.bmj.com/content/349/bmj.g7608.full.pdf+html

McInnes, Colin. "The Many Meanings of Health Security." In *Routledge Handbook of Global Health Security*, edited by Simon Rushton and Jeremy Youde, 7–17. Abingdon: Routledge, 2015.

McInnes, Colin. "HIV/AIDS and Security." *International Affairs* 82, no. 2 (2006): 315–326.

McInnes, Colin, and Simon Rushton. "HIV/AIDS and Securitization Theory." *European Journal of International Relations* 19, no. 1 (2011): 115–138.

McInnes, Colin, and Kelley Lee. "Health, Security and Foreign Policy." *Review of International Studies* 32, no. 1 (2006): 5–23.

Moran, Nuala. 2015. "Chimerix, Toyama Drugs, Whole Blood and Plasma in First Ebola Clinical Trials." *BioWorld*. November 19, 2014.

NIH. "Liberia–US Clinical Research Partnership opens Trial to test Ebola Treatments." February 27, 2015. http://www.nih.gov/news/health/feb2015/niaid-27.htm.

NIH. "PREVAIL Phase 2/3 Clinical Trial of Investigational Ebola Vaccines." February 2, 2015. http://www.niaid.nih.gov/news/QA/Pages/EbolaVaxresultsQA.aspx.

Nunes, Joao. "The Politics of Health Security." In *Routledge Handbook of Global Health Security*, edited by Simon Rushton and Jeremy Youde, 60–70. Abingdon: Routledge, 2015.

PEPFAR. "PEPFAR Funding." June 2015. http://www.pepfar.gov/documents/organization/189671.pdf.

Paul, Steven M., Daniel Sl. Mytelka, Christopher T. Dunwiddie, Charles C. Persinger, Bernard H. Munos, Stacy R. Lindborg, and Aaron L. Schacht. "How to improve R&D Productivity: The Pharmaceutical Industry's Grand Challenge." *Nature Review Drug Discovery* 9 (March 2010): 203–214.

Petryna, A., Andrew Lakoff, and A. Kleinman. *Global Pharmaceuticals: Ethics, Markets, Practices*. Durham, NC: Duke University Press, 2007.

Rid, Annette, and Ezekiel J. Emanuel. "Ethical Considerations of Experimental Interventions in the Ebola Outbreak." *Lancet* 384, no. 9957 (2014): 1896–1899.

Roemer-Mahler, Anne. "The Rise of Companies from Emerging Markets in Global Health Governance: Opportunities and Challenges." *Review of International Studies* 40, no. 5 (2014): 897–918.

Rose, Dale. "How did the Smallpox Vaccination Program come About?" In *Biosecurity Interventions: Global Health and Security in Question*, edited by Andrew Lakoff and Stephen Collier, 89–119. New York: Columbia University Press, 2008.

Rushton, Simon. "Global Health Security: Security for Whom? Security from What?" *Political Studies* 59, no. 4 (2011): 779–796.

Rushton, Simon, and Jeremy Youde (eds.). *Routledge Handbook of Global Health Security*. Abingdon: Routledge, 2014.

Searle, John. *Speech Acts: An Essay in the Philosophy of Language*. Cambridge: Cambridge University Press, 1969.

Singer, Peter. "AIDS and International Security." *Survival* 44, no. 1 (2002): 145–158.

Stein, Sam. 2014. "Ebola Vaccine would likely have been found by now if not for Budget Cuts: NIH Director." *Huffington Post*, October 12.

Stroud, Clare, Lori Nadig, and Bruce M. Altevogt. *Medical Countermeasure Dispensing: Emergency Use Authorization and the Postal Model*. Workshop Summary. Washington, DC: Institute of Medicine. October 22, 2010.

United Nations. S/RES/2177. New York, September 18, 2014.

US Department of Health and Human Services. "Ebola Virus Disease Therapeutics." *Federal Register* 80, no. 77 (2015): 22534–22539.

US Department of Health and Human Services. "Ebola Virus Disease Vaccines." *Federal Register* 10, no. 79 (2014): 73314–73319.

US Department of Health and Human Services. "Testimony of Anthony S. Fauci before the Senate Subcommittee on Bioterrorism and Public Health." February 5, 2005.

US Food and Drug Administration. "Ebola Virus EUA Information". May 6, 2015. http://www.fda.gov/EmergencyPreparedness/Counterterrorism/MedicalCountermeasures/McmlegalRegulatoryandPolicyFramework/ucm182568.htm#ebola

US Food and Drug Administration. *Vaccines and Related Biological Products Advisory Committee Meeting.* FDA Briefing Document. Washington, DC: FDA, May 12, 2015.

Weir, Lorna. "Inventing Global Health Security, 1994–2005." In *Routledge Handbook of Global Health Security*, edited by Simon Rushton and Jeremy Youde, 18–31. Abingdon: Routledge, 2015.

Weir, Lorna, and E. Mykhalovskiy. *Global Public Health Vigilance: Creating a World on Alert.* Abingdon: Routledge, 2010.

Wellcome Trust. "New Trial of TKM-Ebola Treatment to start in Sierra Leone." March 11, 2015.

Wellcome Trust. "Ebola Treatment Trials to be Fast-tracked in West Africa." September 23, 2014.

Wellcome Trust, and CIDRAP. *Recommendations for Accelerating the Development of Ebola Vaccines: Report and Analysis.* Minneapolis, MN: University of Minnesota, February 2015.

White House. "President Bush Signs Project Bioshield Act of 2004." Press release. Washington, DC, July 21, 2004.

White House. "Progress in our Ebola Response at Home and Abroad." Fact Sheet. Washington, DC, February 11, 2015.

World Health Organization (WHO). "African Regulators' Meeting looking to Expedite Approval of Vaccines and Therapies for Ebola." 2015. http://www.who.int/medicines/news/AFR_reg_meet/en.

WHO. "Agenda of the Meeting on Ebola Vaccines Access and Financing." Geneva, October 23, 2014. http://www.who.int/mediacentre/events/2014/agenda-23-october-2014.pdf?ua=1

WHO. "Compassionate Use of Experimental Treatments for Ebola Virus Disease: Outcomes in 14 Patients admitted from August to November, 2014." Geneva, 2015. http://www.who.int/medicines/ebola-treatment/outcomes_experimental_therapies/en/

WHO. "Potential Ebola Therapeutics and Vaccines." Draft background document for participants. September 3, 2014. http://www.who.int/csr/disease/ebola/ebola-new-interventions-02-sep-2014.pdf

WHO. "Ebola Response Roadmap." Geneva, August 28, 2014. http://www.who.int/csr/resources/publications/ebola/response-roadmap/en/

WHO. "Ebola Treatment and Interventions Meetings and Consultations." Geneva, 2015. http://www.who.int/medicines/ebola-treatment/meetings/en/

WHO. *Ethical Considerations for Use of Unregistered Interventions for Ebola Virus Disease (EVD): Summary of the Panel Discussion.* Geneva, August 12, 2014. http://www.who.int/mediacentre/news/statements/2014/ebola-ethical-review-summary/en/

WHO. "Fast-tracking the Development and Prospective Roll-out of Vaccines, Therapies and Diagnostics in Response to Ebola Virus Disease: Special Session of the Executive Board on the Ebola Emergency." EBSS/3/INF./1 and EB136/INF./4. Geneva, January 9, 2015. http://apps.who.int/gb/ebwha/pdf_files/EBSS3/EBSS3_INF1-en.pdf

WHO. *Meeting Summary of the WHO Consultation on Potential Ebola Therapies and Vaccines*, Geneva, 4–5 September 2014. http://apps.who.int/iris/bitstream/10665/136103/1/WHO_EVD_Meet_EMP_14.1_eng.pdf

WHO. Q&A on trial of Ebola Virus Disease vaccine in Guinea. 1 April 2015. http://www.who.int/medicines/ebola-treatment/q_a_vaccine_trial_guinea/en/

WHO. *Second WHO High-level Meeting on Ebola Vaccines Access and Financing.* Summary Report. WHO/EVD/Meet/HIS/15.1. Geneva, January 8, 2015. http://www.who.int/medicines/ebola-treatment/evd_meet15_1eng/en/

WHO. "Statement on the 1st meeting of the IHR Emergency Committee on the 2014 Ebola Outbreak in West Africa." Geneva, August 8, 2014. http://www.who.int/mediacentre/news/statements/2014/ebola-20140808/en/

WHO. *WHO High-level Meeting on Ebola Vaccines Access and Financing.* Summary Report. Geneva, October 23, 2014. http://apps.who.int/iris/bitstream/10665/137184/1/WHO_EVD_Meet_EMP_14.2_eng.pdf?ua=1

WHO. World Health Report. *A Safer Future – Global Public Health Security in the 21st Century*, 2007. Geneva: WHO, 2007. http://apps.who.int/iris/handle/10665/69698

Wilkinson, Annie, and Melissa Leach. "Briefing: Ebola – Myths, Realities and Structural Violence." *African Affairs* 114, no. 454 (2015): 136–148.

Williams, Simon J., Paul Martin, and Jonathan Gabe. "The Pharmaceuticalisation of Society? An Analytical Framework." *Sociology of Health and Illness* 33, no. 5 (2011): 710–725.

Wintour, Patrick. 2014. "David Cameron presses for Indemnities to speed Ebola Vaccinations." *Guardian*, November, 14.

Personal Protective Equipment in the humanitarian governance of Ebola: between individual patient care and global biosecurity

Polly Pallister-Wilkins

Department of Politics, University of Amsterdam, The Netherlands

ABSTRACT
This article focuses on the use of Personal Protective Equipment in humanitarianism. It takes the recent Ebola outbreak as a case through which to explore the role of objects in saving individual lives *and* protecting populations. The argument underlines the importance of PPE in mediating between individual patient care and biosecurity. In addition it questions the preoccupation with technical fixes; challenges dominant perceptions about the subject of humanitarianism being the victims of disaster; traces the production of a particular politics of life; and explores the individualisation of risk and concomitant processes of labour discipline in the everyday lives of humanitarian workers.

Introduction

> Rubber gloves were nearly as scarce as doctors in this part of rural Liberia, so Melvin Korkor would swaddle his hands in plastic grocery bags to deliver babies. His staff didn't bother even with those when a woman in her 30s stopped by complaining of a headache. Five nurses, a lab technician – then a local woman who was helping out – cared for her with their bare hands. Within weeks, all of them died. The woman with the headache, they learned too late, had Ebola. (Sergeant Kollie Town, Liberia, August 2014)[1]

Personal Protective Equipment (PPE) has come to symbolise the recent Ebola outbreak in West Africa. Images of humanitarian workers clad in plastic clothing with their faces obscured by masks and goggles have become an easy visual cue for the virus itself and the complexities of the public health and biosecurity response. Meanwhile, international humanitarian agencies trumpet the necessity of PPE and offer web-based interactive tours of what exactly PPE is and how much it costs.[2] This is set against a backdrop of Ebola-affected regions lacking in the most basic equipment, local infrastructures struggling to cope and local health workers having to use plastic bags for protection. All of which, in turn, has necessitated outside, international intervention by those with the capacity and importantly the equipment to facilitate 'safe' intervention.

There is a long history of actions designed around the moral imperative to save lives and reduce suffering using tools, technologies, techniques and instruments to make a difference to life-saving endeavours. It extends from Florence Nightingale's famous use of lamps in the hospital wards of the Crimean War, the British Navy's post-abolition use of gunboats to police the Transatlantic Slave Trade,[3] the use of quarantine to combat disease,[4] and the use of urban planning, mapping and statistics in the governance and ultimate eradication of cholera in European towns to the more recent heraldry of drones and satellite surveillance systems alongside 'simpler' technologies such as the Mid-Upper Arm Circumference (MUAC) band, Plumpy'nut and the Peepoo in humanitarian efforts guided by the logics of patient-level care and the wider well-being of populations.[5] This historical symbiosis of technologies, or what Tom Scott-Smith has called 'humanitarian objects',[6] with humanitarian rationalities concerned with saving lives has been underexplored in studies of humanitarian action. Yet, as we can see, objects play and have played a central role in humanitarianism – or practices that display humanitarian logics – over the years.

With this in mind this article focuses on the role of PPE as a mediating device in human-itarian action. It takes the recent outbreak of Ebola in West Africa and elsewhere, in which the use of PPE has been of critical importance in the facilitation of intervention, as a case study through which to explore the intersection of humanitarian and biosecurity actions and the role of objects, or what I will call 'devices',[7] in mediating such actions. These actions include both individual patient care and corresponding global health management where, the article argues, PPE works to mediate the relationship between the act of individual care giving by humanitarian workers and the management of the spread of the disease at local, national and global levels. This relationship and its tensions have been notably highlighted by the criticisms of some practitioners within Médecins Sans Frontières (MSF) and made public when an internal letter was published in the French newspaper *Libération*.[8] The critics claimed concerns over the risks to humanitarian workers were placed above medical prac-titioners' responsibilities to provide the best possible care to their patients. These criticisms were revisited by MSF in its own Ebola report published in the spring of 2015. In this report, *Ebola: Pushed to the Limit and Beyond*, the concerns over providing individual patient care remain but are joined by competing responsibilities for staff safety and the centrality of human resources in tackling the virus.[9]

Considering the centrality of PPE in facilitating and mediating the response, the argument takes seriously and aims to contribute to the debates around the reliance on 'technological fixes' and 'technological fetishism' in humanitarian practice.[10] The argument builds on and complicates these debates, focusing on 'how matter comes to matter' in on-the-ground humanitarian practice and its interface with wider systems of global health security.[11] In the process it offers a counter-case to those instances where technology is assumed to be a 'fix' alone and focuses more on how technology comes to play a mediating role. Further, starting the analysis with PPE itself facilitates an exploration of the politics of devices and their role in (re)producing social and structural inequalities between lives and in the provi-sion of health care.

The article proceeds as follows: it starts with a discussion of humanitarianism's dual role as a provider of individualised patient care and a biosecurity actor in the global health response. It then moves on to consider recent discussions around the role of material objects and tech-nologies in humanitarianism, introducing an analytic of the 'device' as a way of exploring the productive work that humanitarian objects do. What follows moves beyond a Foucauldian biopolitical approach to humanitarian action by considering Didier Fassin's arguments concerning the 'politics of life' as a useful way to discern the ways in which humanitarian action produces particular lives that are worthy of being saved or sacrificed.[12] After this, the article goes on to tackle the substantive empirical investigation of PPE, exploring the mediating role it plays in managing the continuum of risk as humanitarians move between the demands of individual patient care and responsibility for wider biosecurity.

Biomedicine, biosecurity, devices and the politics of life

Humanitarianism as a technique of government and as a practice centres on the preservation of human life;[13] one of the principle ways humanitarian values come to be performed is through medical intervention of some kind. This action is often simultaneously concentrated on the individual patient and the well-being of the wider population. Such tension makes up a central part of humanitarianism as a value system, a technique of government and a practice, and is inherent within the commitment to seeing humanity – a universal subject – as being made up of equivalent individuals. In the provision of medical care this tension is ably captured by what Andrew Lakoff has termed humanitarian biomedicine and global health security, and what this article calls biosecurity.

Lakoff's discussion of the humanitarian biomedicine and biosecurity approaches is concentrated on how both have contrasting views of health care provision on a global scale based on practices developed in national approaches to public health management. Humanitarian biomedicine is concentrated on providing medical care in contexts of insufficient health infrastructure, where 'human suffering demands an urgent and immediate response outside the framework of state sovereignty'.[14] In contrast, biosecurity is concentrated on the health and well-being of the population at a 'global' level and 'comes from the recognition that existing national public health systems are inadequate for the potentially catastrophic threat of emerging and re-emerging infectious diseases'.[15] According to Lakoff, both biomedical and biosecurity responses rest on normative and technical elements but they have very different views on the social aspects of health care provision and the technical means of achieving it.[16] Biosecurity focuses on creating 'pre-emptive' systems capable of managing 'emerging infectious' diseases at the level of populations and combines a range of technical aspects concerned with 'surveillance, immediate alerts and immediate responses to disease outbreaks' especially, in the global context, when the disease has crossed international borders.[17] Humanitarian biomedicine, in contrast, while appearing to be more patient-centred, relies on a range of technical interventions such as drugs, vaccines and various objects used to manage public health, such as bed nets to prevent malaria or, in the case of this article, PPE.[18]

In exploring the particular role of 'objects' in humanitarian practice, Peter Redfield's work on MSF's use of the 'humanitarian kit' traces the relationship between humanitarian sensibilities and the material world. In doing this Redfield has been keen to emphasise that humanitarian practice itself offers a 'unique vantage point that alters the field of assumptions surrounding biological emergencies,'[19] while the perspective of humanitarian responses from agencies such as MSF does a number of things to our ideas of human security more generally:

> First, it shifts the focus one step away from the nation state, given that intergovernmental and nongovernmental entities play significant roles in defining and enacting humanitarian projects. Second, it also moves concerns about people and things one step closer to the domain of

ethics, to the extent that humanitarian conceptions of suffering commonly and overtly mobilise discourses about good, evil, and moral obligation. And finally, if the horizon is truly global, it both enlarges and diminishes the sense of infrastructure involved, amplifying the degree of mobility essential to achieving care from a distance even as it reduces the sense of 'life' to a minimal proportion of needs.[20]

So humanitarian's symbiosis with the material world of objects brings normative and political questions into discussions about the productive nature of such objects. Meanwhile it makes us cognisant of the spatio-temporal reach of such practices, suggesting they are simultaneously local and global, happening at the level of local public health management, for example, and at the global level of biosecurity.

In addition, Tom Scott-Smith has recently explored the role of what he terms 'humanitarian objects' in the management of malnutrition emergencies. Examining the use of Plumpy'nut and MUAC bands, Scott-Smith argues that in such instances these objects have become fetishised and 'divorced from their contested origins, credited with magical powers and increasingly seen as indispensable in inflexible approaches to relief'.[21] Such an argument is a useful starting point for considering the role of objects, urging caution as opposed to hasty judgments about the importance and positive role of objects in humanitarian practice. Further, Scott-Smith suggests humanitarian objects should be considered whole, with histories that place them in complex sociologies and processes of production. As such, the rush to fetishise humanitarian objects works to conceal both their origins and their effects.

These recent explorations of humanitarianism and the material used in its practices have tended to focus on those objects used by or on the victims of disaster or disease, such as MSF's 'kit', and those designed to make humanitarian work easier, quicker and more efficient. This has led to the charge of 'fetishism', where objects are 'presented as a miraculous curative' or a 'standardised intervention'.[22] In the case of PPE any fetishisation of the plastic suit, rubber boots, gloves, goggles and face masks that make up this ensemble would conceal both the history of PPE in military responses to chemical and biological warfare and the wide-ranging effects PPE has on the provisions of individual patient care and the governance of biosecurity in the present. However, a charge of fetishisation cannot be levelled at the object of this article in the same way. PPE's important role in facilitating human action while mediating between the care of individual patients and the management of wider biosecurity at local, national and global levels means that it cannot be characterised as a 'technical fix' alone, even while it was concomitantly presented as central in the response to Ebola.

Considering both the productive nature of objects and the problems of fetishisation, the question then becomes how objects in certain instances make humanitarian actions possible and what work they do. This is where turning to devices is useful. Recent work advancing the analytic of devices helps us trace the importance of objects without effacing the often long-running socio-political techniques or rationalities they are created by, work with, or work to bring into being.[23] Importantly this enables the avoidance of privileging either the social or the technical. Instead it facilitates questions about the ways certain modes of government, certain sensibilities, structural conditions and social hierarchies are constituted through their relations with objects and how certain objects come to be constituted through particular social relations.

In working through the facilitation of humanitarian action made possible by the specificities of PPE it is important that we think not only about the role of devices, but also about what kind of human action is made possible and what kind of social relations are rendered visible and enacted by PPE. In this instance, the Foucauldian biopolitics of humanitarian bio-medicine and biosecurity are analytically insufficient for capturing the values and meanings that are and come to be attached to human life here.[24] In addition to being a biopolitics of socio-techniques concerned with the regulation and well-being of populations, humanitarian intervention is:

> [a] politics of life as it takes as its object the saving of individuals, which presupposes not only risking others but also making a selection of which existences it is possible or legitimate to save. It is also a politics of life in that it takes as its object the defence of causes, which presupposes not only leaving other causes aside but also producing public representations of the human beings to be defended.[25]

The question then becomes: 'what sort of life is implicitly (or even explicitly) taken into account in the political work of humanitarian intervention?'[26]

A particular politics of life is not only rendered starkly visible through an investigation of PPE but is also produced and consolidated through the provision, use and focus on PPE in the recent Ebola outbreak. This, along with an exploration of the other ways PPE comes to play a mediating role between local biomedical responses and global biosecurity, as well as managing the continuum of risk, will be examined in the following section. The section will focus on the ways in which the specific characteristics of the virus interact with the specifics of PPE to determine medical intervention, advancing the idea of PPE as an individuated barrier device, exploring what this means for the individual humanitarian workers who had to work with PPE and the wider humanitarian systems in which such care was administered. It also discusses the ways in which a politics of life is produced and consolidated among local and international health workers involved in the humanitarian response, throwing into stark relief the simultaneous discrepancy between the biomedical response and biosecurity concerns.

In addition to these explorations, the analysis will aim to further the debates around the role of devices in humanitarian practice, discussing the ways in which PPE is more than a 'technological fix', centred as it is on facilitating human interaction and mediating different responses to risk. It focuses on the continuum of risk and the humanitarian worker as the potential subject that is simultaneously both *at risk* and *a risk*. Here the role of PPE as an individuated device performing biosecurity at the personal as well as the global level will be worked through before attention is turned to the disciplinary effects of PPE and the way the 'personal' in Personal Protective Equipment works to individualise the management of risk and bring ideas around labour discipline into the humanitarian field. Throughout, the analysis draws on the testimonies, reflections and critiques of practitioners engaged in the humanitarian and medical response to Ebola, focusing on their experiences of using PPE and the wider structures and politics in which their interventions were situated.

Personal Protective Equipment facilitating and mediating the management of Ebola

'You can't stop Ebola without staff, stuff, space and systems.'[27] According to Paul Farmer, anthropologist, medical practitioner and co-founder of Partners in Health,[28] 'stopping transmission' was the first step in governing the virus, bringing it under control and ultimately ending the pandemic. 'Transmission is person to person, in the absence of an effective medical system, it occurs wherever care is given: in households, clinics, and hospitals, and where the dead are tended'; this requires 'uninterrupted supplies of personal protective equipment'.[29] Thus the focus of the following section is on the relationship between staff and stuff.[30]

This focus on PPE is not without foundation. The particular characteristics of Ebola, 'multiplying as the patient declines and increasingly oozing out in bodily fluids', places caregivers at particular risk of catching the virus and/or becoming vectors of transmission,[31] revealing the continuum of risk and how 'care itself has become a source of existential insecurity'.[32] These particular characteristics of the virus are important to consider when working through why PPE played such a central mediating role. Ebola is not an airborne virus, but is transmitted via bodily fluids: blood, urine, breast milk, sweat, tears, vomit, semen and diarrhoea. This results in the particular characteristics of PPE as an individuated, bodily barrier which, if used correctly, prevents health care workers coming into contact with the bodily fluids of patients.

The mode of transmission is also an important factor in understanding how health care workers are not only *at risk* of falling ill themselves but are also *a risk* as potential vectors of transmission. As MSF's report into their Ebola response makes clear: 'In Ebola outbreaks, health facilities without proper infection control often act as multiplying chambers for the virus, and become dangerous places for both health workers and patients'.[33] This risk of infection and the possibilities of transmission result in humanitarians being 'scared of Ebola as it's something about the way it is emitted – through the blood, sweat and tears of human beings'.[34]

Barrier devices

Building on this fear, this section analyses the role of PPE at the level of the virus itself and how PPE facilitates the intervention of humanitarian assistance while also managing the continuum of risk. In her work on governing 'pathogenic circulation' Nadine Voelkner draws our attention to the 'double bind' of circulation for human security. According to Voelkner, circulation is necessary for health security but concomitantly a possible source of risk.[35] Further, in exploring how this 'double bind' is managed, Voelkner argues for the performative role of material objects. PPE is designed to perform security by preventing bad circulation – the transmission of the Ebola virus through bodily fluids – and enabling good circulation – the life-giving forces needed by the caregiver, such as oxygen. As such, PPE is a selectively permeable barrier working at both the bodily level of the individual and also at the molecular level, distinguishing between 'bad' liquids and 'good' gases. This is not an inconsequential distinction but forms an integral part of how PPE works as a life-saving device that takes account of the individual risks faced by the health care worker and the wider risks of transmission that such workers are partly responsible for.

In a recent intervention into caring as an existential act of insecurity, Sung-Joon Park and René Umlauf pointed to the way 'protective gear allows for hermetic isolation of the caregiving individual'.[36] While the identification of care giving as a source of existential insecurity and of PPE's isolating role is accurate here, the characterisation of protective gear as *hermetic* isolation reproduces similar mainstream logics around other forms of barrier, focusing on the blockading actions of barrier devices at the expense – in the most extreme of cases – of mischaracterisation of the device itself.[37] No barrier designed for wider techniques of government concerned with biopolitical logics can ever perform 'hermetic isolation' when circulation is a central life-force. Instead barriers work to mediate between levels of risk. For example, specially constructed infectious disease isolation wards still allow for the movement of people, caregivers in this instance, as well as things: medicines, food, water and oxygen. These movements are tightly controlled and filtered according to calculations of risk but these units do not prevent movement. The same is true of PPE itself, designed as it is to stop the transmission of Ebola and other viruses contained in bodily fluids. It does not seal the wearer in but facilitates good, life-giving circulation through the use of permeable facemasks allowing for the movement of gases – oxygen in and carbon dioxide out – without which the wearer would die. Thus Redfield's more accurate description of PPE as a 'second skin' better captures its particular characteristic as a selectively permeable membrane.[38]

The focus on the passing of gasses through the facemasks of PPE is not a small observation, as it is often the facial areas where PPE is vulnerable as a form of protection and where transmission is most likely to occur. By having to allow for circulation of oxygen and carbon dioxide, PPE has an in-built weakness and can itself become a site of transmission. The need to consider the well-being of the body inside the PPE alongside the ability of the device to stop transmission is highlighted by the secondary ways that PPE, while acting as a device for securing the individual against the spread of particular liquid-borne pathogens, can itself also be a risk to the well-being of the wearer. In such a way PPE becomes a double-sided device or a 'double-bind'.[39] Adam Levine, an emergency medicine specialist treating Ebola sufferers in Liberia shows how PPE can become a risk to health and the ability to provide patient care while recounting a story of having to rehydrate an Ebola patient by feeding him rehydration fluids by the capful: 'Only a few hundred more capfuls to rehydrate him, but I know that in the stifling heat I am not going to last much longer in my full PPE'.[40] As a result, most experts do not think that caregivers should spend more than two to three hours in PPE for their own health and to be able to provide care safely.

That being said, when one considers the role of PPE in facilitating individual patient care, it does in certain ways become a barrier mediating between health care workers and their patients, as shown by the experiences of Levine above and outlined by Hilde De Clerck, a doctor with MSF:

> We have to move and breathe slowly due to the overpowering heat, limiting us to spending an hour maximum inside at a time. Inside the high-risk zone, I have to plan the most crucial activities I can squeeze into an hour. It's frustrating and upsetting that I can't spend unlimited time with my patients or connect with them as I usually would, with a smile or a comforting human touch.[41]

Here PPE may be a selectively permeable barrier but the suits, face masks and goggles act as a barrier between the medical practitioner and the patient, limiting time, physical contact and emotional connections.[42] This physical isolation from patients is a source of much discomfort for humanitarians. Furthermore it is difficult to identify the individuals inside the suits, as faces become obscured and bodies become encased in plastic 'space suits'. Humanitarians have attempted to deal with this de-personalisation for both themselves and their patients by writing their names on their suits, most usually on their foreheads in recognition of the importance of the facial area and eye contact in forging personal connections.

In addition to the discomfort with physical and emotional isolation, and the problems of overheating and dehydration, PPE also causes problems for the wearer's ability to deliver patient-centred care by restricting movement. Frederique Jacquerioz, a doctor and researcher, told the American Society of Tropical Medicine and Hygiene's annual meeting in 2014 that PPE hindered ease of movement and that movement in the suit was itself an acquired skill, 'not something that can be learned in 20 minutes'.[43] These concerns were also echoed by MSF when faced with time constraints in training new, inexperienced staff in the realities of working with Ebola.[44] In addition, PPE hampers existing skills, making it difficult to listen to the lungs or to put in an IV drip.[45]

That people have to remove PPE – and have to do this so regularly in tropical conditions – causes additional problems, as the removal of the suits becomes a major source of potential transmission. This along with the problem of overheating, where workers lose up to 1.5 litres of sweat per hour, and other problems with 'regular' PPE have been recognised by experts tasked with managing the biosecurity response to Ebola, such as the US Centers for Disease Control and Prevention (CDC) and USAID. These problems include 28 possible points of transmission where the barrier functions of PPE are thought to break down around 'seam zones'. Additionally the time it takes for removal – up to 20 minutes and involving up to 31 steps – has been acknowledged as a weakness in the effectiveness of PPE. A focus on these weaknesses shows how PPE becomes a point of tension itself. Through its work mediating different levels of risk it is also a 'double bind', leading to calls for a technological fix.

Some of those concerned with the technology of global health management believe that PPE can be made to work better to manage the tensions its 'double bind' character produces in practice. Such potential technological fixes have been suggested through the 'Fighting Ebola: a Grand Challenge for Development' competition run and financed by USAID.[46] One of the winners of the competition was the Johns Hopkins Center for Bioengineering Innovation and Design, in conjunction with the international health organisation JHPIEGO, which designed a new PPE suit 'purposefully designed to address safety and climate issues now putting health workers at risk'.[47] Here the suit becomes 'fetishised' as the 'thing' that needs fixing, while the wider underlying structural factors of the Ebola pandemic go unaddressed. Attention is focused on creating the perfect suit to manage this and future outbreaks, instead of addressing the inadequacies of health care systems unable to cope with treating Ebola. In addition, such technological fixes fail to address the already existing problems of inadequate PPE provision. In the recent Ebola pandemic local health care workers were reduced to using plastic bags, and even international humanitarian agencies were unable to provide adequate and effective protection for local health care workers outside the specially built Ebola Treatment Centres.

Protecting and producing the humanitarian subject

The body inside the PPE cannot be ignored. This section will examine PPE's role in the production of the humanitarian worker as the subject of protection. Here attention will be paid to the importance of the protection of 'human resources' and the responsibility of humanitarian agencies for the protection of their staff on both ethical and practical grounds. Through this focus on 'human resources' and the protection of personnel we witness the production and consolidation of a politics of life between those who were accorded the protection of full PPE and those who had to make do with homespun, *ad hoc* solutions, such as plastic bags, or simply go without. In the process the section highlights PPE's involvement in wider postcolonial relations and political economies of inequality. In the Ebola outbreak, however, this politics of life was not a politics of neat categories between those lives risked and those saved. Instead, echoing the blurred boundaries of postcolonial relations that challenge the neat categories of 'self' and 'other', the politics of life enacted by PPE's mediation of a continuum of risk produced a context-specific and relationally contingent politics of life.

As much humanitarian action occurs within a continuum of risk where its subjects are both *at* risk and *a* risk, where they may move between the two and may be both simultaneously, the governance of Ebola and the difference made by PPE in the performance of such interventions complicates the issue of who is the subject of such protection. With humanitarianism's focus on protecting both the individual and the wider population, the subject is usually presumed to be the 'victim(s)' of natural disasters, disease and conflict. However, it has also been recognised that the humanitarian is also at risk through the practice of saving lives, particularly in situations of violent conflict.[48] The performance of PPE speaks to this, because the *person* in the *person*al protective equipment is the humanitarian worker and not the Ebola sufferer. Through being worn on the body of the humanitarian worker, PPE enables said worker to carry out humanitarian tasks and produces the worker as the principal subject of protection.

'Everything needed to be done by someone and on a massive scale.'[49] So having enough staff and protecting them from infection was of critical importance. The issues of human resources and the protection of staff were critical in two ways: so that there were enough people to carry out life-saving tasks; and to avoid deterring potential volunteers.[50] Here the role of PPE in protecting and enabling comes to the fore in the central role that human resources played in many organisations' ability to respond effectively and safely to the pandemic. The specific experiences of MSF in this regard are illuminating, where again and again the need for staff, their protection, not deterring new volunteers through fear of the virus and the limitations that these created all affected the response. Lindis Hurum, MSF's Emergency Coordinator in Monrovia in August 2014, had this to say:

> we are not without limits. And we've reached our limit. It's very frustrating, because I see the huge needs but I simply don't have the human resources. We have the money thanks to our donors. We have the will. We certainly have motivation, but I don't have enough people to deal with this.[51]

'MSF does not have an Ebola army with a warehouse of personnel on standby. We rely on the availability and commitment of our volunteers.'[52] In addition, MSF felt it was 'under pressure to set an example and show it was possible to treat Ebola safely, in an effort to mobilise others to intervene. If we took even more risks and too many staff fell ill, we'd be unable to maintain trust with our teams or recruit new volunteers'.[53] Furthermore, like other humanitarian organisations, MSF had a duty of care to its staff and volunteers. 'Our duty for our staff is certainly crucial...Though we have invested heavily In personal protective equipment, training and security protocols, we have painfully learned there is never zero risk.'[54]

When we consider the idea of risk as a continuum rather than a binary relationship, the humanitarian community can no longer be cast solely in the privileged position of saviour. The specific nature of the Ebola virus and the role of PPE in countering it ask us to recast the humanitarian net to include the humanitarian community itself as not only the providers of protection but also the subjects of protection. In turn, this works in part to privilege issues of the security of particular individuals above and before issues of humanity as a whole and forces us to ask questions about whose security is being considered. It also works, in practice, to entrench the structural privileges of international agencies over more local responses, often along racial lines, while simultaneously working to efface Ebola's victims. Such an observation is not surprising, when the security of populations clashes with issues of individual security, raising as it does so ethical and risk-based calculations, especially in the field of humanitarianism where – at least in theory – every individual is said to have equal humanity. In other words, these tensions are of particular ethical concern for the humanitarian community itself.

> But in a public health emergency of this scale and danger, patient communication and coun-selling can be brushed aside under the pretext of urgency. Ebola patients can be considered mere disease-carriers rather than complicated, emotional human beings.[55]

That being said, the production of the humanitarian worker as the subject raises additional ethical questions around a politics of life and the production of particular 'hierarchies of humanity' and moral economies. This was starkly illuminated when 'the realisation dawned that Ebola could cross the ocean. When Ebola became an international security threat, and no longer a humanitarian crisis affecting a handful of poor countries in West Africa',[56] and a belated global biosecurity response was mobilised. This response was mostly restricted to supporting coordination and logistics and included the building of medical facilities for treating healthcare workers while ignoring the provision of direct medical assistance to local populations.[57]

However, even with this focus on protecting the humanitarian workers, not everyone was the subject of protection. Instead, in certain instances already existing structural and racial hierarchies between international humanitarian workers and local health workers treating Ebola were reproduced. As Paul Farmer argues, effective PPE is not and was not available to every clinician or to those – usually women – attempting to care for sick family members at home.[58] In an attempt to address this inadequacy of equipment and the risks to those caring for their families and communities at home, away from the infection controls offered at Ebola Treatment Centres, MSF distributed 600,000 'home disinfection kits' in Monrovia in order to reduce infection risk, while knowing that 'these kits were not the solution'.[59] In contrast, those staff affiliated with international agencies had access to equipment such as PPE and medical facilities to treat them if they fell ill. Many international staff were evacuated back to North America and Europe for treatment in state-of-the-art infectious disease units such as those at the Emory University Hospital in Atlanta and the Royal Free Hospital in London, while nearly 500 local medical workers lost their lives, starkly highlighting the structural differences in public health provision. Not only were Western medical and humanitarian workers treated in state-of-the-art units, but they were also the recipients of treatments unavailable in West Africa. In Western hospitals patients were tended to by many clinicians 24 hours a day, while those who fell ill in West Africa were most often treated by their families at home or in Ebola Treatment Centres, where health care workers could only spend a few minutes with each patient and in certain instances were forced to institute drastic systems of triage and limit who they could admit. This 'meant dead bodies in the homes and lying in the street, sick people unable to get a bed and spreading it to their loved ones and only being able to offer very basic palliative care'.[60] Thus the humanitarian subject was also within specific contexts and relationships a racialised humanitarian subject, echoing Fassin's argu-ments around the differing moral economies attached to values of life for international and local humanitarian workers.[61]

Personal to global protection equipment

The lack of PPE in the zones of the Ebola outbreak highlights the spatio-temporal logics of a technocratic approach to global health that seeks to govern through vertical interven-tions, technological fixes, 'benchmarking progress' and circumventing 'the messy realities of international politics and local infrastructures…for more effective results'.[62] Throughout this article it has been argued that PPE mediates the relationship between providing a humanitarian biomedical response and managing global biosecurity. This section turns to this relationship in specific detail, exploring how in the process PPE acts as a barrier device between the personal, local and global, and between the ability to provide individual patient-centred care and the ability to manage biosecurity on a global scale. This in turn uncovers tensions between the two approaches outlined by Lakoff in empirical practice, drawing our attention to 'an impossible tension between curbing the spread of the disease, and providing the best clinical care to each patient'.[63] Such tensions generated hard-hitting critiques from within organisations,[64] as well as between those practitioners present on the ground and those such as the CDC who were concerned with managing the pandemic and protecting populations.[65] What an analysis of PPE and the work it does enables us to see is that, in practice, these tensions are mediated and managed through an imbrication of human action and technologies that leave wider structural causes and inequalities unresolved.

By recasting the individual biosecurity of the humanitarian worker as the subject and policing their individual body PPE highlights the personal in biosecurity, but moreover PPE works to police the exterior or the wider population by managing the individual biosecurity of humanitarian workers. By policing the individual body of the humanitarian and the centrality of circulation across space – individual to local to global – in humanitarian responses to Ebola, PPE also works to police the exterior and the security of the wider population. As the humanitarian response to Ebola has been an international one, workers move from areas of infection to other parts of the globe in line with long-standing forms of humanitarian practice. This means they are a risk for transmitting the virus not only in Ebola-affected regions of West Africa, but across the planet. Consequently humanitarian workers must not only be protected by PPE to save their own lives and so that they can perform humanitarian biomedicine, but, as a potential vector of transmission, they must also be protected so that they do not become risks to wider populations.

Such logics were on display in the responses to those humanitarian workers who were evacuated to Spain, the USA and the UK in 2014 to receive treatment. Their returns sparked nationally focused concerns about borders, quarantines and flight bans. When Craig Spencer, a doctor who had volunteered for MSF in Guéckédou, Guinea, tested positive for Ebola on 23 October 2014 in New York City, after a period of self-monitoring, there were subsequent orders from the governors of New York and New Jersey for the routine quarantining of returning humanitarian workers that resulted in nurse Kaci Hickox being detained at Newark airport.[66] These calls for flight bans, border closures and the enactment of quarantines all failed to consider the necessity of mobility and human resources for an effective response to Ebola. Hickox criticised her detention on the grounds that it would deter people from volunteering with organisations like MSF and carrying out much needed work to fight the disease.[67] Additionally, like much of the Ebola response that saw other medical services scaled back or stopped completely, the calls for quarantines and flight bans also failed to consider the wider security of the populations of Guinea, Liberia and Sierra Leone, with their already fragile economies.

While, as we have seen, PPE mediates the relationship between providing humanitarian biomedicine based on individualised patient-care and wider biosecurity, the case of Craig Spencer also highlights the ways in which individual humanitarian workers were made responsible not only for their own biosecurity but for the biosecurity of whole populations.

Through PPE being worn on the body of the individual caregiver, risk, both personal and potentially global, is individuated and embodied at the level of the humanitarian worker and, crucially, is determined by how well they use their PPE. As such, PPE speaks to previous debates around the incorporation of citizens and individuals into the performance of security. However, previous debates have tended to focus on individuals reporting suspicions to institutions of authority, such as UK-based campaigns around reporting potential terrorists and irregular migrants, turning citizens into informants encouraged to police their societies.[68] The individualisation and embodiment of risk in the PPE that adorns humanitarian workers casts them as both informant *and* policeman by enjoining them in a variety of spatial settings to self-monitor, police their bodies and notify the relevant authorities when they detect any change in their body temperature, as indeed was the case with Craig Spencer in New York. Crucially this policing and reporting is not concerned with suspicions of others, but suspicions of the self as a potential biosecurity risk.

This is not therefore just about individual bodies being the subject of potential global (in)security, but the subject of security being the self and that same self being responsible for ensuring his/her own security and that of others. As such, processes of discipline and labour play a role in the relationship between humanitarians, their PPE, their capacity to perform individual patient care and the global human biosecurity assemblage of which they are a part. The humanitarian worker must be properly trained in using PPE for it to work effectively, as without proper training PPE can become a hazard, offering as it does a false sense of security. Here the cases of Nina Pham and Amber Joy Vinson, the two nurses who contracted Ebola at the Texas Health Presbyterian Hospital in Dallas where they encountered Thomas Eric Duncan, the USA's first Ebola fatality, are instructive. Pham and Vinson were the first two people to contract Ebola in the USA (Duncan had contracted the virus in Liberia) and controversy raged over whether they had received adequate training in using PPE safely, amid continually changing Ebola protocols at the Dallas hospital. Bonnie Costello from the largest nurses union in the USA, National Nurses United, accused the hospital of scapegoating Pham,[69] while others reported that Pham and Vinson had not had access to any PPE when first encountering Duncan. In handling questions around the transmission of the virus, Tom Frieden, the director of the CDC, emphasised the importance of using PPE safely, in particular the importance of removing the equipment – above all gloves – correctly.[70] Meanwhile, in the case of Pauline Cafferkey, a British Save the Children worker who contracted Ebola while working in Sierra Leone, Michael von Bertele, the charity's humanitarian director, said:

> It's really important for us to try and understand whether it was a failure of training, of protection, of procedure, or indeed whether she contracted it in some incidental contact within the community, because our workers don't just work inside the red zone, which is a very high-risk area, they do also have contact – although we are very, very careful in briefing people to avoid personal contact – outside of the treatment centre.[71]

In these cases it is clear that caregivers in the process of carrying out their duties of employment are disciplined into behaving correctly in order to ensure their own and others' security. And yet even here we see a global health approach that privileges a 'technological fix' for the problems of discipline and the risk individual mistakes in removing PPE can pose. A case in point is the aforementioned new PPE designed by Johns Hopkins to mitigate the risks of heat, as it is also designed to lessen the potential risks in removing the suit. As the Johns Hopkins Ebola Hub says:

The Johns Hopkins prototype is designed to do a better job than current garments in keeping health care workers from coming in contact with Ebola patients' contagious body fluids, both during treatment and while removing a soiled suit.[72]

Such a 'technological fix', while being attentive to the previous deficiencies and weaknesses of PPE, and to the fallibility of its human subjects, creates a suit that circumvents and makes no attempt to address the messy political and structural realities and inequalities that underpin local health care provision in West Africa.

Conclusion

This article has explored the intersections and symbioses of the human and non-human in processes of governance using the symbiotic and historical relationship between humanitarian practice – as a field constituted around the human[73] – and technology, devices and material in performing both individual patient care and biosecurity. In advancing the analytic of the device it has argued for understanding how PPE mediates between on-the-ground humanitarian biomedicine and global biosecurity. PPE here is an important risk-mediator where its wearers are both *at* risk of catching the virus and simultaneously *a* risk as a possible transmission vector. Through tracing the work PPE does as a humanitarian device, the continuum of risk faced by many involved in the humanitarian response to Ebola, and the dual role they played, has been highlighted. In exploring how PPE facilitates wider humanitarian techniques, the article has traced the messy networks and worlds produced and consolidated through the use of PPE in the governance of Ebola. It has extended the analytic of barriers concerned with governing circulation to encompass barriers at the level of the individual human body.

Meanwhile, it has shown how PPE also challenges the primacy of biopolitics in a biosecurity response concerned with protecting populations by exploring PPE's role in producing and consolidating a particular politics of life. Here PPE privileges the humanitarian as the risky subject and therefore the subject of protection, recalibrating the relationship between victim and saviour in humanitarian practice and reproducing pre-existing racial and socioeconomic hierarchies between a technically capable West and countries lacking in even the most basic of resources. An analysis of the politics of life produced by PPE leads to much wider questions around *whose* security was being managed and whose security was being disregarded in the humanitarian biomedical response to Ebola, with attempts to provide patient-centred care while also pre-emptively managing the biosecurity of those populations not affected by the pandemic. The biopolitics of biosecurity, concerned with technical fixes and management systems, is also unsettled through the individualisation of risk and issues of discipline and labour.

In doing this, the article has argued that, while humanitarian practice has the tendency to fetishise objects in the pursuit of technical fixes for complex emergencies, objects cannot be considered solely in this vein. PPE works to complicate the idea of the technological fix by making its case as a necessary facilitator of life-saving interventions, while also having its own faults technologically fixed for improved efficiency and risk management. In uncovering what work PPE does, an additional empirical case has been offered, to add to those offered previously by Redfield and Scott-Smith, to highlight the complex sociologies of devices used in humanitarian practice and wider biosecurity.

Disclosure statement

No potential conflict of interest was reported by the author.

Acknowledgements

I would like to thank the reviewers and editors for their engagement with this piece and the insightful comments and suggestions. I would like to thank those members of MSF-Holland and those in the Operational Centre in Amsterdam who shared their experiences and insights with me and listened to my arguments. Thanks must go to Alison Howell, Lee Seymour and those present at the 'Humanitarianism and Technology: Agents, Actions and Orders' panel held during the 2015 ISA conference in New Orleans, where this article was first presented. In addition, thanks to those at the 'The Ontological Politics of Security: Materialism and Discontents' panel of the 2015 EISA conference in Sicily for their comments, questions and suggestions, with special thanks to Rocco Bellanova.

Notes

1. Hinshaw, "Ebola Virus."
2. See MSF's interactive tour of PPE: http://www.msf.org/article/interactive-learn-about-our-ebola-protective-equipment.
3. Blackburn, "Gunboat Abolitionism."
4. Turner, "The Enclave Society," 290–291.
5. Redfield, "Bioexpectations"; and Scott-Smith, "The Fetishism of Humanitarian Objects."
6. Scott-Smith, "The Fetishism of Humanitarian Objects."
7. Amicelle et al., "Questioning Security Devices."
8. "Ebola: A Challenge to our Humanitarian Identity – A Letter to the MSF Movement," an internal letter written by nine MSF practitioners to the movement in December, 2014. http://www.youscribe.com/BookReader/IframeEmbed?productId=2541547&width=auto&height=auto&startPage=1&displayMode=scroll&documentId=2622078&fullscreen=1&token=aJNTPzsW88Pb%2bKLv2wQI6egMIN58L6IVJM wGsoZGeNEuOQVCugGs1DfeITN6jz6ulJnT99yY6KhGt13Mn8XtnQ%3d%3d. The letter appeared in *Libération*, February 3, 2015 . http://www.liberation.fr/terre/2015/02/03/parfois-le-traitement-symptomatique-a-ete-neglige-voire-oublie_1194960.
9. MSF, *Ebola*.
10. Abdelnour and Saeed, "Technologizing Humanitarian Space"; and Scott-Smith, "The Fetishism of Humanitarian Objects."
11. Barad, "Getting Real," 108.
12. Fassin, "Humanitarianism as a Politics of Life."
13. Barnett and Weiss, *Humanitarianism in Question*.
14. Lakoff, "Two Regimes of Global Health," 64.
15. Lakoff, "Two Regimes of Global Health," 63.

16. Lakoff, "Two Regimes of Global Health," 59.
17. Lakoff, "Two Regimes of Global Health," 67.
18. Ibid.
19. Redfield, "Vital Mobility," 147.
20. Redfield, "Vital Mobility," 148.
21. Scott-Smith, "The Fetishism of Humanitarian Objects," 914.
22. Ibid.
23. Amicelle et al., "Questioning Security Devices."
24. Foucault, "The Birth of Biopolitics."
25. Fassin, "Humanitarianism as a Politics of Life," 501.
26. Ibid.
27. Farmer, "Diary," 39.
28. http://www.pih.org/.
29. Farmer, "Diary," 39.
30. However, I do not discount the role of space, such as in the creation of Ebola treatment centres that make use of a range of devices seeking to manage the circulation of patients, staff and systems of triage, and the wider systems of logistics governing the response to the pandemic, or the longer-term viable health systems needed to address the structural factors underpinning the specifics of this Ebola outbreak.
31. Redfield, "Medical Vulnerability."
32. Park and Umlauf, "Caring as Existential Insecurity."
33. MSF, Ebola, 7.
34. Dr. Javid Abdelmoneim, MSF doctor in Sierra Leone, quoted in MSF, Ebola, 17 .
35. Voelkner, "Managing Pathogenic Circulation," 240.
36. Park and Umlauf, "Caring as Existential Insecurity," 3.
37. For more on barriers as more than blockading technologies and as selectively permeable membranes, see Pallister-Wilkins, "Bridging the Divide."
38. Redfield, "Vital Mobility."
39. Voelkner, "Managing Pathogenic Circulation."
40. Farmer, "Diary."
41. MSF, Ebola, 17.
42. Dr. Hilde De Clerck, see note 12 above, 17.
43. Radin, "Frozen by the Hot Zone."
44. MSF, Ebola, 9.
45. Intravenous rehydration through the use of IVs in treating Ebola patients is a source of much disagreement within the medical and humanitarian world.
46. See USAID, Fighting Ebola: A Grand Challenge for Development, 2014, http://www.usaid.gov/news-information/press-releases/dec-12-2014-united-states-announces-results-grand-challenge-fight-ebola.
47. See John Hopkins' Ebola Hub: http://hub.jhu.edu/2014/12/12/ebola-suit-design-funding.
48. Fassin, "Humanitarian Reason."
49. Dr Jean-Clément Cabrol, MSF Director of Operations, quoted in MSF, Ebola, 12.
50. De Clerck, Ibid.
51. Lindis Hurum, quoted in MSF, Ebola, 10.
52. Brice de le Vingne, MSF director of operations, quoted in MSF, Ebola, 9.
53. Hurum, Ibid.
54. Henry Gray, MSF emergency coordinator, quoted in MSF, Ebola, 17.
55. Frankfurter, "The Danger." Frankfurter was a health worker in Sierra Leone.
56. Dr Joanne Liu, MSF international president, quoted in MSF, Pushed to the Limit, 11.
57. MSF, Ebola, 14.
58. Farmer, "Diary," 39.
59. Anna Halford, MSF coordinator for distribution, quoted in MSF, Ebola, 18.
60. Rosa Crestani, MSF Ebola task force coordinator, quoted in MSF, Ebola, 10.
61. Farmer, "Diary," 39.

62. Beisel, "On Gloves," 2.
63. MSF, *Ebola*, 19.
64. See note 10 above.
65. Over, "CDC vs Médecins Sans Frontières."
66. Gambino, "Craig Spencer declared Free of Ebola"; and Lakoff, "Timeline."
67. Gambino, "Craig Spencer declared Free of Ebola."
68. Vaughan-Williams, "Borderwork beyond Inside/Outside?"
69. "US CDC Head Criticized."
70. Goodwyn, "Was CDC too Quick?"
71. Halliday, "Scottish Ebola Case."
72. See note 38 above.
73. Watson, "The 'Human' as Referent Object?"

Bibliography

Abdelnour, Samer, and Akbar M. Saeed. "Technologizing Humanitarian Space: Darfur Advocacy and the Rape-stove Panacea." *International Political Sociology* 8, no. 2 (2014): 145–163.

Amicelle, Anthony, Claudia Aradau, and Julien Jeandesboz. "Questioning Security Devices: Performativity, Resistance, Politics." *Security Dialogue* 46, no. 4 (2015): 293–306.

Barad, Karen. "Getting Real: Technoscientific Practices and the Materialization of Reality." *Differences: A Journal of Feminist Cultural Studies* 10, no. 2 (1998): 87–128.

Barnett, Michael, and Thomas C. Weiss eds. *Humanitarianism in Question: Politics, Power, Ethics*. Ithaca, NY: Cornell University Press, 2008.

Beisel, Uli. "On Gloves, Rubber and the Spatio-temporal Logics of Global Health." *Somatosphere*, 2014. http://somatosphere.net/2014/10/rubber-gloves-global-health.html.

Blackburn, Robin. "Gunboat Abolitionism." *New Left Review* 87 (2014): 143–152.

Farmer, Paul. 2014. "Diary: Ebola." *London Review of Books*, October Article History 23 . http://www.lrb.co.uk/v36/n20/paul-farmer/diary.

Fassin, Didier. *Humanitarian Reason: A Moral History of the Present*. Berkeley: University of California Press, 2012.

Fassin, Didier. "Humanitarianism as a Politics of Life." *Public Culture* 19, no. 3 (2007): 499–520.

Foucault, Michel. *The Birth of Biopolitics: Lectures at the Collège de France 1978–1979*. Basingstoke: Palgrave Macmillan, 2008.

Frankfurter, Raphael. "The Danger of losing sight of Ebola Victims' Humanity." *The Atlantic*, August 22, 2014. http://www.theatlantic.com/health/archive/2014/08/the-danger-in-losing-sight-of-ebola-victims-humanity/378945/.

Gambino, Lauren. 2014. "Craig Spencer declared Free of Ebola, says he is 'Living Example' of how Virus Protocols Work." *Guardian*, November Article History 11 , http://www.theguardian.com/us-news/2014/nov/11/no-ebola-america-craig-spencer-leaves-hospital.

Goodwyn, Wade. "Was CDC too quick to blame Dallas Nurses in Care of Ebola Patient?" National Public Radio, October 24, 2014. http://www.npr.org/2014/10/24/358574357/was-cdc-too-quick-to-blame-dallas-nurses-in-care-of-ebola-patient.

Halliday, Josh. 2014. "Scottish Ebola case triggers Save the Children Investigation." *Guardian*, December Article History 31 . http://www.theguardian.com/world/2014/dec/31/scottish-ebola-case-save-children-investigation-pauline-cafferkey.

Hinshaw, Drew. 2014. "Ebola Virus: For Want of Gloves, Doctors Die." *Wall Street Journal*, August 16. http://www.wsj.com/articles/ebola-doctors-with-no-rubber-gloves-1408142137.

Lakoff, Andrew. "Timeline: Ebola 2014." *Limn* 5 (2015). http://limn.it/timeline-ebola-2014/.

Lakoff, Andrew. "Two Regimes of Global Health." *Humanity: An International Journal of Human Rights* 1, no. 1 (2010): 59–79.

Médecins Sans Frontières (MSF). *Ebola: Pushed to the Limit and Beyond – A Critical Analysis of the Global Ebola Response one Year into the Deadliest Outbreak in History*. 2015. https://www.doctorswithoutborders.org/sites/usa/files/msf143061.pdf.

Pallister-Wilkins, Polly. "Bridging the Divide: Middle Eastern Walls and Fences and the Spatial Governance of Problem Populations." *Geopolitics* 20, no. 2 (2015): 438–459.

Park, Sung-Joon, and René Umlauf. "Caring as Existential Insecurity: Quarantine, Care, and Human Insecurity in the Ebola Crisis." *Somatosphere*, 2014. http://somatosphere.net/2014/11/caring-as-existential-insecurity.html.

Over, Mead. "CDC vs. Médecins Sans Frontières on Ebola: Is the Perfect the Enemy of the Good?" Center for Global Development, September 25, 2014. http://www.cgdev.org/blog/cdc-vs-medecins-sans-frontieres-ebola-perfect-enemy-good.

Radin, Joanna. "Frozen by the Hot Zone." *Limn* 5 (2015). http://limn.it/frozen-by-the-hot-zone/.

Redfield, Peter. "Medical Vulnerability, or Where there is no Kit." *Limn* 5 (2015). http://limn.it/medical-vulnerability-or-where-there-is-no-kit/.

Redfield, Peter. "Bioexpectations: Life Technologies as Humanitarian Goods." *Public Culture* 24, no. 1 (2012): 157–184.

Redfield, Peter. "Vital Mobility and the Humanitarian Kit." In *Biosecurity Interventions: Global Health and Security in Question*, edited by Andrew Lakoff and Stephen J Collier, 147–171. New York: Columbia University Press, 2008.

Scott-Smith, Tom. "The Fetishism of Humanitarian Objects and the Management of Malnutrition in Emergencies." *Third World Quarterly* 34, no. 5 (2013): 914–928.

Turner, Bryan S. "The Enclave Society: Towards a Sociology of Immobility." *European Journal of Social Theory* 10, no. 2 (2007): 287–304.

"US CDC Head criticized for blaming 'Protocol Breach' as Nurse gets Ebola." Reuters, October 13, 2014. http://www.reuters.com/article/2014/10/13/us-health-ebola-usa-nurse-idUSKCN0I206820141013.

Vaughan-Williams, Nick. "Borderwork beyond Inside/Outside? Frontex, the Citizen-detective and the War on Terror." *Space and Polity* 12, no. 1 (2008): 63–79.

Voelkner, Nadine. "Managing Pathogenic Circulation: Human Security and the Migrant Health Assemblage in Thailand." *Security Dialogue* 42, no. 3 (2011): 239–259.

Watson, Scott. "The 'Human' as Referent Object Humanitarianism as Securitization." *Security Dialogue* 42, no. 1 (2012): 3–20.

Ebola, gender and conspicuously invisible women in global health governance

Sophie Harman

School of Politics and International Relations, Queen Mary University of London, UK

ABSTRACT

The international response to Ebola brings into stark contention the conspicuous invisibility of women and gender in global health governance. Developing feminist research on gender blindness, care and male bias, this article uses Ebola as a case to explore how global health rests on the conspicuous free labour of women in formal and informal care roles, yet renders women invisible in policy and practice. The article does so by demonstrating the conspicuous invisibility of women and gender in narratives on Ebola, emergency and long-term strategies to contain the disease, and in the health system strengthening plans of the World Health Organization and World Bank.

The international response to and rhetoric surround Ebola Virus Disease (Ebola) in Guinea, Liberia and Sierra Leone in 2014 brings into stark contention a central paradox in global health governance: the conspicuous invisibility of women and gender. On the one hand, women such as World Health Organization (WHO) Director General Margaret Chan and Médecins San Frontières (MSF) International President Joanne Liu have been conspicuously visible in the Ebola response, while actors such as Melinda Gates have a high profile in promoting women's reproductive health issues. On the other hand, the differing impacts of the disease on women and men, the gendered role of women as carers, and the role of women in health systems in West Africa have been invisible. Other than a handful of high-profile women leading global institutions, women are conspicuously invisible in global health governance: people working in global health are aware of and see women in care roles that underpin health systems, yet they are invisible in global health strategy, policy or practice. Women are only made visible through motherhood. The problem here is not only the conspicuous invisibility of women but that of gender, as global health policy and practice ignores and subsequently reinforces gendered norms of care and social reproduction. Ebola provides an insightful case study in which to demonstrate the conspicuous invisibility of women and gendered care roles in emergency and long-term global health policy and practice. This article will demonstrate that gender and women are conspicuously invisible at every point in the international response to the outbreak: first, with regard to data on the number of males and females contracting and dying from Ebola; second, in the lack of any discussion on gender as an analytical lens in the emergency and long-term response; third, in the little critical engagement on gender and Ebola in wider academic debates on the response; and, finally, in the complete absence of discussion as to the role of social reproduction and women in the care economy in strategies to strengthen health systems.

The article develops its argument by first situating the concept of conspicuous invisibility within wider feminist debate on gender blindness in international policy making, care and social reproduction. It then provides an overview of the literature on Ebola from January 2014 to January 2015 to demonstrate how the 'crisis' has been represented by key opinion and knowledge formers in global health governance. The inclusion of women and gender in the response to Ebola is then reviewed with reference to initiatives from the World Bank and WHO as two of the key leaders in the response. The article goes on to explore discussions over the long-term strategy towards health system strengthening by the Bank and WHO to show how the role of women in the care economy is invisible at every stage of the planning process. It then considers what could be done differently as a basis for thinking about gender in future disease outbreaks and long-term health system strengthening. In conclusion, the article argues that, should women and issues of gender remain invisible, health systems will remain weak, precarious and dependent on the resilience of women to address deadly viruses such as Ebola. This will be to the detriment of women's health and well-being, and will reinforce gender assumptions and the conspicuous invisibility of women in care.

Gender, care and social reproduction

Care is a critical issue of inquiry for scholars of feminist political economy and public health with regard to women's under-valued, often unpaid labour in the care economy and the burden of social reproduction roles in the family and community. The burden of care-giving at multiple levels, public and private, is highly feminised. Studies show that the burden of care falls to women across a range of incomes, education and welfare systems.[1] Feminised burden of care can be explained by the gender norms and expectations of women as a gender with regard to social reproduction in the family and wider communities in which they live. Adopting Rai's definition, 'social reproduction' refers to biological reproduction, unpaid production in the home of good and services, and the reproduction of culture and ideology, notably the expectation that women will suspend periods of employment for biological reproduction.[2] Such roles are under-valued or assumed in society and international public policy making and tend to be unpaid or low paid. Women are overly represented in this low/unpaid reproductive economy but under-represented in the paid productive economy, which economists, policy makers and society recognise and value.[3] The feminised unpaid reproductive care economy 'acts as a "shock absorber" in periods of crisis', by taking on the care and welfare functions when the state, employer or individual can no longer pay for them.[4] The ability of the individual or state to address such welfare and care provisioning can have a direct impact on intersectional inequalities and risk vulnerability across gender, race, class and geography.[5] Women absorb the burden of care through self-exploitation (leading to direct and indirect health impacts on women as a gender), reliance on family, or outsourcing care roles to poorer women.[6]

According to feminist research, the performance of women in social reproduction and care roles is either assumed or ignored in the design of public policies.[7] Care roles and social reproduction are commonly naturalised in public policy in such a way that the cost of care is unacknowledged or assumed. Such a lack of engagement with the gendered dimensions of care can be explained by the presence of what Elson terms 'male bias' in the policy process. According to Elson, male bias is not deliberate but is a blindness to the economic structures 'that operate in favour of men as a gender, and against women as a gender, not that all men are biased against women'.[8] Elson argues for the need to move away from the emphasis on 'women in development' that generalises women and makes them the problem, instead of looking at the structural constraints and injustice afforded to them on account of their gender. Elson emphasises the need for gender-aware and gender-visible policy that recognises conscious and unconscious bias in the policy process.[9] On account of women's over-representation in the reproductive sector and the lack of social and financial value placed on such roles, feminist political economists argue that the unpaid care economy must become a highly visible part of policy making.[10]

The formal and informal care economy and assumptions of gender in the policy-making process are vital, yet often overlooked, components of global health. Provision of care, healthcare and reproduction of healthy bodies is a core part of social reproduction and social reproduction is integral to the functioning of health systems: care in the home and the community, provision of infant and child health, and expectations that such care roles are given to women as a gender. Women perform these social reproduction roles in a way that underpins health systems and through labour that is normally unpaid. The formal care economy is also highly feminised, with healthcare being a core driver of skilled female migration.[11]

The gendered dimensions of care and burden of care in public health have long been recognised by prominent scholars such as Lesley Doyal;[12] they have gained increased attention with regard to HIV/AIDS. The HIV/AIDS pandemic has drawn attention to gender and sexuality,[13] gender, risk, and structural violence,[14] gender, conflict and HIV/AIDS,[15] governance,[16] and the feminised response to the disease that has highlighted the care roles of women, particularly grandmothers.[17] Such attention has been reflected by increased prominence of gender issues in institutions such as the Joint United Nations Programme of HIV/AIDS (UNAIDS) and flagship reports such as Women and Health by the WHO, which recognise the feminised burden of care, the structural limitations to why women do (not) access key health services, and the gendered mortality rates regarding children and AIDS.[18] Such recognition is to be welcomed. However, there is much to suggest that such recognition is isolated to key reports and sectors of these institutions and does not cut across a range of health issues or pandemic outbreaks. Increasingly gender issues have been reduced to the issues of maternal (and at times, reproductive) health strategies that, while of great importance, are evoked by health actors as evidence of doing gender.[19] Studies on key global health issues such as the WHO's work on the social determinants of health have shown how such work 'is at odds' with contemporary work on gender and women's health.[20] Contemporary feminist theory and debate, the role of the informal and formal care economy, and issues of intersectionality all remain absent from global health strategies or are instrumentalised in such a way that women deliver on wider health goals and targets. This is a central paradox in global health: women are conspicuous in the delivery of care and thus the delivery of health, but are invisible to the institutions and policies that design and implement global health strategies.

Adopting the intent of feminist political economy to recognise reproduction in our understanding of the dynamics of international policy and economic structures, this paper uses the concept of 'conspicuous invisibility' to demonstrate how women and gender have been left out of the 2014 Ebola 'crisis' and wider long-term strategies of health systems resilience. The conspicuous invisibility of women in global health governance confirms what we know about gender assumptions and male bias in international public policy making, but also extends our knowledge to show how women's care roles can be such a conspicuous essential of everyday healthcare yet be wilfully invisible from discussion or strategy on global health.

Depicting the Ebola 'crisis'

Research and opinion pieces are critical signifiers in global health policy, and thus integral to understanding policy responses to Ebola and the role of women and gender within global health. Scholarly research and opinion pieces in flagship publications such as the *Lancet* and the *New England Journal of Medicine* have core advocacy and policy-shaping functions in global health. They publish research from policy makers working in institutions such as the World Bank and they provide the research that underpins evidence-based policy making. It was in 2014 that Ebola was confirmed to be a 'public health emergency of international concern',[21] the result of which was much scholarly debate in the correspondence pages and opinion pieces of noted journals over what had led Ebola to become an emergency, how the international response had functioned, and the future needs of the health systems in the three countries hit by it. Four key narratives framed such debate. These four narratives have been identified by an extensive literature review through a RefWorks database search of articles, correspondence and opinion pieces on 'Ebola' in the fields of public health, politics and social sciences from January 2014 to February 2015. The RefWorks search generated 2311 possible scholarly publications on Ebola for the time period: the abstracts for each of these papers were reviewed and any duplications in the search, clinical or biomedical papers were then discounted. This reduced the relevant literature to 61 articles. Each article was read to note the main content of the argument and see if any reference was made to gender, women or men, male or female, and verified by a word search using these terms. The categorisation of each of the four frames became apparent, as many of the papers were arguing similar points and spoke to each other. Earlier papers focused on the US response and the need for a vaccine, later papers discussed the failure of the international community. Women and gender are, on the whole, absent from the framing of the crisis.

The first narrative focuses on the response of the US government to the outbreak,[22] and on the perceived utility and ethics of quarantine for those personnel returning from West Africa, particularly those that volunteered in the Ebola response. Much of this debate is critical of the use of excessive quarantine measures, which were seen to act as a potential deterrent to volunteers, and were ineffectual given that an individual is not infectious until they show symptoms of Ebola.[23] Authors such as Hankivsky have highlighted the racial metaphors evident in this narrative and how intersectional axes of privilege – eg race, gender, class, sexuality – structure the perceptions of disease in the USA.[24] Gender here is thus considered as part of a wider intersectional lens for understanding not only perceptions of Ebola but how such analysis needs to be integrated in thinking about future processes of global health governance.

The second narrative surrounds the need for vaccines and treatment for Ebola and the wider ethical debate over the use of randomised controlled trials and of unproven treatment in an emergency health context.[25] Part of this narrative engages in advocacy over the need and urgency of a vaccine and timely intervention based on epidemiological modelling.[26]

This advocacy positions the response to Ebola as an ethical obligation of the global public health community. Such an ethical obligation takes a public health approach to delivering on Ebola treatment that seeks to bring health provision to all; thus gender is not highlighted as a concern within this.

The third narrative centres on how the Ebola crisis in West Africa is an emergency and was a 'perfect storm' arising from under-funded health systems and failing post-conflict public infrastructure that has been undermined by structural adjustment programmes and international capital flight.[27] A vocal proponent of this 'perfect storm' narrative is Peter Piot, Director of the London School of Hygiene and Tropical Medicine, who co-discovered Ebola in 1976.[28] This narrative primarily concentrates on the domestic infrastructures within Guinea, Liberia and Sierra Leone, how domestic governments were slow to act, and the problems of burial practices and relationships with healthcare workers that made preventative behavioural change difficult.[29] The explanation here was that health systems had been a neglected part of global and domestic health policy strategies and that, given the lack of clinicians, hospitals, primary treatment centres, educational and training facilities, laboratories, drug procurement facilities and cold chain supplies required for a functioning health system, these countries were particularly susceptible to disease outbreaks. For the 'perfect storm' narrative the core solution to preventing the impact and rapid spread of outbreaks such as Ebola is to build strong health systems.[30] The role of women as informal carers within the health sector and their relationship to the bodies and burial practices of the dead are not acknowledged within this debate. Their role is conspicuously invisible in the need to rebuild health systems and care for the children who have been orphaned by the disease. This is a core omission in the debate on health systems reform in the post-Ebola process.

The fourth narrative is around the international response to the outbreak and the perceived failure of key institutions such as the WHO to respond in a timely and sufficient manner.[31] This narrative provides an overview of the response in 2014, urges the international community to do more and commit more funds, and emphasises the need for greater coordination.[32] A key undercurrent of the narrative is the perceived failure of the WHO. The Ebola outbreak happened when the WHO was mid-way through an extended consultation on institutional reform. Such reform has been the result of external challenges to its mandate on account of a growth of institutions working on global health issues, such as the World Bank and Global Fund to Fight AIDS, Tuberculosis and Malaria, as well as internal problems of a lack of core financing and leadership divisions that have historically plagued the running of the institution.[33] A core part of this narrative, developed by global health lawyer Lawrence Gostin, is the role of the 2005 International Health Regulations (IHRs). The IHRs are a global tool with which to protect and prevent the spread of disease and provide a public health response to any outbreak. The failure to fully equip states to deliver on the core requirements of disease surveillance under the IHRs was seen as a key problem in the mismanagement of Ebola; thus for the future the narrative here is for the international community to be responsible for investing in and strengthening the IHRs in low- and middle-income countries.[34] The central focus of this narrative is to learn the lessons of the past as a means of greater and more directed investment in health in the future. However, similarly to the first narrative there is very little on the need to consider gender as an analytical concern in the implementation of the IHRs. Of the articles surveyed, only two acknowledge the care roles of women, one by the public health advocate Farmer and another by Martin-Moreno.[35] These two articles position women as a risk category because of their role as caregivers in the family and as primary healthcare providers. This is an important acknowledgment; however, the gender structures that reproduce norms of women as maternal carers and the future role of global health policy in reproducing such norms are not considered. Moreover, given the wealth of correspondence and opinion pieces on Ebola in 2014, two sentences acknowledging women as maternal caregivers being disproportionately affected by the outbreak shows the otherwise invisibility of women and the gendered impacts of the outbreak.

Of all the papers reviewed only one focused explicitly on women and one on gender. The first is a piece of correspondence in the *Lancet* that highlights the impact the Ebola outbreak has been having on maternal and newborn child services, stigma and the vulnerability of women as primary caregivers. Menendez et al note that Ebola 'is exacerbating problems that have persisted for decades' yet the main argument of the letter is that the global response needs to safeguard women's and children's maternal and newborn child health services rather than to address the gendered aspect of care.[36] The second paper contributes to wider discussion over the lack of funding for health systems by the international development community and reinforces concern over the increase in maternal mortality, suggesting Ebola presents a dual crisis: that of the disease itself and that of maternal and newborn child death.[37] The paper acknowledges the care dynamics that underpin the health systems of the three countries in question and argues for the need to address the structural dynamics of such systems. Both of these pieces, though short briefing interventions, highlight important issues concerning women and gender but do not fully engage with the way these issues are being considered within the wider response. They are isolated as stand-alone pieces and not fully integrated within the mainstream narratives on Ebola and show that the only (narrow) space women occupy within this debate is with reference to their role as mothers.

The narratives that have emerged in reaction to the Ebola response have not fully addressed how women may be disproportionately infected and affected by the disease and the gendered dynamics of health system resilience and of access to and provision of care and treatment. Where gender has been considered, it has been reduced to women as a vulnerable risk group in their role as carers or as mothers accessing maternal and newborn child health services. The Ebola crisis is not depicted as a gendered crisis, nor are women a particular analytical concern in the response with regard either to short-term issues of how to stop the spread of Ebola or to long-term strategies of how to develop resilient health systems. The construction of these narratives and the framing of women and gender within them are important, as they both reflect and set the wider debate for international public policy on Ebola and demonstrate the invisibility of women and issues of gender in global health opinion and research.

Gender and emergency policy: the Ebola response

The lack of engagement with gender and women in discussions around the Ebola response is reflected in international public policy strategies. These strategies, developed by institutions such as the WHO and World Bank, rarely involve how the short- and long-term effects of Ebola may affect women and men differently and do not include any acknowledgement of gender as a factor in how care is produced and consumed. Institutions such as UN Women and the African Development Bank have engaged the issue of gender when discussing both the short-and long-term response and impact of Ebola. However, these institutions based such discussions on unconfirmed data that do not correspond with official WHO epidemiological data on the epidemic. This section reviews the international policy response to Ebola to show, first, how women and gender are invisible in the short- and medium-term policy response.

As the leading UN agency on health, the WHO had a core role in the Ebola response. The WHO Ebola Response Roadmap was the flagship coordination document of the international response to Ebola; it had the stated purpose of assisting government and building on 'country-specific realities to guide response efforts and align implementation activities across different sectors of government and international partners'.[38] The Roadmap included a set of priority activities as part of each of its three objectives.[39] 'The needs of women' are highlighted within one sentence, alongside those of vulnerable groups such as cleaners in the 20-page document. There is no elaboration on what the 'needs' of women are beyond them constituting 'a significant proportion of care providers'.[40] The 'needs' of women are not listed anywhere else in the Roadmap as a priority activity and there are no gender disaggregated indicators or metrics in its monitoring and evaluation framework. This is a notable omission, as a failure to measure the potentially different impact and death from Ebola on women and men suggests WHO did not recognise or was not concerned with how gender can affect disease transmission and treatment.

WHO did not publish data on confirmed and probable Ebola cases disaggregated by sex until its 17th Situation Report in December 2015 – one year on from the first suspected Ebola case in Guinea.[41] WHO's *One Year into the Ebola Epidemic* report only mentions women at the very end: 'Given the fear and stigma associated with Ebola, people who survive the disease, especially women and children, need psycho-social support and counselling services as well as material support.'[42] However, it does not explain why women as a gender require such services especially more than men as a gender. The report tells the story of Ebola in 2014, and highlights the cultural and health systems aspects to its spread, but gender is not considered anywhere in the document.

Since the outbreak of Ebola the World Bank has played a key role in galvanising resources for the response and for reviewing the economic impact of the disease on Guinea, Liberia and Sierra Leone. As of February 2015 the Bank had committed US$1 billion of International Development Agency (IDA) and International Finance Corporation (IFC) funds to its Ebola Recovery and Reconstruction Trust Fund, making it a significant player in the immediate response and long-term recovery.[43] The focus of the Bank was to highlight how unprepared the three countries in West Africa and global health institutions were in responding to Ebola and the potential short- and long-term economic losses to these countries.[44] The Bank saw women as particularly vulnerable to such economic losses as they work in informal, self-employed jobs. One World Bank study in Liberia suggests that, since the outbreak, '60 percent of women are not currently working, compared with 40 percent of men; and women have been consistently more likely to be out of work compared with men'.[45] The Bank does not have comparable studies for Sierra Leone and Guinea, but suggested such a vulnerable trend would be similar in Sierra Leone.[46] For that country a Bank report notes, 'Gender impacts are inconclusive'; there is some evidence of a decline in post-natal services in Freetown but not in the rest of the country. [47]

The World Bank's consideration of gender is limited to two small sections of country reports on the socioeconomics impacts of Ebola. Neither gender, women, nor men had been mentioned in any of the Bank's multiple press releases or in President Jim Kim's statements or speeches on Ebola as of February 2015. The World Bank's report, *The Economic Impact of the 2014 Ebola Epidemic*, received considerable attention, given the estimated restrictions on growth on account of Ebola.[48] The report detailed the potential impacts of Ebola on aspects of the economy such as mining, agriculture, services and food prices but did not discuss potential gendered impacts or the role of women within these economies. The issue of gender was not systematically included in each round of the country-specific studies on the socioeconomic impact of Ebola. Hence the Bank has not fully considered the gendered impacts of Ebola on Guinea's, Liberia's and Sierra Leone's health systems and economy.

The only institutions to note concern over the gendered aspects of Ebola have been UN Women and the African Development Bank. A blog by the African Development Bank Special Envoy on Gender highlights restrictions on women's access to health services and the effect of Ebola on their employment, given the impact on the agricultural and tourism sectors, and on the informal economy in which women work. The over-arching argument of this gender-approach is to think about the long-term effects of Ebola on the working lives and livelihoods of women. However, the most interesting element of the blog is the citation of *Washington Post* data suggesting women made up 52% of deaths from Ebola in Sierra Leone, 55% in Guinea and 75% in Liberia.[49] The data used in this blog entry were similarly cited in UN Women's Inter-Agency Standing Committee 'Gender Alert' on the disease.[50] This alert used historical evidence to highlight the primary care roles of women in the formal health sector and informally within the family and communities in which they live, and the increased risk to pregnant women given their heightened contact with health services. Accompanying the issues raised in the alert were a number of action points that provide helpful tools for international policy and strategy.

Importantly, however, once WHO had stratified data by male and female in December 2014, it turned out that the data cited in the UN Women and African Development Bank papers were inaccurate (significantly so with respect to Liberia) and evidence from research in the three countries suggests assumptions about body-washing made by UN Women (ie that women wash both male and female dead bodies) to be incorrect (in most countries it is customary for men to wash male dead bodies and women to wash female dead bodies).[51] After stratifying the data on cumulative confirmed and probable cases, 'the number of cases in males and females is about the same' and has continued to be the same in all reports published up to January 2015. [52] One could therefore argue that there is no gender disparity in the number of people dying and infected with Ebola, there is no gender difference in who is washing the bodies, and hence it is not an issue of concern or priority in the global response to Ebola.

Discrepancy over the data is problematic for the visibility of women and gender for several reasons. First, there is much to suggest that such data are inconclusive. The WHO acknowledges that confirmed and suspected cases are estimates and could be two to four times higher that the situation reports suggest.[53] Given the infrastructural problems of the health systems in Guinea, Liberia and Sierra Leone, mapping the outbreak and confirming Ebola cases has been particularly difficult. The small number of laboratories, problems with information management between IT services and the health sector, and stigma and secrecy within communities that lead people to hide or dispose of the dead themselves without reporting them can each cause problems in tracking and recording confirmed and suspected cases. Second, the research that is disseminated and published by the World Bank and WHO tends to be based on quantitative estimates and does not take into consideration on-the-ground qualitative studies that may tell a different tale, particularly when it comes to gender sensitivities, hierarchies and the different health, social and economic impacts of

Ebola on men and women. Third, the publication of conflicting data by UN Women can be used to discredit the institution and, in so doing, the need to ask questions of gender in the Ebola response. Therefore, while the WHO data suggests no gender difference in confirmed and suspected cases of Ebola, this pertains to one (albeit important) aspect of the disease, rests on estimates that are difficult to make, and does not employ a range of research methods to address various aspects of impact that cannot be quantified. In sum, just because delayed data suggest no difference in male and female confirmed and suspected cases of Ebola, this does not mean gender is not an issue with regard to the disease.

The data and evidence collated on Ebola by leading institutions such as the WHO and World Bank did not systematically take gender into account and did not see the impacts on men as a gender and on women as a gender as potentially different or of concern. The conspicuous invisibility of women and gender has precluded any systematic and continued research on potential gender difference by the WHO and World Bank not only in confirmed and suspected cases but in terms of the wider socioeconomic impacts on men and women. This is an important omission in both the response to Ebola and the position of women in global health governance: it assumes that there is no gender bias in the delivery and uptake of health services and that gender is not of concern or consideration in public health emergencies.

Gender and long-term strategy: health systems

If gender was not a concern in the immediate, emergency response to Ebola, it is important to consider whether women and gender remain conspicuously invisible in long-term strategies of health system strengthening. One of the core priorities emerging from the Ebola response is the need to strengthen health systems in low- and middle-income countries. According to the WHO, there are five central elements to a functioning health system: leadership, information systems, health workforce, financing, supplies and service delivery.[54] As the previous sections have demonstrated, part of the blame for the spread of Ebola has been on weak country health systems that were ill-equipped to address the outbreak. In a similar pattern to the absence of women or gender in the framing of the Ebola outbreak, those that have used Ebola as a basis to argue for further health system strengthening and commitment to the IHRs do not say anything about gender within this process.[55] Strategies to address and strengthen health systems focus on the formal economy and government practices; however, such systems also depend on an informal care economy. Weak health systems are often underpinned by an informal care economy made up of voluntary carers working with community-based groups, non-governmental organisations, or independently in response to the needs of the community and carers working in extended families. These roles tend to be occupied by women. However, because these roles are informal and assumed as a result of gender norms over what women's work is and what men's work is, such care roles are conspicuously invisible in international public policy making: people know they exist, that women are over-represented in them, yet women are invisible in global health planning, strategy and implementation beyond the role of women as mothers.

As with the emergency response to Ebola, global strategies for health system strengthening firmly locate women as mothers. This is particularly the case in the WHO's Framework for Action on strengthening health systems, 'Everybody's Business'.[56] Gender within the action plan is framed in the wider context of the WHO's commitment to human rights and the 'gender mix' of the health labour of different countries. Gender is acknowledged in three parts of the document:

> in many countries, groups such as the poor – and too often women more than men – migrants and the mentally ill are largely invisible to decision-makers.

> WHO will increase its support for realistic, national health workforce strategies and plans for workforce development. These will consider the range, skill-mix and gender balance of health workers.

> Medium-term Strategic Objective: 'To address the underlying social and economic determinants of health through policies and programmes that enhance health equity and integrate pro-poor gender-responsive and human-rights based approaches.[57]

What these three excerpts suggest is that, while the WHO acknowledges gender difference in the health workforce, it does so within the wider context of human rights for all and places the emphasis for action on member states. The document does not stipulate what a gender-responsive health system would look like or the role of the WHO in articulating this or partnering with countries to develop this. The focus on gender in the action plan is very much on formal health workers, with no reference to the informal care economy or gender difference within it. Gender is seen as a barrier to accessing health services, particularly with reference to maternal health, but gender is invisible with reference to how health services are underpinned by the free labour of women. Gender only appears in the IHRs with reference to accounting for the concerns of travellers with regard to gender, ethnicity, religion and sociocultural factors: there is no reference to gender, feminised care or the informal role of women in health system strengthening.[58] Thus gender is assumed as an issue that affects the formal labour of health workers and access to health services and it is assumed that states are aware of this and will both articulate and action gender-responsive health systems.

The World Bank's strategy for health, nutrition and population 'Healthy Development' incorporates gender as an indicator of health disparities and constraints. Here the Bank emphasises the need for states to disaggregate priority indicators by gender and age and commits to increased support for countries to identify health systems constraints, including gender, income and geography.[59] This, however, is only a minor part of the strategy. The main gendered focus is on reproductive and maternal health services and maternal mortality, where the strategy outlines a set of indicators on contraceptive access and safe delivery. The Bank emphasises the need to improve health services to meet the needs of women because:

> Women endure a disproportionate burden of poor sexual and reproductive health. Their full and equal participation in development is contingent in accessing sexual and reproductive health care, including the ability to make voluntary and informed decisions about fertility.[60]

The position of gender within the Bank's strategy is therefore to improve women's maternal health as an instrumental means to enable their participation in delivering development. Nowhere in the document does the Bank acknowledge what women's role in development is, or the gendered aspects of women's labour in delivering on key health and development priorities such as Millennium Development Goal (MDG)2 'Reduce Child Mortality' and MDG4 'Achieve Universal Primary Education'. The role of women in underpinning key development goals and health system targets and indicators is assumed by institutions such as the Bank or seen as something they need to be healthy to do. In this sense women's health is not seen as an end it self but as a means for them to perform social obligations and functions to deliver development expected of them as a gender.

The instrumental framing of women in the Bank's strategy and the focus on maternal health in both the WHO's and Bank's strategies is unsurprising. Women have long been positioned in instrumental roles in international development, typified by what Chant depicts as 'the feminisation of poverty alleviation'.[61] What is important here is that institutions do not challenge or acknowledge the role of women as a gender in providing free, elastic labour that underpins functioning health systems. The informal care economy is conspicuously invisible and women's health is framed with regard to this invisibility: women are only visible in global health policy as mothers. In making women visible as mothers global health institutions reproduce gender norms of social reproduction. The reproduction of such norms may have direct impacts on women's health – as primary carers and first responders to people sick with highly infectious diseases such as Ebola – and indirect impacts on ill health of women from the burden of care, employment and family responsibilities. Hence conspicuous invisibility not only shows a wilful blindness on the part of these institutions but exacerbates the vulnerability of women in society and their susceptibility to infectious diseases such as Ebola.

Making women and gender conspicuously visible in global health

There is an argument that suggests the failure to recognise women and issues of gender in the Ebola response was not wilful blindness but born out of the emergency situation those combating the epidemic found themselves in. Ebola spread rapidly and the early days of the response were a confused and desperate time, particularly in countries such as Sierra Leone and Guinea. In these countries the immediate response was crisis management conducted by a sporadic group of committed people rather than a systematic and well-resourced operation. Part of the problem of the conspicuous invisibility of women in the Ebola response was the lack of any professional crisis management in the early stages of the outbreak that may have recognised the need to raise questions of gender. However, this only explains part of the story, as women remained conspicuously invisible from policy and practice as such expertise arrived. The story of Ebola shows that, when a health emergency arises, questions of gender are forgotten and at best viewed as a side issue. Therefore the first recommendation that can be made is to build gender-awareness and planning into operational responses to complex health emergencies. This awareness should begin with the basic question of gender and feminist studies, which asks 'Where are the women?' when formulating a plan of action. Epidemiological data need to be disaggregated by gender from the outset. Community mobilisers need to be both male and female. Any framework for action has to understand the formal and informal roles of men and women in the local care economy. Gender affects health crises as they happen and therefore needs to be addressed as a health crisis unravels, not after the event as part of the lessons learned, to be ignored.

The second recommendation is that those who deliver responses to public health emergencies of international concern – the health sector, humanitarian agencies and, in this instance, domestic and foreign militaries – need to both be aware of the effect of gender on health outcomes and crisis management and to know how to ask questions that make women and their needs visible in response planning. As responses to health issues increasingly involve actors from the security sector, it is not enough for the gender experts of health institutions alone to be trained in such issues. The security sector, especially those military actors involved in the Ebola response in Sierra Leone, have a tendency not only to overlook issues of gender difference in how men and women experience disease, but to reproduce gender norms in masculinised spaces of decision making and implementation.[62] Women need to be conspicuously visible in the minds of all actors responding to health emergencies.

The third recommendation is to put gender and the informal economy at the forefront of debates on health system strengthening. The first step here is to ask where the men and women are in health systems in both the formal and informal delivery of healthcare. The second step is then to identify how health systems can be adapted to meet the different needs of men and women, particularly in resource-poor settings. The third step is to ensure that women and gender are not isolated just in the areas of reproductive, maternal and newborn child health but are systematically addressed across the health sector. This requires a consistent challenge of asking where the women are in health systems and strategies and in financing for health system strengthening at every stage of the policy process – from design to implementation. Such questions have to be asked by everyone involved in health policy and planning, not just by gender specialists within specific institutions, as they can be systematically ignored, isolated or instrumentalised as evidence that gender was considered in the health policy process. These steps will provide a simple basis from which more systematic and long-term change towards gender equality in global health governance, both in crisis management and in everyday health systems, can be made.

Conclusion: conspicuously invisible women and global health governance

Women are conspicuously invisible in global health governance: everyone knows they are there and that they do the majority of the care work, but they remain invisible in global health policy. The 2014 Ebola outbreak provides an acute case study on conspicuous invisibility, where issues of women and gender have been invisible in both the emergency response and in long-term planning on health system resilience. The short- and long-term responses to Ebola show that the male bias is very much present in thinking about disease outbreaks: there is little to no discussion about gendered impacts of the disease in framing the crisis, data disaggregated by sex were late in coming, and no strategy includes gender indicators. This could in part be explained by the lack of evidence to suggest that Ebola is a gendered disease with regard to mortality and infection and, indeed, the data (however flawed) would suggest there is not a case to be made here. However, focusing on the data alone misses the wider point: this does not explain the lack of gendered concerns with regard to the care and treatment of people with Ebola and the feminised care economy that underpins the health systems that are key to preventing an outbreak of such magnitude happening again. Women are only made visible in the Ebola response and wider strategies of global health as mothers.

This paper furthers understanding of gender and women in global governance and global health in two key ways. First, the article has built on feminist research on gender blindness and the male bias to highlight an area of concern where women are conspicuously present in a number of core roles yet remain invisible to policy makers. These roles are hidden in plain sight of those working in global health. Global health governance at best takes women's care and social reproduction roles as a given, but at worst engages in policy practices and strategies that keep these roles invisible to debate, knowledge creation and policy. Second, the Ebola outbreak and response is indicative of how care is unaddressed in global health governance. Care underpins various dimensions of economies and societies, but none as plain as the delivery of health and well-being. Depicting women as conspicuously invisible highlights the tension between health and care in global health, and between knowing that women conspicuously underpin health systems through care roles and rendering women invisible in global health governance so as not to take any measures to recognise or address such roles.

In conclusion the 'perfect storm' of post-conflict, lack of health system investment, and a weak WHO that led to the unprecedented Ebola outbreak in 2014 misses out a crucial part of the storm: the free, supposedly elastic work of women that underpins health systems through social and primary health care roles. To develop resilient health systems, global health policy makers and scholars need to not only think about how gender acts as a barrier to health services and as an enabler of poor health but also about how global health strategies reproduce social and health care burdens on women as a gender. A start would be to make visible the conspicuous feminised nature of care, to consider gender in emergency and long-term health strategies, to recognise and place value on care roles that are very much a part of health systems and, crucially, to ask where the women are in emergency and long-term health systems policy and planning. Until care is valued and gender and women are made visible beyond issues of maternal health, health crises will continue to test health systems that rest on feminised care provision and will exacerbate the poor health of women. Health systems are not only built on leadership, information systems, health workforce, financing, supplies and service delivery, but on the free labour of women in social reproduction and care.

Disclosure statement

No potential conflict of interest was reported by the author.

Acknowledgements

Thanks and acknowledgment to James Dunkerley for helping me to articulate 'conspicuously invisible'. Thanks to the reviewers, to Simon Rushton for his editorial comments, and to the audience at the 'Ebola' panels at the 2015 BISA Annual Conference for their questions and suggestions on an earlier draft of the paper.

Notes

1. See, for example, Madorin et al., "Advanced Economy"; and Palriwala and Neetha, "Between the State, Market and Family."
2. Rai et al., *Depletion and Social Reproduction*.

3. Rai and Waylen, "Feminist Political Economy."
4. Razavi and Staab, "Introduction"; and Elson, "Economic Crises."
5. See, for example, Young et al., *Questioning Financial Governance*.
6. Razavi, "Addressing/Reforming Care."
7. Razavi and Staab, "Introduction."
8. Elson, "Male Bias in the Development Process," 3.
9. Elson, "Male Bias in the Development Process."
10. Rai and Waylen, "Feminist Political Economy."
11. Yeates, "Women's Migration."
12. See, for example, Doyal, *What Makes Women Sick*.
13. Baylies and Bujra, *AIDS, Sexuality and Gender*; and Doyal et al., *AIDS*.
14. Anderson, *Gender, HIV and Risk*.
15. Seckinelgin, *International Security*.
16. Griffin, *Gendering the World Bank*.
17. Razavi and Staab, "Introduction"; Harman, "The Dual Feminisation"; and Anderson, "Infectious Women."
18. WHO, *Women and Health*.
19. Harman, "Women and the MDGs."
20. Bates et al., "Gender and Health Inequities"; Springer et al., "Introduction"; and Springer et al., "Beyond a Catalogue of Differences."
21. WHO, "Six Months after the Ebola Outbreak was Declared."
22. Gostin et al., "The President's National Security Agenda," 27–28.
23. Drazen et al., "Editorial"; "Ebola, Quarantine and the Law," 5–6; and "Editorial: Rationality and Co-ordination," 1163.
24. Alcabes, "Race and Panic"; Dionne and Seay, "Perceptions about Ebola in America," 6–7; and Hankivsky, "Intersectionality and Ebola," 14–15.
25. Friedrich, "Potential Therapies," 1503; Trad et al., "Ebola in West Africa," 779; Kass, "Ebola, Ethics and Public Health," 744–745; and Gupta, 'Rethinking the Development of Ebola Treatments," e563–564.
26. Kanapathipillai et al., "Ebola Vaccine"; Fisman and Tuite, "Ebola"; and Galuani et al., "Ebola Vaccination."
27. O'Hare, "Weak Health Systems and Ebola"; Ross et al., "Are we ready for a Global Pandemic?"
28. Piot, "Editorial"; and Piot et al., "Ebola in West Africa."
29. Salmon et al., "Community-based care of Ebola Virus Disease."
30. Kieny and Doulo, "Beyond Health Systems."
31. Youde, "The World Health Organisation"; and Busby and Grepin, "What accounts for the World Health Organization's Failure?," 12–13.
32. Trad et al., 'Editorial'; Gostin, "The Ebola Epidemic"; Baden et al., "Editorial"; Mullan, "Editorial"; "Overview of Ebola Virus Disease"; Martin-Moreno et al., "Ebola"; and "Editorial: Ebola – A Failure."
33. Harman, *Is Time up for WHO?*
34. Gostin, "Ebola"; Gostin and Friedman, "Ebola"; and "Editorial: Ebola – What Lessons?"
35. Farmer, "The Largest ever Epidemic"; and Martin-Moreno, "The International Ebola Response."
36. Menendez et al., "Ebola Crisis," e130.
37. Diggins and Mills, *The Pathology of Inequality*.
38. WHO, "Ebola Response Roadmap," 4.
39. WHO, "Ebola Response Roadmap."
40. Ibid., 10.
41. WHO, "WHO Situation Reports."
42. WHO, *One Year into Ebola Epidemic*, 50.
43. World Bank, "Ebola Response Factsheet."
44. World Bank, 'Press Release'; World Bank, "Ebola"; and World Bank, "Ebola Hampering Household Economies."
45. World Bank, "Ebola Hampering Household Economies"; and World Bank, "The Socioeconomic Impacts of Ebola."

46. World Bank, "The Socio-economic Impacts of Ebola."
47. Ibid., 13.
48. World Bank, *The Economic Impact of the 2014 Ebola Epidemic*.
49. Fraser-Moleketi, "Ebola."
50. UN Women Inter-Agency Standing Committee, "Humanitarian Crisis in West Africa," 2.
51. Richards and Yei-Mokuwa, "Burial Practices."
52. WHO, "WHO Situation Reports."
53. WHO, "Ebola Response Roadmap."
54. WHO, "Key Components."
55. Gostin, "Ebola"; Gostin and Friedman, "Ebola"; and "Editorial: Ebola - What Lessons?"
56. WHO, *Everybody's Business*.
57. Ibid., 8, 17, 38.
58. WHO, *International Health Regulations*.
59. World Bank, *Healthy Development*.
60. Ibid., 88.
61. Chant, "Rethinking the 'Feminisation of Poverty.'"
62. Kamradt-Scott et al., "Saving Lives," 16.

Bibliography

Alcabes, Philip. "Race and Panic: America confronts Ebola." *Chronicle of Higher Education* 61, no. 9 (2014).

Anderson, Emma-Louise. "Infectious Women: Gendered Bodies and HIV in Malawi." *International Feminist Journal of Politics* 14, no. 2 (2014): 267–287.

Anderson, Emma-Louise. *Gender, HIV and Risk: Navigating Structural Violence*. Basingstoke: Palgrave, 2015.

Baden, Lindsey R., Rupa Kanapathipillai, Edward W. Campion, Stephen Morrisey, Eric J. Rubin, and Jeffrey M. Drazen. "Editorial: Ebola – An Ongoing Crisis." *New England Journal of Medicine* 371 (2014): 1458–1459.

Bates, Lisa, Olena Havinsky, and Kristen Springer. "Gender and Health Inequities: A Comment on the Final Report of the WHO Commission on the Social Determinants of Health." *Social Science and Medicine* 69 (2009): 1002–1004.

Baylies, Carolyn, and Janet Bujra. *AIDS, Sexuality and Gender in Africa: Collective Strategies and Struggles in Tanzania and Zambia*. Abingdon: Routledge, 2000.

Busby, Joshua, and Karen A. Grepin. "What accounts for the World Health Organization's Failure on Ebola?" *Political Science and Politics* 48, no. 1 (2015): 12–13.

Chant, Sylvia. "Rethinking the 'Feminisation of Poverty' in Relation to Aggregate Gender Indices." *Journal of International Development* 7, no. 2 (2006): 201–220.

Diggins, Jennifer, and Elizabeth Mills. *The Pathology of Inequality: Gender and Ebola in West Africa*. IDS Practice Paper in Brief. Brighton: Institute of Development Studies, 2015.

Dionne, Kim Yi, and Laura Seay. "Perceptions about Ebola in America: Othering and the Role of Knowledge about Africa." *Political Science and Politics* 48, no. 1 (2015): 6–7.

Doyal, Lesley. *What Makes Women Sick: Gender and the Political Economy of Health*. Basingstoke: Palgrave, 1995.

Doyal, Lesley, Jennie Naidoo, and Tamsin Wilton eds. *AIDS: Setting a Feminist Agenda*. London: Taylor and Francis, 1994.

Drazen, Jeffrey M., Rupa Kanapathipillai, Edward M. Campion, Eric J. Rubin, Scott M. Hammer, Stephen Morissey, and Lindsey Baden. "Editorial: Ebola and Quarantine." *New England Journal of Medicine* 371 (2014): 2029–2030.

"Ebola, Quarantine and the Law." *The Hastings Center* 45, no. 1 (2015): 5–6.

"Editorial: Ebola – A Failure of International Collective Action." *Lancet* 384, no. 9944 (2014): 637.

"Editorial: Ebola – What Lessons for the International Health Regulations?" *Lancet* 384, no. 9951 (2014): 1321.

"Editorial: Rationality and Co-ordination for Ebola Outbreak in West Africa." *Lancet Infectious Diseases* 14, no. 12 (2014): 1163.

Elson, Diane. "Male Bias in the Development Process: An Overview." In *Male Bias in the Development Process*, edited by Diane Elson, 1–28, 2nd ed., Manchester, NH: Manchester University Press, 1995.

Elson, Diane. "Economic Crises from the 1980s to the 2010s: A Gender Analysis." In *New Frontiers in Feminist Political Economy*, edited by Shirin Rai and Georgina Waylen, 189–212. London: Routledge, 2014.

Farmer, Paul. "The Largest ever Epidemic of Ebola." *Reproductive Health Matters* 22, no. 44 (2014): 157–162.

Fisman, David, and Tuite, Ashleigh. "Ebola: No Time to Waste." *Lancet Infectious Diseases* 14, no. 12 (2014): 1164–1165.

Fraser-Moleketi, Geraldine. "Ebola: The Need for a Gendered Approach." 2014. www.adfb.org/en/blogs/measuring-the-pulse-of-economic-transformation-in-west-africa/post/ebola-the-need-for-a-gendered-approach-13472/.

Friedrich, M. J. "Potential Therapies and Vaccines to Combat Ebola." *Journal of the American Medical Association* 312, no. 15 (2014): 1503.

Galuani, Alison P., Martial L. Ndeffo-Mbah, Natasha Wenzel, and James E. Childs. "Ebola Vaccination: If not Now, When?" *Annals of Internal Medicine* 161, no. 10 (2014): 749–750.

Gostin, Lawrence O. "Ebola: Towards an International Health Systems Understanding." *Lancet* 384, no. 9951 (2014): e49–51.

Gostin, Lawrence O., and Eric A. Friedman. "Ebola: A Crisis of Global Health Leadership." *Lancet* 384, no. 9951 (2014): 1323–1325.

Gostin, Lawrence O., Daniel Lucey, and Alexandra Phelan. "The Ebola Epidemic: A Global Health Emergency." *Journal of the American Medical Association* 312, no. 11 (2014).

Gostin, Lawrence O., Henry A. Waxman, and William Foege. "The President's National Security Agenda: Curtailing Ebola, Safeguarding the Future." *Journal of the American Medical Association* 313, no. 1 (2015): 27–28.

Griffin, Penny. *Gendering the World Bank: Neoliberalism and the Gendered Foundations of Global Governance*. Basingstoke: Palgrave, 2009.

Gupta, Rajesh. "Rethinking the Development of Ebola Treatments." *Lancet Global Health* 2, no. 10 (2014): e563–564.

Hankivsky, Olena. "Intersectionality and Ebola." *Political Science and Politics* 48, no. 1 (2015): 14–15.

Harman, Sophie. "The Dual Feminisation of HIV/AIDS." *Globalizations* 8, no. 2 (2011).

Harman, Sophie. "Women and the MDGs: Too Little, too Late, too Gendered." In *The Millennium Development Goals and Beyond: Global Development after 2015*, edited by Rorden Wilkinson and David Hulme, 84–101. London: Routledge, 2012.

Harman, Sophie. *Is Time up for WHO? Reform, Resilience and Global Health Governance*. FUNDS Briefing No. 17, May 2014. http://futureun.org/media/archive1/briefings/FUNDSBriefing17-WHO-Harman.pdf.

Kamradt-Scott, Adam, Sophie Harman, Clare Wenham, and Frank Smith III. *Saving Lives: The Civil–Military Response to the 2014 Ebola Outbreak in West Africa*. Sydney: University of Sydney, 2015. http://sydney.edu.au/mbi/news/2015/savinglives.php.

Kanapathipillai, Rupa, Ana Maria Henao Restrepo, Patricia Fast, David Wood, Christopher Dye, Marie-Poole Kieny, and Vasee Moothy. "Ebola Vaccine – An Urgent International Priority." *New England Journal of Medicine* 371 (2014): 2249–2251.

Kieny, Marie-Paule, and Delanyo Doulo. "Beyond Health Systems: A New Agenda for Resilient Health Systems." *Lancet* 385, no. 9963 (2015): 91–92.

Kass, Nancy. "Ebola, Ethics and Public Health: What Next?" *Annals of Internal Medicine* 161, no. 10 (2014): 744–745.

Madorin, Mascha, Brigitte Schnegg, and Nadia Baghdadi. "Advanced Economy, Modern Welfare State and Traditional Care Regimes: The Case of Switzerland." In *Global Variations in the Political and Social Economy of Care: Worlds Apart*, edited by Shahra Razavi and Silke Staab, 43–60. London: Routledge, 2012.

Martin-Moreno, Jose M. "The International Ebola Response: Heroes and Bystanders in the Chronicle of an Epidemic Foretold." *Journal of Public Health* 36, no. 4 (2014): 525–526.

Martin-Moreno, Jose M., Walter Ricciardi, Vesna Bjegovic-Mikanovic, Peggy Maguire, and Martin McKee. "Ebola: An Open Letter to European Governments." *Lancet* 384, no. 9950 (2014): 1259.

Menendez, Clara, Anna Lucas, Khatia Munguambe, and Ana Langer. "Ebola Crisis: The Unequal Impact on Women and Children's Health." *Lancet Global Health* 3, no. 3 (2015): e130.

Mullan, Zoe. "Editorial: Ebola - The Missing Link." *Lancet Global Health* 2, no. 10 (2014).

O'Hare, Bernadette. "Weak Health Systems and Ebola." *Lancet Global Health* 3, no. 2 (2015): e71–72.

"Overview of Ebola Virus Disease in 2014." *Journal of the Chinese Medical Association* 78, no. 1 (2015): 51–55.

Palriwala, Rajni, and N. Neetha. "Between the State, Market and Family: Structures, Policies and Practices of Care in India." In *Global Variations in the Political and Social Economy of Care: Worlds Apart*, edited by Shahra Razavi and Silke Staab, 176–197. London: Routledge, 2012.

Piot, Peter. "Editorial: Ebola's Perfect Storm." *Science* 345, no. 6202 (2014): 1221.

Piot, Peter. "Jean-Jacques Muyemba, and W. John Edmunds. "Ebola in West Africa: From Disease Outbreak to Humanitarian Crisis"." *Lancet Infectious Diseases* 14, no. 11 (2014): 1034–1035.

Rai, Shirin, Catherine Hoskyns, and Dania Thomas. *Depletion and Social Reproduction*. CSGR Working Paper 274/11. 2007. http://www2.warwick.ac.uk/fac/soc/csgr/research/workingpapers/2011/27411.pdf.

Rai, Shirin, and Georgina Waylen. "Feminist Political Economy: Looking Back, Looking Forward." In *New Frontiers in Feminist Political Economy*, edited by Shirin Rai and Georgina Waylen, 1–18. London: Routledge, 2014.

Razavi, Shahra. "Addressing/Reforming Care, but on whose Terms?" In *New Frontiers in Feminist Political Economy*, edited by Shirin Rai and Georgina Waylen, 114–134. London: Routledge, 2014.

Razavi, Shahra, and Silke Staab. "Introduction: Global Variations in the Political and Social Economy of Care – Worlds Apart?" In *Global Variations in the Political and Social Economy of Care: Worlds Apart*, edited by Shahra Razavi and Silke Staab, 1–25. London: Routledge, 2012.

Richards, Paul, and Esther Yei-Mokuwa. "Burial Practices." *FutureLearn/LSHTM: Ebola in Context*. 2015. https://www.futurelearn.com/courses/ebola-in-context/steps/24959/progress.

Ross, Allen G. P., Remigio M. Olveda, and Li Yuesheng. "Are we ready for a Global Pandemic of Ebola Virus?" *International Journal of Infectious Diseases* 28 (2014): 217–218.

Salmon, Sharon, Mary-Louise McLaws, and Dale Fisher. "Community-based care of Ebola Virus Disease in West Africa." *Lancet Infectious Diseases* 15, no. 2 (2015): 151–152.

Seckinelgin, Hakan. *International Security, Conflict and Gender: 'HIV/AIDS is Another War'*. London: Routledge, 2012.

Springer, Kristen, Olena Havinsky, and Lisa Bates. "Introduction: Gender and Health – Relational, Intersectional, and Biosocial Approaches." *Social Science and Medicine* 74 (2012): 1661–1666.

Springer, Kristen, Jeanne Stellman, and Rebecca Jordan-Young. "Beyond a Catalogue of Differences: a Theoretical Frame and Good Practice Guidelines for Researching Sex/Gender in Human Health." *Social Science and Medicine* 74 (2012): 1817–1824.

Trad, Mohammed-Ali, Dale Andrew Fisher, and Paul Anantharajah Tambyah. "Ebola in West Africa." *Lancet Infectious Diseases* 14, no. 9 (2014): 779.

UN Women Inter-Agency Standing Committee. "Humanitarian Crisis in West Africa (Ebola): Gender Alert." 2014. http://www.unwomen.org/en/news/stories/2014/9/gender-alert-ebola-west-africa.

World Bank. "Ebola hampering Household Economies across Liberia and Sierra Leone." 2015. http://www.worldbank.org/en/news/press-release/2015/01/12/ebola-hampering-household-economies-liberia-sierra-leone.

World Bank. "Ebola: Most African Countries avoid Major Economic Loss but Impact on Guinea, Liberia, Sierra Leone remains Crippling." January 20, 2015. http://www.worldbank.org/en/news/press-release/2015/01/20/ebola-most-african-countries-avoid-major-economic-loss-but-impact-on-guinea-liberia-sierra-leone-remains-crippling.

World Bank. "Ebola Response Factsheet." 2015. http://www.worldbank.org/en/topic/health/brief/world-bank-group-ebola-fact-sheet.

World Bank. *The Economic Impact of the 2014 Ebola Epidemic: Short and Medium Term Estimates for Guinea, Liberia, and Sierra Leone*. Washington, DC: World Bank, 2014. http://documents.worldbank.

org/curated/en/2014/09/20214465/economic-impact-2014-ebola-epidemic-short-medium-term-estimates-guinea-liberia-sierra-leone.

World Bank. *Healthy Development: The World Bank Strategy for Health, Nutrition and Populations Results*. Washington, DC: World Bank, 2007.

World Bank. "Press Release: World Bank Group President – World is 'Dangerously Under-prepared for Future Pandemics." 2015. http://www.worldbank.org/en/news/press-release/2015/01/27/world-bank-group-president-world-dangerously-unprepared-future-pandemics.

World Bank. "The Socioeconomic Impacts of Ebola in Liberia – Round 3." 2015. http://www.worldbank.org/content/dam/Worldbank/document/Poverty%20documents/SocioEconomic%20Impacts%20of%20Ebola%20in%20Liberia,%20Jan%2012%20%28final%29.pdf.

World Health Organization (WHO). "Ebola Response Roadmap." 2014. http://www.who.int/csr/resources/publications/ebola/response-roadmap/en/.

WHO. *Everybody's Business: Strengthening Health Systems to improve Health Outcomes: WHO's Framework for Action*. Geneva: WHO, 2007.

WHO. *International Health Regulations*. Geneva: WHO, 2005. http://whqlibdoc.who.int/publications/2008/9789241580410_eng.pdf?ua=1.

WHO. "Key Components of a Well Functioning Health System." 2010. http://www.who.int/healthsystems/EN_HSSkeycomponents.pdf.

WHO. *One Year into Ebola Epidemic: A Deadly, Tenacious and Unforgiving Virus*. Geneva: WHO, 2015.

WHO. "Six Months after the Ebola Outbreak was Declared: What happens when a Deadly Virus hits the Destitute?" 2014. http://www.who.int/csr/disease/ebola/ebola-6-months/en/.

WHO. "WHO Situation Reports: 17 December 2014." 2014. www.who.int/csr/disease/ebola/situaton-reports/archive.en.

WHO. *Women and Health: Today's Evidence, Tomorrow's Agenda*. Geneva: WHO, 2009.

Yeates, Nicola. "Women's Migration, Social Reproduction and Care." In *The Gendered Impacts of Liberalization: Towards 'Embedded Liberalism'?*, edited by Shahra Razavi. London: Routledge, 2009.

Youde, Jeremy. "The World Health Organisation and Responses to Global Health Emergencies." *Political Science and Politics* 48, no. 1 (2015): 11–12.

Young, Brigitte, Isabella Bakker, and Diane Elson (eds.). *Questioning Financial Governance from a Feminist Perspective*. London: Routledge, 2011.

Ebola and the production of neglect in global health

João Nunes

Department of Politics, University of York, UK

ABSTRACT

This article argues that the 2014 Ebola outbreak in West Africa reinscribed the neglect that has surrounded this disease. The argument develops theoretical tools for understanding how neglect is produced in global health. Arguing that neglect is connected with the production of harm and vulnerability, it stresses the importance of emotions in issue-prioritisation in global health. Focusing on the dynamics of abjection, the article shows how the 2014 Ebola outbreak was framed as a (racialised) African problem and obfuscated by a political and media spectacle. The result was the preference for short-term crisis-management responses that detracted from long-term structural solutions.

The Legbala River has its source in a plateau in the northern part of what is now the Democratic Republic of Congo. It runs westwards, joining the Dua River to form the Mongala, which then merges into the Congo. Since the colonial era the Legbala has been known by another name. In 1939 Belgian africanists wrote about this region, stating – in the matter-of-fact tone of empire – that only in the 'mouths of indigenes' would you hear the word 'Legbala': 'in the geographical language we call it Ebola'.[1] This could well be another story of colonial erasure, were it not for the outbreak, in 1976, of an acute form of haemorrhagic fever in this region. Peter Piot, a scientist then working for the Antwerp Institute of Tropical Medicine, identified the disease and named it after the river – even though the outbreak had originated in a village called Yambuku, 60 miles away.[2] In 2014 'Ebola' became a globally recognised word after another outbreak reached epidemic proportions.

What's in a(n erased) name? Perhaps it is not so important when we consider the human suffering caused by the latest outbreak of the Ebola virus, which at the time of writing (October 2015) was still ongoing in Guinea and Sierra Leone after claiming more than 11,000 lives – although the real figures are estimated to be two to three times higher. Nonetheless, this erasure is not insignificant. It can be seen as a metaphor for the ways in which the realities of the global South have been interpreted and addressed: violently suppressed during the colonial era and still mis-recognised. Systematic mis-recognition has led to forgetting or to the imposition of narratives that do not correspond to actual lived experiences. This in turn has had an impact upon how injustices and suffering are dealt with.

Erasure and forgetting may seem unlikely starting points for an analysis of the recent Ebola outbreak. After all, in recent months Ebola has commanded great media scrutiny and public attention, leading to the mobilisation of vast human, material and financial resources from a broad range of international actors. Nonetheless, once we go beyond the 'sound and fury' of headlines, deeper layers of forgetting begin to reveal themselves. This article argues that media attention and a momentary political anxiety over a particular issue do not necessarily mean that the issue is being adequately addressed. In fact, media and political spectacles can be detrimental to addressing the complex nature of health issues. In the case of Ebola the spectacle ultimately reflected and exacerbated the neglect that has historically surrounded this disease, as well as the needs and vulnerabilities of the populations that have been most affected by it.

The complex pattern of neglect in the case of Ebola must be understood alongside a broader analysis of existing global health governance mechanisms. This argument thus begins by exploring how health issues emerge as something to be governed (or ignored) at the international level. It then investigates the meaning of neglect and how it is produced, arguing that it emerges in the context of power-laden global structures and relations. Because of its deeply political character, neglect may persist under many guises and may assume a structural nature – that is, one that exists independently of moments or cycles of attention. Cultural factors are paramount in this story, and the article makes the case for the importance of emotions, and not simply interests, in the definition of health policies and priorities. Specifically my argument links neglect with an affective process of abjection. Applying these ideas to the case of Ebola, the article argues that the disease was framed as an exotic and racialised phenomenon, in addition to being enveloped in a media and political spectacle that resulted overwhelmingly in a short-term, 'crisis management' modality of response. Meanwhile, deep-seated neglect continued.

Neglect and the politics of global health

How do health issues become matters of international political concern? Inversely, how do they fail to emerge as significant? Since at least the 19th century the world has witnessed the development of rules, regimes and institutions seeking to govern health at the international level.[3] More recently scholars and policy makers have begun to speak of 'global health governance', defined as the set of 'collaborative activities among states, IGOs, and NGOs that seek to influence the character of particular international problems'.[4]

The idea of global health governance signals an overwhelmingly optimistic outlook regarding the world's ability to recognise and tackle issues through increased international cooperation, coordination and consensus. For some, stumbling-blocks like insufficient coordination, inadequate allocation of resources or new demands mean that governance periodically readjusts itself in a 'punctuated equilibrium'.[5] Put differently, governance adapts and transforms itself in order better to respond to external shocks. For others, governance develops along a 'challenge–response–innovation' continuum with three components: 'physical challenges to health, governance responses to these challenges, and the innovation called forth and needed in the face of new challenges when the old responses failed'.[6] These visions share a belief in the incremental development of cooperative mechanisms, supported by enhanced regulation, standardisation of procedures, and scientific and technological progress.

This optimistic view has clashed with glaring failures: acute inequalities in health provision, groups excluded from access to healthcare and huge discrepancies in health indicators.[7] One of the ways in which failure reveals itself is neglect, that is, the persistence of issue-areas that are given less attention (by policy makers, funders, the media or the public) than would be expected, given their actual burden on individuals and societies. Neglect also pertains to the systematic exclusion of certain groups – defined in terms of gender, age, race, sexual orientation or class – from the highest standards of healthcare available in a given society. Neglect shows that, for all its sophistication, global health governance is still unable to identify and tackle the problems faced by a significant percentage of the world's population – particularly the poor and underprivileged.

Neglect is often assumed to be an epiphenomenon of the interests of powerful actors and donors. These interests shape incentives to commit funding and resources, thus helping to determine what is present (and absent) in the agenda. In this sense neglect is a function of marginality and lack of power – it is determined by the relative position of the state, region or group in question within global political and economic structures. While this view can be helpful when explaining the reasons why certain issues end up being neglected, it does not tell us much about how interests are formed in the global health agenda. What are the political, social and cultural processes that enable actors' interests to be defined in such a way that certain issues and groups end up being overlooked or inadequately addressed? As Simon Rushton and Owain Williams have put it:

> what the literature has not generally done is to interrogate the reasons why these failures continue to be reproduced...The literature frequently tends to jump from describing the institutional architecture to the 'end product' of a policy process without really addressing what structures and determines the policy process.[8]

The question is not simply about identifying the interests that are supposedly at the root of neglect, but rather about probing into the practices of mis-recognition and erasure that enable these interests to be formed. In other words, understanding neglect requires one to consider the politics of problem definition, that is, the processes through which certain issues become problems while others do not.

As Murray Edelman has argued, 'problems' are not self-evident realities but rather 'ambiguous claims' advanced by different groups, 'each eager to pursue courses of action and call them solutions'.[9] These claims are themselves underpinned by narratives that structure reality in certain ways. Donald A Schön and Martin Rein have used the term 'frame' to refer to these narratives, conceiving policy debates as 'disputes in which the contending parties hold conflicting frames', the latter determining 'what counts as a fact and what arguments are taken to be relevant and compelling'.[10] Frames shape the nature of 'problems' and 'solutions' by ordering reality in a certain way; they 'select for attention a few salient features and relations from what would otherwise be an overwhelmingly complex reality. They give these elements a coherent organization, and they describe what is wrong with the present situation in such a way as to set the direction for its future transformation.'[11]

Interests, then, should not be taken as given. It is true that frames may be used to advance interests, but frames also shape interests. According to Schön and Rein, 'it is the frames held by the actors that determine what they see as *being* in their interests...[t]heir problem formulations and preferred solutions are grounded in different problem-setting stories rooted in different frames'.[12]

The corollary is that problem definition is not merely a value-neutral exercise of identifying self-evident problems. Problems emerge as significant not just because they are 'there', but also because they reinforce assumptions about what is important. Policy choices 'are always statements of values, even if some value positions are so dominant that their influence goes unexamined or so unrepresented that their neglect goes unnoticed'.[13] For Edelman problem definitions create or reinforce 'beliefs about the relative importance of events and objects', with the result that they end up constructing 'areas of immunity from concern'.[14] Considering the processes of framing and problem definition that give rise to certain policy decisions thus allows one to discern how other areas suffer from an absence of policy.

Colin McInnes and Kelley Lee have used framing to look at global health, arguing that visions of the latter reflect 'a particular dominant narrative or set of narratives emphasizing certain types of risks, the interests of certain population groups, the way in which the global nature of the problem is defined, and the need for certain high-level political responses'.[15] A similar point is made by Rushton and Williams, who have suggested that health policies result from the interaction of frames (the 'cognitive foreground') and paradigms, or broad sets of meanings and beliefs from which actors draw when framing health issues (the 'cognitive background'). They write:

> In framing an issue, in a particular way, an actor…connects it with a set of deeper paradigms that form the ideational underpinnings of global health governance. These paradigms influence (often unconsciously) the ways in which actors think and talk about global health problems.[16]

Importantly Rushton and Williams recognise the role of agency and power in this process and argue that the distribution of material and ideational resources affects the capability to frame health problems.

The idea of framing has also been used to study issue prioritisation in global health. Here, Jeremy Shiffman has argued that the ascendance of an issue in the scale of priorities depends, first, on 'ideational portrayal', that is, on the effective communication of the importance of a certain issue 'in ways that appeal to political leaders' social values and concepts of reality'. Second, institutions are required that can promote and sustain such portrayals.[17] In previous work Shiffman and Smith identified a number of factors shaping prioritisation, organising them into four categories: (1) the power of the actors putting forward a particular issue as a health priority (which includes their cohesion, the level of mobilisation around the issue and the existence of strong leadership and sustaining institutions); (2) the strength of the ideas, that is, their internal coherence and resonance; (3) the political context, which includes propitious moments for these ideas to be mobilised, as well as a structural context in which they can be mobilised and received; and (4) the characteristics of the issue, and the possibility of making a credible case for its severity and for the effectiveness of the measures to address it.[18]

By revealing health agendas as sites of framing and political contestation, this literature has begun to unpack interests and policy agendas in global health. It provides tools for the analysis of issue prioritisation, allowing for an assessment of how certain issues receive attention. More needs to be said, however, about the 'dark side' of agenda setting: the processes by which issues are left out and made invisible. In order to explore this dimension, the meaning of neglect must first be clarified.

The meaning of neglect: harm and vulnerability

Neglect is a layered concept, which includes not simply the disregard of a certain issue, but also the failure to care in an adequate way – even if such issue is not completely disregarded. In turn, 'to care' may mean different things. On the one hand, it can denote a feeling of empathy: seeing a certain problem as something important, something that matters not just for oneself but also for others. On the other hand, 'to care' can also mean to act in a way that effectively tackles the problem. As a result, neglect can pertain to different situations: a situation in which the issue is simply disregarded (neglect by invisibility); another in which the issue is regarded but not considered important (neglect by apathy); and yet another in which the issue is considered important but decisive action to address it is not undertaken, either because actors with the ability to shape outcomes are not willing to act (neglect by inaction) or are not acting adequately (neglect by incompetence).

It thus becomes clear that neglect is more than just the invisibility of an issue. It is also about a moral landscape in which that issue is deemed something that does not matter, and about a political arena in which effective solutions are not imagined and mobilised. By placing neglect within a moral and political context this understanding also allows us to reach an important preliminary conclusion: neglect does not just happen; it is made to happen. At the crux of the production of neglect it is always possible to locate human agency and choices. Issues are rendered invisible in certain ways, by certain actors following certain purposes. Along similar lines neglect by apathy is the result of processes that shape the sphere of moral obligation – apathy is in fact a denial of empathy and a failure to care about the plight of others. In turn, neglect by inaction is not simply absence of action – rather, it can more aptly be described as denial of response. Finally, neglect by incompetence also forces us to consider how resources are allocated and to question why adequate responses are not devised or applied.

As has been mentioned, neglect pertains not simply to particular diseases, but also to determinants (economic, social and infrastructural) and to groups. A disease may be considered neglected when it is not studied well enough, for example, or when decisive steps are not taken to address it (neglected tropical diseases would be an example). A determinant is neglected when its role in outbreaks, disease incidence or people's ability to deal with the occurrence of disease is not recognised or addressed (for instance, the quality of health-systems). A group is neglected when it is systematically placed in a position of vulnerability to disease, or is excluded from high-quality and affordable healthcare (for example, undocumented migrants).

In sum, neglect can be defined as a sustained process of making invisible a problem or condition and/or the denial of resources necessary to understand or address it – this being at odds with the burden that this problem or condition has on individuals and societies. Neglect may happen as a combined effect of the actions and inactions of different actors: policy makers, donors, the media and the general public.

This discussion points to the importance of seeing neglect as intertwined with broader dynamics of harm and vulnerability. On the one hand, neglect is a form of harm and also acts as a multiplier of harm. Harm is conceived here as more than a physical injury – that is, the occurrence of a particular disease and its lasting effects. Harm also pertains to other kinds of injuries. One of these is psychological harm related to the stigmatisation of and disrespect for the dignity of those suffering from neglected health problems. It is also possible to speak of a public dimension of harm, which pertains to damage being done to the very institutions that are responsible for avoiding harm. In this sense neglect reinforces public harm by leading to the absence of adequate mechanisms and institutions that can prevent and tackle certain diseases. Finally, we can talk of structural harm in relation to neglect: this pertains to situations when groups are neglected not exactly by the absence of rules and institutions, but rather by the fact that existing ones are skewed and place groups in positions of subordination or disadvantage.[19]

On the other hand, neglect is connected with vulnerability: a group's or individual's susceptibility to harm, but also the inability to 'bounce back' and deal with harm. Neglect is an important factor in the reproduction of vulnerabilities because it entails differentiated exposure to disease and an unequal distribution of capabilities to deal with it. The neglect of a certain disease may lead to fewer resources being available for prevention and cure, and therefore to immediate vulnerabilities, that is, to more people being exposed. Vulnerability may also be potential, when individuals or groups are socially and economically positioned in such a way that their health is prone to being inordinately affected by the slightest changes in circumstances and by decisions they cannot control or predict. These potential vulnerabilities go a long way in determining the incidence of a disease and its ability to decisively damage – or even cut short – the lives of those affected.[20]

It becomes clear that neglect involves the existence of groups that are systematically privileged in relation to others, and the presence of unequal relationships. Importantly, because neglect materialises in both immediate and more structural forms of harm and vulnerability, overcoming neglect necessarily encompasses more than superficial attention. Such attention can only be expected to manage or contain immediate forms of harm and vulnerability, while leaving deeper problems intact.

The production of neglect: abjection

This article has emphasised the importance of the ideas that construct health problems in certain ways, while foreclosing other kinds of framing. Understanding the production of neglect requires an engagement with the broad political imagination in which certain policy options emerge as possible and desirable. Common explanations of neglect, focused as they are on rational actors that bring their (predefined) interests to the table in a strategic effort to maximise their own utility, often overlook an important dimension of the political imagination that enables neglect. This dimension is affect.

Emotions play an important role in world politics.[21] Neta C. Crawford has argued that the role of emotions can be witnessed at different levels. On the one hand, emotions affect actors' perceptions of others' motives, thus shaping the content of relations. On the other hand, emotions also have effects at the level of cognition, that is, on actors' definitions of their interests and courses of action. This is because emotions influence the processes through which actors gather and process information about their environment; their calculation of risks, costs and benefits; and their ability and receptivity to dialogue with other actors.[22]

Research on emotions usually considers engagement, that is, how actors establish relations within an affective context. The analysis suggested here is somewhat different: it assesses how emotions foster non-engagement or disengagement. Crucial for an affective analysis of neglect is abjection, defined as the act of casting away something or someone, but also as the process of debasing or rendering despicable. 'Abjection' refers to the dynamics through which certain groups are framed or emerge as alien (that is, outside the sphere of moral obligation); disgusting (triggering an unpleasant emotional reaction); and beyond any possibility of improvement. Abjection is an unavoidable feature of the cultural context in which certain groups are made invisible and some actors become emotionally desensitised to the needs and suffering of less privileged others. This understanding of abjection allows us to place the focal point squarely on groups: it is not simply about neglected issues, but also about the invisibility of certain groups as they are affected by these issues.

Julia Kristeva engaged with the concept of abjection while discussing subject-formation. Departing from other psychoanalytical writers, she argues that our subjectivity – sense of self – is sustained not by desire but by the exclusion of others. Nonetheless, exclusion is not the same as objectification, since between the subject and the object there is still a bond of desire. The relation between the subject and the abject is more complex than that. Kristeva writes:

> There looms, within abjection, one of those violent, dark revolts of being, directed against a threat that seems to emanate from an exorbitant outside or inside...It beseeches, worries, and fascinates desire, which, nevertheless, does not let itself be seduced.[23]

Abjection is presented as an ambiguous fascination, insofar as the abject is something that simultaneously beckons and repels. As Kristeva notes:

> abjection is above all ambiguity. Because, while releasing a hold, it does not radically cut off the subject from what threatens it…But also because abjection itself is a composite of judgment and affect, of condemnation and yearning.[24]

The abject, then, lies at the margins of the self and emerges as its opposite. However, the abject is not completely separable because it permanently unsettles and threatens to disrupt the integrity of the self. As Iris Marion Young put it, the abject 'provokes fear and loathing because it exposes the border between self and other as constituted and fragile, and threatens to dissolve the subject by dissolving the border'.[25]

The importance of abjection to an analysis of neglect can be gleaned in Young's account of the mechanisms of oppression, which for her is 'enacted through a body aesthetic, through nervousness and avoidance'.[26] According to Young, instances of oppression like racism and sexism persist, despite the adoption of anti-discrimination laws, by becoming embodied and unconscious. In her words:

> oppression persists in our society partly through interactive habits, unconscious assumptions and stereotypes, and group-related feelings of nervousness and aversion. Group oppressions are enacted in this society not primarily in official laws and policies but in informal, often unnoticed and unreflective speech, bodily reactions to others, conventional practices of everyday interaction and evaluation, aesthetic judgments, and the jokes, images, and stereotypes pervading the mass media.[27]

For Young interactions between groups are underpinned by emotional dynamics of attraction and aversion. Specifically, oppression is supported by a process through which certain groups are rendered abject – that is, different, alien and loathsome. She writes:

> When the dominant culture defines some groups as different, as the Other, the members of those groups are imprisoned in their bodies. Dominant discourse defines them in terms of bodily characteristics, and constructs those bodies as ugly, dirty, defiled, impure, contaminated, or sick.[28]

In sum, when thinking about neglect in global health, one must engage with the cultural and emotional processes through which interests are defined together with an anxiety over (certain kinds of) groups and bodies. These groups and bodies are not simply marginalised or excluded. They are portrayed as morally tainted and a source of moral pollution. They are also considered irredeemable, beyond possibilities of improvement. Taken together, these features mean that abject groups are placed outside the sphere of moral concern.

Framing Ebola: security and crisis

The neglected, then, is the abject. It may be invisible but it is not totally absent. In fact, the neglected can be present – albeit in specific ways. The 2014 Ebola outbreak can be seen as a powerful illustration of how neglect yields a particularly complex combination of visibility and invisibility. At first glance this would seem to be an issue that emerged out of neglect. But once we go beneath the veneer of superficial attention, neglect begins to reveal itself in its multifaceted nature.

The Ebola outbreak began in December 2013 in Guinea, with the World Health Organization (WHO) officially notified in March 2014.[29] Following international pressure the WHO declared Ebola a 'public health emergency of international concern' in August of that year.[30] The following month Médecins sans Frontières made an appeal for a robust civilian and military intervention to tackle the epidemic.[31] This framing of the outbreak raises a number of questions. To begin with there was insufficient recognition on the part of the media, the public and even certain policy-making sectors that this was not a 'new' or 'unprecedented' challenge. Even though Ebola was, up until recently, a minor issue on the global health agenda, it is far from new. Between 1976 and 2012 there were 28 reported outbreaks of the virus in several African countries – namely Cote D'Ivoire, Democratic Republic of Congo, Gabon, South Africa, Sudan and Uganda. As a result of systematic underreporting, it is almost certain that the total of 2387 cases and 1590 deaths in these outbreaks is but a portion of the actual number of casualties.[32] Ebola has been a recurrent problem in some regions of the African continent in the past few decades – more precisely, it has been allowed to remain a problem.

Even though the WHO knew of this long history of Ebola outbreaks, it ended up framing the outbreak using the same tools used for dealing with 'emerging infectious diseases'. By declaring the outbreak a public health emergency the WHO was doing more than just describing a problem – it was inscribing Ebola as a particular kind of problem. The figure of the 'public health emergency of international concern' is part of the 2005 International Health Regulations and typifies a novel way of approaching health issues in the international sphere. In this new reasoning the focus is placed not on actual diseases but more precisely on 'events' that can constitute future risks. As Lorna Weir and Eric Mykhalovskiy have argued, we have witnessed a 'fundamental shift from surveillance of the certain to vigilance of public health risk'.[33] This introduces a strong 'interpretive dimension' into the reporting of health issues, which are conceived as 'both known and unknown'.[34] There was not only a strong subjective dimension in the framing of Ebola, but also the recognition that what mattered in the response was not simply what was happening on the ground, but also what could be envisaged to happen – the scenarios that were developed around the disease.

In practice Ebola was framed as an emerging crisis and configured as a risky event that demanded the calculation of an unknown future. This happened to the detriment of seeing the outbreak from a broader perspective, that is, as the result of a series of events and conditions that stretched out into past choices and inaction. Seeing Ebola as an emerging crisis hindered a comprehensive engagement with the conditions that gave rise to the problem in the first place. What of the social and economic conditions that have turned Ebola into an endemic feature of this region? And the weak and inefficient health systems that have rendered some West African countries unable to cope?[35] And the low levels of trust between politicians and the public, which, at least in the case of Liberia, seem to have considerably weakened the ability of health authorities to alter the trajectory of the epidemic?[36] Finally, what about the global context in which the outbreak emerged, and the structural inequalities therein?[37] These questions were not given sufficient attention and arguably are not receiving sufficient attention now, as the world turns to the development of pharmacological 'magic bullets' in the form of vaccines.

The reduction of Ebola to a discrete crisis event – and a risk potentially leading to a catastrophic scenario – was heightened by the underlying process of securitisation that was visible in the call for military intervention. According to the securitisation perspective, an issue is securitised when it is framed or emerges as an existential threat demanding extraordinary (normally undemocratic) measures.[38] The securitisation narrative is underpinned by a fear-based imaginary, which is concerned with the protection of the integrity of the political body in the face of exogenous elements. The presence of a securitisation modality goes a long way in explaining the preoccupation with securing borders, controlling international circulation and establishing sanitary cordons that characterised the response to the outbreak – which in turn echoes a long tradition of demarcation and self/other distinctions in the history of international health.[39]

The securitised modality of response interacted with the crisis narrative in the framing of the outbreak. The crisis narrative overlaps with securitisation because the presence of an existential threat is also assumed. However, whereas securitisation is underpinned by the externalisation of threat (disease is something foreign to the political body that must be contained and kept at bay), the crisis narrative is more strongly focused on internal elements. Narratives of internal decay, degeneracy or vulnerability – and the anxiety they create – are an intrinsic element of the crisis narrative.[40] In the case of Ebola this took the form of an anxiety about the uncontrollable nature of existing social and economic processes. The threat was not simply Ebola but also the inherent vulnerabilities in the globalised world – particularly in its more developed regions – with complex networks in which humans, non-humans, goods and information circulate at great speed.

In sum, the framing of the Ebola outbreak contributed to rendering the phenomenon visible in certain – and very limited – ways. Both narratives were markedly solipsist: while in the securitisation frame the primary concern was the protection of the (Western) self *vis-à-vis* a threatening other, in the crisis frame the emphasis was laid on the inherent vulnerability of the self, which left it exposed to disruption. In both cases the regions, populations and individuals that were mostly affected by the disease were merely the background, or secondary characters, in a narrative about the West and its travails. Neglect thus manifested itself in the invisibility of the groups most affected by the disease, as well as of the social and economic conditions that made the outbreak possible.

Ebola and the faces of abjection

The framing of the Ebola outbreak laid out the conditions for the abjection of certain groups. The same process that briefly brought the populations in West Africa into the limelight also shaped the limited ways in which they were seen: helpless victims, anonymous faces arousing momentary pity, distant others in wretched lands, reiterations of a familiar story of 'African despair'.

To start with, the framing of Ebola obfuscated the gendered nature of the problem. As Sophie Harman argues in her contribution to this special issue, women have been 'conspicuously invisible' in the framing and in responses to the outbreak. A similar point has been made by Olena Hankisvky, who has called for the recognition of inter-sectionality in the analysis of Ebola. She writes:

> the dynamics of the epidemic cannot be reduced to single foci or explanatory factors. Geography (including urban/rural location), race, gender, and socioeconomic status operate together in a synergistic fashion to shape the experiences of those affected.[41]

The perspectives of feminism and inter-sectionality question the quality of attention that Ebola received, allowing us to recognise how superficial it actually was. They highlight the extent to which the framing and coverage of the outbreak were not able conceive its victims as something other than an undifferentiated mass. Concrete experiences, specific vulnerabilities and their social, economic and cultural background were largely overlooked.

In addition to this, there are elements to suggest that abjection was also present in the constitution of certain groups and practices as alien, exotic and disgusting. In August 2014 the American weekly news magazine *Newsweek* ran as its cover story an alarmist account of the evolving Ebola outbreak. Instead of privileging the unfolding human suffering in West Africa, the magazine chose to focus on the dangers of the import of 'bushmeat' into the USA and Europe, the 'secret' trade in monkey meat that could become Ebola's 'backdoor' into the West. A similar story appeared in news outlets in the UK and Sweden. Ebola was thus linked to backward African practices that were deemed exotic and disgusting.[42] This corresponds to a broader process of racialisation of this disease, which cannot be separated from the ensuing stigmatisation of West Africans living in the West. As Kim Yi Dionne and Laura Seay have noted:

> the Ebola outbreak highlights ethnocentric and xenophobic understandings of Africa. Current American reactions continue a long history of viewing Africans and the African continent as a diseased, monolithic place. Framing Ebola as a disease that affects 'others' has a negative impact on attitudes toward immigrants as well as public health responses.[43]

The framing of Ebola in the Western media cannot be separated from a persistent anxiety over certain kinds of groups, their supposedly different and disgusting behaviour, and the threat they present to the integrity of the political community. This was supported by an underlying narrative of the African continent as a place of 'tragedy', despair and helplessness, about which little could be done except for preventing problems from spilling over to more ordered regions of the world. The same forces that attracted the attention of the West ultimately led to aversion.

In a clear instance of abjection, then, Ebola was framed as a racialised African problem deriving from backward practices and requiring a mixture of surveillance and containment. This happened to the detriment of seeing the outbreak as a problem of global health governance – of inequality, injustice and the systematic reproduction of the vulnerability of certain groups. Neglect thus manifested itself in the re-inscription of the conditions for apathy and inaction. As populations in West Africa were placed outside the sphere of sustained moral concern, the framing of Ebola led to the denial of action that could address the deep-seated structures that were at the root of the problem.

The spectacle of Ebola

By resulting in the abjection of West African populations the framing of Ebola led to a modality of response based on crisis management: emergency preparedness, surveillance, control and containment. This reactive, short-term approach was made possible by the very nature of the media cycle: noise followed by boredom, hysteria followed by apathy, feeding off the short attention span of contemporary consumer societies organised around 'the production and consumption of images, commodities, and staged events'.[44] As Douglas Kellner has noted, the advent of 24/7 news channels has meant increasing competition for ratings and advertising. This has forced information to be more exciting, more visual, fusing codes of entertainment into journalism. News coverage of events thus becomes more sensationalist; at the same time it becomes superficial and short-termist, as high ratings require sources of excitement to be permanently recycled. It comes as no surprise that in Western media the Ebola outbreak ended up being treated as a staged event, a dramatic occurrence punctuated by ritualistic moments: images from infirmary wards, nameless individuals in mourning, the health workers in biohazard suits, the rioting crowds, sombre declarations in Washington and Geneva, the arrival of Western personnel. This is a familiar narrative, repeated countless times in news and films, and discarded as soon as its attention-grabbing effect starts to wear off.

This is also an age of social media, and social networking platforms like Twitter, Facebook and Instagram contributed to the visibility of Ebola. Once again, one needs to consider the kind of visibility that was afforded by these platforms, and to question the extent to which such visibility was in fact a form of obfuscation and abjection. A study of images posted in November 2014 with the 'Ebola' tag found that images on Instagram overwhelmingly treated Ebola as joke material (42%) or were unrelated to the disease (36% of images tagged 'Ebola' featured other things, such as motorbikes). On Flickr the situation was somewhat different, with a greater attention to health professionals (46%) but scarce attention given to images containing factual information (6%).[45] This survey provides further indication that Ebola became visible in ways that did not increase public awareness and engagement with the problem, but rather enabled its appropriation as a form of self-validation and entertainment.

Guy Debord's writings on 'the spectacle' add an important political edge to this discussion of visibility enmeshed with distraction. Debord defined the spectacle not simply as the accumulation and consumption of images, but rather as 'a social relation among people, mediated by images'.[46] On the one hand, the spectacle says more about the dominant order that it does about the people and problems it refers to: as Debord put it, the spectacle is 'the existing order's uninterrupted discourse about itself, its laudatory monologue'.[47] On the other hand, the spectacle shapes how this dominant order engages with its 'others'. The correlative of the spectacle is the spectator – a passive, reactive and indifferent consumer of marketable images.[48] The excitement created around issues, by depending upon the repetition (and eventually discarding) of familiar tropes, becomes a veneer for banalisation and forgetting.

This does not mean that the spectacle does not have political effects. Banalisation becomes a depoliticising tool that obfuscates the reproduction of unequal relations and ultimately serves the interests of privileged groups. As Debord notes, the spectacle becomes a tool for domination:

> The society which carries the spectacle does not dominate the underdeveloped regions by its economic hegemony alone. It dominates them *as the society of the spectacle*.[49]

Spectacles may be staged events but their effects are very real for the individuals affected inasmuch as they help to shape their position *vis-à-vis* those actors with the capacity to shape outcomes.

In the case of Ebola the spectacle reinforced the different modalities of neglect mentioned above: invisibility, apathy, inaction and incompetence. The outbreak was made invisible by a ready-made narrative that said more about the developed world, its anxieties and needs, than about the actual disease and the populations suffering from it. The effect of framing Ebola through the prism of a spectacle was, paradoxically, that the problem receded in the midst of a succession of images. The spectacle may have brought Ebola to our screens, but it presented the outbreak as a theatrical event and a spectator sport. While making us feel that we were face to face with it, it also created a reassuring separation. Thus, in addition to perpetuating apathy and inaction, the spectacle has foreclosed the development of adequate competences and long-term strategies for preventing and dealing with future outbreaks.

Conclusion

Ebola is neglected. The 2014 outbreak in West Africa signified the re-inscription and entrenchment of this neglect. This article has explored Ebola from the standpoint of neglect in global health, embedding the latter in the context of political structures and relations. It has also argued that neglect should not be considered mere invisibility, but rather a process of making something invisible and denying an adequate response.

The standpoint of neglect is important because it helps us understand how Ebola was made invisible and why the response to this outbreak was inadequate. The argument has emphasised the importance of the affective dimension, focusing in particular on the dynamics of abjection – a mixture of attraction and repudiation – which accompanies neglect and which was present in the case of Ebola. The article has shown that the neglect of Ebola was paradoxically exacerbated by an intertwined narrative of security and crisis. This was supported by its framing as a media and political spectacle.

Understanding neglect can have a positive impact in responses to future outbreaks. Coming to terms with the complex processes through which neglect is produced is crucial for developing adequate response mechanisms. These certainly require short-term strategies aimed at containing crises but they also need to include the broader social, political and economic transformations that a lasting solution to the problem requires. This is why we need alternative framings of Ebola that consider power inequalities, the relations between groups and the production of harm, vulnerability and structural violence in the international sphere.[50] We also need to highlight the persistence of 'mutually reinforcing systems of colonialism, racism, neoliberalism, globalism, imperialism, xenophobia, and sexism'.[51] These decisively shape perceptions of health problems and of the moral worth of certain regions and groups – thereby affecting the incidence of disease and conditioning responses to it.

This article began with the story of a misnamed river, a metaphor of erasure. Unlike the river, the Ebola epidemic is not a natural phenomenon but a human-made one. Certainly, the virus is a natural entity, but the epidemic was allowed to happen and to develop because of human actions and inactions. A river flows regardless of what we call it, but the trajectory of disease can and does change as a result of words, ideas and choices.

Disclosure statement

No potential conflict of interest was reported by the author.

Funding

Financial support from the Leverhulme Trust (ECF-2012-406) is gratefully acknowledged.

Acknowledgments

For their comments on earlier drafts of this article the author would like to thank Simon Rushton, Anne Roemer-Mahler, Owain Williams, the anonymous reviewers and the participants in the workshop 'Ebola: An International Relations Response', held at the University of Sussex, November 2014.

Notes

1. Tanghe and Vangele, "Region de la Haute Ebola," 61 (my translation).
2. Wordsworth, "How Ebola got its Name."
3. Huber, "The Unification of the Globe by Disease?"; and Fidler "The Globalization of Public Health."
4. Zacher and Keefe, *The Politics of Global Health Governance*, 15.
5. Price-Smith and Huang, "Epidemic of Fear."
6. Cooper et al., "Critical Cases in Global Health Innovation," 7.
7. Farmer, *Pathologies of Power*.
8. Rushton and Williams, "Frames, Paradigms and Power," 152.
9. Edelman, *Constructing the Political Spectacle*, 15.
10. Schön and Rein, *Frame Reflection*, 23.
11. Schön and Rein, *Frame Reflection*, 26.
12. Schön and Rein, *Frame Reflection*, 29 (emphasis in the original).
13. Rochefort and Cobb, *The Politics of Problem Definition*, 8.
14. Edelman, *Constructing the Political Spectacle*, 12.
15. McInnes and Lee, *Global Health and International Relations*, 34.
16. Rushton and Williams, "Frames, Paradigms and Power," 148.
17. Shiffman, "A Social Explanation," 610.
18. Shiffman and Smith, "Generation of Political Priority."
19. Linklater, *The Problem of Harm*, 49–61.
20. Mackenzie et al., "What is Vulnerability?"
21. Mercer, "Human Nature"; and Bleiker and Hutchison, "Fear no More."
22. Crawford, "The Passion of World Politics."
23. Kristeva, *Powers of Horror*, 1.
24. Kristeva, *Powers of Horror*, 9–10.
25. Young, *Justice and the Politics of Difference*, 144.

26. Young, *Justice and the Politics of Difference*, 149.
27. Young, *Justice and the Politics of Difference*, 148.
28. Young, *Justice and the Politics of Difference*, 123.
29. WHO Ebola Response Team, "Ebola Virus Disease in West Africa."
30. WHO, "Statement on the 1st meeting of the IHR Emergency Committee."
31. MSF International President, "United Nations Special Briefing on Ebola."
32. WHO, "Ebola Virus Disease."
33. Weir and Mykhalovskiy, *Global Public Health Vigilance*, 126.
34. Weir and Mykhalovskiy, *Global Public Health Vigilance*, 128, 136.
35. Kruk et al., "What is a Resilient Health System?"
36. Epstein, "Ebola in Liberia."
37. Benatar, "Explaining and responding to the Ebola Epidemic."
38. Buzan et al., *Security*.
39. Martin, *Flexible Bodies*.
40. Hay, "Crisis."
41. Hankivsky, "Intersectionality and Ebola," 14–15.
42. McGovern, "Bushmeat and the Politics of Disgust."
43. Dionne and Seay, "Perceptions about Ebola in America," 6.
44. Kellner, *Media Spectacle and Insurrection*, xiv–xv.
45. Seltzer et al., "The Content of Social Media's Shared Images."
46. Debord, *Society of the Spectacle*, §4.
47. Debord, *Society of the Spectacle*, §24.
48. Kellner, *Media Spectacle and Insurrection*.
49. Debord, *Society of the Spectacle*, §57 (emphasis in the original).
50. Leach, "The Ebola Crisis."
51. Hankivsky, "Intersectionality and Ebola," 15.

Bibliography

Benatar, S. "Explaining and responding to the Ebola Epidemic." *Philosophy, Ethics, and Humanities in Medicine* 10, no. 1 (2015): 1–3.

Bleiker, R., and E. Hutchison. "Fear no More: Emotions and World Politics." *Review of International Studies* 34, no. Supplement 1 (2008): 115–135.

Buzan, B., O. Wæver, and J. de Wilde. *Security: A New Framework for Analysis*. Boulder, CO: Lynne Rienner, 1998.

Cooper, A. F., J. J. Kirton, and M. A. Stevenson. "Critical Cases in Global Health Innovation." In *Innovation in Global Health Governance: Critical Cases*, edited by A. F. Cooper and J. J. Kirton, 3–20. Farnham: Ashgate, 2009.

Crawford, N. C. "The Passion of World Politics: Propositions on Emotion and Emotional Relationships." *International Security* 24, no. 4 (2000): 116–156.

Debord, G. *Society of the Spectacle*. Detroit, MI: Black & Red, 1983.

Dionne, K. Y., and L. Seay. "Perceptions about Ebola in America: Othering and the Role of Knowledge about Africa." *Political Science & Politics* 48, no. 1 (2015): 6–7.

Edelman, Murray. *Constructing the Political Spectacle*. Chicago, IL: University of Chicago Press, 1988.

Epstein, H. "Ebola in Liberia: An Epidemic of Rumors." *New York Review of Books* 61 (2014): 91–94.

Farmer, P. *Pathologies of Power: Health, Human Rights, and the New War on the Poor*. Berkeley, CA: University of California Press, 2003.

Fidler, D. P. "The Globalization of Public Health: The First 100 Years of International Health Diplomacy." *Bulletin of the World Health Organization* 79, no. 9 (2001): 842–849.

Hankivsky, O. "Intersectionality and Ebola." *Political Science & Politics* 48, no. 1 (2015): 14–15.

Hay, C. "Crisis and the Structural Transformation of the State: Interrogating the Process of Change." *British Journal of Politics & International Relations* 1, no. 3 (1999): 317–344.

Huber, V. "The Unification of the Globe by Disease? The International Sanitary Conferences on Cholera, 1851–1894." *Historical Journal* 49, no. 2 (2006): 453–476.

Kellner, D. *Media Spectacle and Insurrection, 2011: From the Arab Uprisings to Occupy Everywhere*. New York: Bloomsbury, 2012.

Kristeva, J. *Powers of Horror: An Essay on Abjection*. New York: Columbia University Press, 1982.

Kruk, M. E., M. Myers, S. T. Varpilah and B. T. Dahn. "What is a Resilient Health System? Lessons from Ebola." *Lancet* 385, no. 9980 (2015): 1910–1912.

Leach, M. "The Ebola Crisis and Post-2015 Development." *Journal of International Development* 27, no. 6 (2015): 816–834.

Linklater, A. *The Problem of Harm in World Politics: Theoretical Investigations*. Cambridge: Cambridge University Press, 2011.

Mackenzie, C., W. Rogers, and S. Dodds. "What is Vulnerability, and Why does it matter for Moral Theory?" In *Vulnerability: New Essays in Ethics and Feminist Philosophy*, edited by C. Mackenzie, W. Rogers and S. Dodds, 1–29. Oxford: Oxford University Press, 2014.

Martin, E. *Flexible Bodies: The Role of Immunity in American Culture from the Days of Polio to the Age of AIDS*. Boston, MA: Beacon Press, 1994.

McGovern, M. "Bushmeat and the Politics of Disgust." *Cultural Anthropology*. 2014. http://www.culanth.org/fieldsights/588-bushmeat-and-the-politics-of-disgust.

McInnes, C., and K. Lee. *Global Health and International Relations*. Cambridge: Polity Press, 2012.

Médecins Sans Frontières (MSF) International President. "United Nations Special Briefing on Ebola." 2014. http://www.msf.org.uk/node/26146.

Mercer, J. "Human Nature and the First Image: Emotion in International Politics." *Journal of International Relations and Development* 9, no. 3 (2006): 288–303.

Price-Smith, A. T., and Y. Huang. "Epidemic of Fear: SARS and the Political Economy of Contagion." In *Innovation in Global Health Governance: Critical Cases*, edited by A. F. Cooper and J. J. Kirton, 23–48. Farnham: Ashgate, 2009.

Rochefort, D. A., and R. W. Cobb. *The Politics of Problem Definition: Shaping the Policy Agenda*. Lawrence: University Press of Kansas, 1994.

Rushton, S., and O. D. Williams. "Frames, Paradigms and Power: Global Health Policy-making under Neoliberalism." *Global Society* 26, no. 2 (2012): 147–167.

Schön, D. A., and M. Rein. *Frame Reflection: Toward the Resolution of Intractable Policy Controversies*. New York: Basic Books, 1994.

Seltzer, E. K., N. S. Jean, E. Kramer-Golinkoff, D. A. Asch and R. M. Merchant. "The Content of Social Media's Shared Images about Ebola: A Retrospective Study." *Public Health* 129, no. 9 (2015): 1273–1277.

Shiffman, J. "A Social Explanation for the Rise and Fall of Global Health Issues." *Bulletin of the World Health Organization* 87, no. 8 (2009): 608–613.

Shiffman, J., and S. Smith. "Generation of Political Priority for Global Health Initiatives: A Framework and Case Study of Maternal Mortality." *Lancet* 370, no. 9595 (2007): 1370–1379.

Tanghe, B., and A. Vangele. "Region de la Haute Ebola: Notes d'histoire (1890–1900)." *Aequatoria* 2, no. 6 (1939): 61–65.

Weir, L., and E. Mykhalovskiy. *Global Public Health Vigilance: Creating a World on Alert*. New York: Routledge, 2010.

Wordsworth, D. "How Ebola got its Name." *The Spectator*, 2014. http://www.spectator.co.uk/life/mind-your-language/9349662/how-ebola-got-its-name/.

World Health Organization (WHO). "Ebola Virus Disease." Fact sheet No. 103. 2015. http://www.who.int/mediacentre/factsheets/fs103/en/.

WHO. "Statement on the 1st Meeting of the IHR Emergency Committee on the 2014 Ebola Outbreak in West Africa." 2014. http://www.who.int/mediacentre/news/statements/2014/ebola-20140808/en/.

WHO Ebola Response Team. "Ebola Virus Disease in West Africa – The First 9 Months of the Epidemic and Forward Projections." *New England Journal of Medicine* 371, no. 16 (2014): 1481–1495.

Young, I. M. *Justice and the Politics of Difference*. Princeton, NJ: Princeton University Press, 2011.

Zacher, M. W., and T. J. Keefe. *The Politics of Global Health Governance: United by Contagion*. Basingstoke: Palgrave Macmillan, 2008.

Index